Study Guide for the

Core Curriculum for Oncology Nursing

Study Guide for the

Core Curriculum for Oncology Nursing

7th Edition

Suzanne M. Mahon, DNS, RN, AOCN®, AGN-BC, FAAN
Professor Emerita
Division of Hematology and Oncology
Saint Louis University
St. Louis, Missouri

Marcelle Kaplan, MS, RN, AOCN®-Emeritus, CBCN®-Emeritus
Oncology Nursing Consultant
Clinical Nurse Specialist
Merrick, Long Island, New York

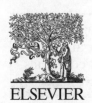

ELSEVIER

Elsevier
3251 Riverport Lane
St. Louis, Missouri 63043

STUDY GUIDE FOR THE CORE CURRICULUM
FOR ONCOLOGY NURSING, SEVENTH EDITION

ISBN: 978-0-323-93052-9

Notice

Practitioners and researchers must always rely on their own experience and knowledge in evaluating and using any information, methods, compounds or experiments described herein. Because of rapid advances in the medical sciences, in particular, independent verification of diagnoses and drug dosages should be made. To the fullest extent of the law, no responsibility is assumed by Elsevier, authors, editors or contributors for any injury and/or damage to persons or property as a matter of products liability, negligence or otherwise, or from any use or operation of any methods, products, instructions, or ideas contained in the material herein.

Executive Content Strategist: Lee Henderson
Content Development Manager: Danielle Frazier
Senior Content Development Specialist: Maria Broeker
Publishing Services Manager: Deepthi Unni
Senior Project Manager: Manchu Mohan

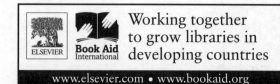

Printed in India
Last digit is the print number: 9 8 7 6 5 4 3 2 1

Preface

The *Study Guide for the Core Curriculum for Oncology Nursing* is a companion to the *Core Curriculum for Oncology Nursing*, Seventh Edition. Each chapter in this new edition of the *Study Guide* has a corresponding chapter in the *Core Curriculum*, reflecting content updates in the practice of oncology nursing since the previous edition. Included in the updates for the *Study Guide*, Seventh Edition are totally new sections with content that is critical to our work, including financial toxicity, social determinants of health, CAR T-cell therapy, and myelofibrosis. Question content, formats, focus, and distribution have been revised to match those of the 2022 OCN® Examination test blueprint, to reflect important changes in cancer treatment and related nursing care, and to reflect the latest research evidence.

In general, oncology nursing certification helps ensure and validate that a nurse has met rigorous requirements for both experience and knowledge in oncology nursing. Specifically, attaining an OCN® credential is a formal recognition of specialized knowledge in oncology nursing. Knowledge in both the science of oncology and in how to best care for patients and families affected by a diagnosis of malignancy is continually evolving. Oncology nurses are continually challenged to keep up with these changes and apply state-of-the-art knowledge to clinical practice. Certification tests this nursing knowledge.

This revised *Study Guide* is the only question-and-answer review book for the OCN® Examination developed in collaboration with the Oncology Nursing Society. The *Study Guide* is a valuable tool for nurses not only to assess their knowledge but also to expand their knowledge base, with the goal of providing excellent clinical care. Each question within the *Study Guide* reflects content that oncology nurses need to understand and apply in their practice to provide safe and effective care.

An answer key with detailed rationales is provided for review and to build on oncology nursing knowledge. The rationale for each question provides information about why a specific answer is the correct choice and also why the other options were either not correct or not the best choice. Review of each rationale provides oncology nurses with an additional educational opportunity to expand their knowledge about the oncology content underlying each question, as well as important related knowledge.

Nurses utilizing this *Study Guide* are encouraged to spend time studying and reflecting on the information provided in the rationale sections and, when indicated, to consult the *Core Curriculum for Oncology Nursing* for additional information.

We would especially like to acknowledge and thank Bill Tony and Dave Burns from the ONS Publications Department for their support and assistance with this edition of the *Study Guide for the Core Curriculum for Oncology Nursing*. Additional thanks go to the staff at Elsevier for their support of this project.

A special thanks and best wishes are extended to all of the nurses taking the step toward certification who will be using this reference as a component of their test preparation. Certification does make a difference. Patients deserve and need nurses who are knowledgeable about the complexities of oncology care.

Suzanne M. Mahon
Marcelle Kaplan

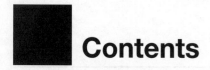

Contents

1 Epidemiology, Prevention, and Health Promotion

1. The oncology nurse is preparing to present a program to the inpatient unit. The nurse discusses that cancer epidemiology is defined as the study of the:
   A. rates of cancer occurrence in a population
   B. number of deaths from cancer in a given time period
   C. distribution and determinants of cancer in a population
   D. most common types of new cancer cases diagnosed each year

2. The oncology nurse is providing a community program on cancer prevention and epidemiology including incidence of major cancers. Which of the following types of cancers have an increasing annual incidence trend in the United States?
   A. Female breast and colon under age 50
   B. Lung and prostate under age 50
   C. Stomach over age 50 and larynx
   D. Kidney and neuroendocrine pancreas

3. The oncology nurse is facilitating a cancer support group. The nurse discusses survivorship and states that there are 16.9 million patients with cancer living as survivors in the United States. A statistical breakdown of cancer survivors reveals:
   A. Almost 64% of survivors are age 65 years or older.
   B. African Americans have higher relative survival rates than whites.
   C. The highest 5-year survival rate is for colon cancer.
   D. Relative survival rates decreased for patients with chronic myeloid leukemia.

4. The oncology nurse is providing a workshop for a large employer to their employees. The nurse discusses disparities. Which of these findings is accurate about disparities in cancer epidemiology among different ethnic groups in the United States?
   A. Asians/Pacific Islanders have the highest incidence and death rates of all groups for kidney cancer.
   B. African American men are more than twice as likely as white men to die from prostate cancer.
   C. Whites have higher mortality rates for colon cancer than African Americans.
   D. Hispanic/Latina women have the lowest incidence rate for cervical cancer but the highest death rate.

5. The oncology nurse refers a current smoker to a tobacco cessation program. Tobacco cessation is an important focus of public health education about cancer prevention in the United States because:
   A. Smokeless tobacco products are an approved alternative to cigarettes.
   B. Adults with a college degree are most likely to use tobacco products.
   C. Tobacco use is the greatest modifiable risk factor for cancer.
   D. Most tobacco users have insurance coverage for cessation programs.

6. The oncology nurse is completing a cancer risk assessment. The nurse discusses that maintaining a healthy weight is considered to be an important strategy in efforts to promote general health in the United States. Overweight populations and people who are obese continue to be one of the largest concerns in promoting general health because:
   A. Obesity and being overweight are responsible for 50% of cancer deaths.
   B. Obesity and being overweight are linked to cancers of the gastrointestinal system.
   C. Obesity and being overweight are associated with increased risk for cancers of the lung.
   D. Obesity and being overweight are associated with approximately 15% of cancers in males and 25% of cancers in females.

7. The oncology nurse is discussing cancer prevention. This includes education about vaccination. For which of the following groups is the vaccination for chemoprevention of the human papilloma virus (HPV) recommended?
   A. Vaccination is recommended for female children only.
   B. Vaccination is recommended for all sexually active adult men and women over the age 26 years.
   C. Vaccination is recommended to be given to girls between the ages of 15 and 18 as a single dose.
   D. Vaccination is recommended to begin in girls and boys aged 9 to 12 years as a two-dose series.

1

8. The oncology nurse is providing education about chemoprevention to a woman receiving care in the high risk breast clinic. The nurse discusses that the United States Federal Drug Administration (FDA) has approved drug treatments to reduce the risk of breast cancer in the general population. These drugs include which one of the following?
   A. Raloxifene
   B. Diethylstilbestrol
   C. Anabolic steroids
   D. Menotropins

9. Ms. P. is a 40-year-old woman, who has identified herself as a smoker, and who is undergoing a preventive cancer risk assessment. A thorough medical history and physical examination is being conducted, and she is being assessed for motivation for preventative behavior as per the health belief model. Which of the following questions should she be asked during the motivation for preventative behavior assessment?
   A. "Do you currently have any medical conditions and what medications for those medical conditions are you currently taking?"
   B. "Have you or anyone in your immediate family ever been diagnosed with cancer?"
   C. "Have you ever undergone treatments for cancer such as chemotherapy, radiation therapy, or immunotherapy?"
   D. "How difficult do you think it will be to decrease your risk for cancer by quitting your smoking habit?"

10. A hospital is planning a community outreach program and the nurse reviews statistics about cancer epidemiology. According to statistics from the American Cancer Society, several factors contribute to cancer mortality in the United States. Factors such as age, gender, geography, and socioeconomic status (SES) play a role in cancer deaths. Regarding socioeconomic status, which of the following is true regarding the cancer mortality in poorer populations?
    A. High SES is associated with increased risk of lung cancer, cervical cancer, stomach cancer, and cancer of the head and neck.
    B. The use of alcohol has increased among poorer populations, leading to a higher rate of cancer mortality.
    C. A higher rate of advanced disease is found at diagnosis among poorer populations and those who live in rural regions than in the rest of the U.S. population.
    D. Low SES is associated with increased risk of breast, prostate, and colon cancers.

11. As of 2016, the FDA classified electronic nicotine delivery systems (ENDS), also known as *e-cigarettes,* as a tobacco product, bringing them under FDA regulation. Of the following statements, the oncology nurse should be aware that which one is true regarding the use of ENDS?
    A. As of 2020, more than 3 million high school age students were identified as e-cigarette users, with a variety of appealing flavors cited as the primary reason for use.
    B. As of 2020, the FDA has approved e-cigarettes as a cessation aid.
    C. Electronic cigarettes are battery-operated devices in which the inhaled vapor is produced from cartridges that contain flavoring and other chemicals, but has not been found to contain any nicotine, like in traditional tobacco products.
    D. Use of e-cigarettes has so far not been linked to leading nonsmokers and children to begin smoking.

12. The oncology nurse is discussing approaches to stopping tobacco products in a tobacco cessation class to smokers. The 5A model to promote smoking cessation is:
    A. Assess Address Assist Affirm Arrange
    B. Ask Advise Assess Assist Arrange
    C. Ask Address Assess Assist Affirm
    D. Address Assess Advise Affirm Assist

13. The oncology nurse is performing a cancer risk assessment which includes assessment for infection. This includes inquiring if the patient has a history of *Helicobacter pylori*, which is associated with:
    A. liver cancer
    B. non-Hodgkin lymphoma
    C. stomach cancer
    D. pancreatic cancer

14. The nurse is proposing that the institution provide educational programs for employers on cancer risks, prevention, and screening. Each program will be tailored to the risks encountered by different occupations. An occupation associated with an increased risk of developing prostate cancer is:
    A. steel workers
    B. rubber workers
    C. chemical workers
    D. miners

15. The oncology nurse is discussing cancer prevention with a patient. Current American Cancer Society recommendations for physical activity to reduce the risk of developing cancer include:
    A. 60 to 90 minutes of low-intensity exercise daily for adults
    B. 150 to 300 minutes of moderate-intensity activity per week for adults
    C. 45 to 60 minutes of moderate-intensity activity 3 days per week for children
    D. 20 to 30 minutes of low-intensity activity daily for children

2 Screening and Early Detection

1. A new fecal occult blood test screening designed to correctly identify the presence of colon cancer is an example of the test's:
   A. reliability
   B. negative predictive value
   C. sensitivity
   D. specificity

2. A 27-year-old female comes to the gynecology clinic for her routine cervical cancer screening. The oncology nurse expects that she will be screened with which screening test recommended for her age group?
   A. Pap test every 3 years
   B. Human papillomavirus (HPV) test with Pap test every 5 years
   C. HPV test with Pap test every 3 years
   D. Screening would not be recommended if she has been vaccinated

3. The oncology nurse is teaching a class of community women about screening guidelines for breast cancer. The nurse should explain that which of the following are included in the recommended screening guidelines for women 45 years of age and older with an average risk of breast cancer?
   A. Clinical breast exam every 6 to 12 months
   B. Begin taking chemoprevention agents
   C. Annual breast MRI
   D. Annual mammography

4. A 76-year-old white male with a history of diabetes and 30-pack-year history of smoking and no family history of prostate cancer asks the nurse whether he should be screened for prostate cancer. Which one of the following replies is the best response for the nurse to give?
   A. "Screening with a PSA test is recommended annually."
   B. "Screening is not recommended at your age."
   C. "Screening should only be done in men with a family history of prostate cancer."
   D. "Screening with a digital rectal examination is recommended annually."

5. A 62-year-old woman with a 22-pack-year smoking history asks the nurse if she should be screened for lung cancer. According to the recommendations of the United States Preventive Services Task Force (USPSTF), the nurse should reply that:
   A. lung cancer screening is not recommended
   B. low-dose computed tomography (LDCT) is recommended
   C. sputum cytology with or without chest x-ray is recommended
   D. chest radiography is recommended every 5 years

6. Which of the following explanations about cancer screening tests should the oncology nurse provide to a general audience? "Cancer screening tests are:
   A. always safe and not harmful if only done annually."
   B. diagnostic tests to find out what is the cause of certain symptoms."
   C. designed to detect the presence of early disease in healthy individuals.
   D. offer a cure which may otherwise not be found if it were not done."

7. A mother brings her 12-year-old son to the doctor for his annual checkup and is told that he should receive an HPV vaccine. The nurse explains that HPV vaccination in a 12-year-old male is an example of:
   A. primary prevention
   B. secondary prevention
   C. tertiary prevention
   D. quaternary prevention

8. The oncology clinical nurse specialist is providing an inservice about cancer epidemiology to the nursing staff on the oncology unit. The nurse explains that the percentage of persons who screen positive and actually have the disease is referred to as:
   A. positive predictive value
   B. negative predictive value
   C. sensitivity
   D. specificity

9. An institution is developing wellness programs and the oncology nurse is gathering data to justify the program. According to the American Cancer Society in 2022 there are over 4 million women living with breast cancer in the United States. This is an example of:
   A. incidence
   B. mortality
   C. epidemiology
   D. prevalence

10. When reviewing cancer-related symptoms, the nurse understands that which one of the following would be considered constitutional?
   A. Fatigue, malaise, recent weight gain or weight loss
   B. Dyspnea, orthopnea, and chest pain
   C. Increased urination, thirst, and perspiration
   D. Joint stiffness, vertigo, limited movement

11. J.L. is a 55-year-old African American female who calls to make an appointment for breast cancer screening. She is asymptomatic without a personal history of breast cancer or breast implants. She will be scheduled for which one of the following types of procedures?
   A. Breast ultrasound
   B. Screening mammogram
   C. Breast MRI
   D. Diagnostic mammogram

12. The nurse is educating a 44-year-old male about colorectal cancer screening. This education should include:
   A. Risk of bleeding with colonoscopy is 7%.
   B. A benefit of colonoscopy is that precancerous lesions can be visualized and removed during the examination.
   C. Evidence suggests that colonoscopy improves mortality over fecal-based tests.
   D. Colon screening should start at age 50 in persons of average risk.

3 Survivorship

1. The oncology nurse is leading a cancer support group and is discussing survivorship. In relation to cancer survivorship, the term survivor refers to which one of the following?
   A. Anyone with a cancer diagnosis, as well as their family and significant others
   B. Someone who is greater than 5 years from a cancer diagnosis
   C. Anyone who is given the diagnosis of an early-stage cancer
   D. An individual diagnosed at age 50 years or younger

2. An important component of survivorship care that the oncology nurse must understand regarding long-term and late effects is that:
   A. Long-term effects are those that begin at least one year after treatment completion.
   B. The first year after treatment is the most critical for treatment sequelae development.
   C. Late effects may manifest months or years later depending on treatment exposures.
   D. Adolescent and young adult (AYA) survivors are at lower risk for significant late effects.

3. T.R. is a 35-year-old female patient, who was treated for Hodgkin lymphoma at the age of 25, and received mantle field irradiation. Which one of the following should be reviewed by the health care team with the patient regarding her screening?
   A. Screening for second malignancy is not needed until age >40 years old.
   B. Annual mammogram, breast MRI, or both are recommended.
   C. A PET scan is indicated to screen for second malignancies.
   D. Factors such as lifestyle behaviors need not be addressed.

4. J.C. is a 47-year-old male patient, and a prostate cancer survivor of 3 years. He arrives at his 6-month post-treatment follow-up with his health care team. After the appointment is complete, and he is about to leave, J.C. asks if he is allowed to schedule a follow-up appointment with his local urologist. The oncology nurse's response is based on which one of the following?
   A. J.C. no longer needs follow-up care for this diagnosis if he is showing no new signs or symptoms or evidence of recurrence.
   B. A survivorship care plan might be useful to his local provider, and can be shared with the provider if the provider requests it.
   C. A local provider can assume care with a coordinated transition of care, with recommendations for disease surveillance, potential late treatment effects, and health promotion.
   D. His post-treatment care can only be provided by cancer specialists, and the oncology nurse advises that J.C. must continue his care with the clinic he has been visiting for at least the next 10 years.

5. The oncology nurse is helping to develop a survivorship clinic. Which one of the following statements best describes psychosocial considerations for cancer survivors?
   A. Screening tools to assess anxiety or depression are of limited value and should be avoided.
   B. Frequent changes in occupation or living arrangements should generally be viewed as positive signs of adaptation.
   C. Symptoms such as anxiety and depression may be indicative of post-treatment issues such as pain, fatigue, and insomnia.
   D. Personal questions can be difficult for both the patient and the health care provider, and may detract from more important aspects of the visit.

6. Mr. S. is a 75-year-old colon cancer survivor. Previously, he had led an active lifestyle, participating in a regular exercise routine, and had been an avid golfer and was in a bowling league. He states his intention to restart exercising again. His oncology nurse should advise which one of the following regimens?
   A. If he maintains a healthy body mass index (BMI), light-intensity exercise once a week can be beneficial.
   B. If he wants to begin exercising again, 150 minutes of moderate-intensity or 75 minutes of vigorous-intensity exercise per week is recommended.
   C. When preparing to exercise or when recovering from exercise, he should be aware that stretching can often lead to strained muscles.
   D. Rest, rather than exercising, is recommended for the first-year post treatment to promote continued healing, especially for patients >60 years of age.

7. As part of preventative and ongoing treatment and follow-up, oncology nurses frequently counsel patients about healthy weight management with the understanding that which one of the following is true?
   A. Fast foods are acceptable in moderation once goal weight is achieved.
   B. Portion control is only relevant for weight loss, not ongoing weight maintenance.
   C. Routine weight checks can be discouraging, and should be avoided.
   D. A plant-based diet contributes to achieving and maintaining healthy weight.

8. When caring for AYA survivors, the oncology nurse understands that which one of the following is true?
   A. A younger age at diagnosis places survivors at lower risk for physical and psychosocial sequalae.
   B. Younger survivors generally have greater access to insurance coverage based on their age and limited health care needs.
   C. Limited financial resources may result in prioritization of expenses such as paying rent instead of filling medication prescriptions.
   D. Cognitive impairment does not typically impact ability to manage high school or college courses.

9. An institution is preparing to launch a new survivorship program. An oncology nurse is assigned to prepare for the launch and, during her preparation, she correctly recognizes that:
   A. General counseling topics such as sun protection and safe sex need not be incorporated in the visits.
   B. Immunization recommendations for both children and adults should be included.
   C. Sun protection recommendations should be addressed only with AYA patients who have received mantle-field radiotherapy for Hodgkin lymphoma.
   D. Information on safe amounts of tobacco or vaping products should be included.

10. In preparing for delivery of survivorship care over the next decade, oncology nurses should recognize that:
    A. The number of cancer survivors is expected to remain stable for the next 8 to 10 years.
    B. The population of cancer survivors are expected to number more than 22.1 million persons by the year 2030.
    C. Cancer diagnoses are expected to decrease significantly in patients who are 64 years and older.
    D. The expected increase in the oncology workforce will continue to meet the needs of survivors.

11. R.J. is a 30-year-old patient, who has a 10-year history of osteosarcoma that was treated with chemotherapy and surgery. At a follow-up appointment, R.J. reports symptoms of new onset dyspnea and lower extremity edema. When considering the next steps, the oncology nurse correctly recognizes which one of the following?
    A. These symptoms are not related to R. J.'s disease and treatment.
    B. The patient is too young to consider cardiac etiology, unless there is a strong family history.
    C. Close monitoring of these symptoms over the coming months is recommended.
    D. The patient should be referred to a cardiologist for further evaluation.

12. T.L. is a 40-year-old patient, who has a history of testicular cancer. He calls in to the oncology clinic to state that he had been doing well up until this past week. He is now dreading his survivorship appointment and reports feeling increasingly anxious about his upcoming visit. Hearing his concerns, the oncology nurse taking his call correctly understands that which one of the following is true?
    A. The patient should be referred to psychiatry for evaluation prior to his visit.
    B. The symptoms he is reporting are common around the time of scans and appointments, and he is encouraged to keep his appointment.
    C. Postponing the visit to a future date will help him to overcome these feelings.
    D. Anxiety and fear of recurrence in survivors actually help to promote vigilance and compliance with follow-up recommendations.

4 Palliative and End-of-Life Care

1. A. E., a patient with advanced colon cancer, asks the oncology nurse to explain palliative care. Which one of the following statements, if made by the nurse, best describes the concept of palliative care? "Palliative care:
   A. focuses on improving the quality of life for the patient."
   B. focuses on treating the cancer with the fewest number of severe side effects."
   C. is delivered by a specialized physician rather than by a health care team."
   D. provides care to the dying patient at end of life."

2. The oncology nurse explains to A. E.'s spouse that in order to access Medicare hospice benefits, A. E. must have an estimated life expectancy of less than:
   A. 3 months
   B. 4 months
   C. 6 months
   D. 12 months

3. The oncology nurse understands that tertiary palliative care refers to which one of the following?
   A. Care provided by a rural palliative care team
   B. Basic palliative care principles carried out by a home health nurse
   C. Care for the most complex cases
   D. Care provided in a cancer center with palliative care certification

4. The oncology nurse instructs the family of a seriously ill patient that certification of prognosis must be provided for hospice care by which one of the following combination of staff members?
   A. Referring physician and social work supervisor
   B. Pastor and hospice medical director
   C. Referring physician and hospice medical director
   D. Hospice medical director and insurance adjuster

5. Both as a philosophy of care and as a regulated insurance benefit, hospice care is a model of high-quality, compassionate care. When a patient signs up for hospice care, the oncology nurse provides education so that the patient understands they are agreeing to which one of the following?
   A. Chemotherapy if the doctor thinks it is an option
   B. Transferring care to a different oncologist
   C. Cessation of aggressive therapy
   D. Intubation for respiratory distress

6. Physicians are often overly optimistic when anticipating life expectancy for patients with terminal or advanced disease, and usually overestimate survival time of their patients by a factor of which one of the following?
   A. Two
   B. Three
   C. Four
   D. Five

7. Unfortunately, it is common for hospice care referrals to occur quite late in the trajectory of a patient's illness. The oncology nurse is aware that the median number of days a patient lives while on hospice care, according to 2019 data by the National Hospice and Palliative Care Association, is which one of the following?
   A. 7
   B. 12
   C. 18
   D. 26

8. From the United Kingdom to the United States, the hospice movement began with pioneers such as Dame Cicely Saunders and Dr. Florence Wald, RN, leading the way for the care of the terminally ill. The roots of the modern hospice movement can be traced to which one of the following time periods?
   A. 1960's in England
   B. 1970's in Scotland
   C. 1980's in the United States
   D. 1990's in Germany

9. The process of dying can be a traumatic and painful experience for any family dealing with the illness and associated suffering of a loved one, even a loved one who is elderly or has been experiencing the trajectory of a long illness. Tho oncology nurse should explain to the patient and family that which one of the following entities is responsible for assisting the family through the dying process and grieving period?
   A. It is the responsibility of extended family members only.
   B. It is the responsibility of the psychotherapist of the patient.
   C. It is the responsibility of the RN who attends to the patient at home.
   D. It is the responsibility of the whole interdisciplinary hospice team.

10. The tool that was developed and adopted by the National Hospice and Palliative Care Organization in 2007 to assess the sociocultural needs of the patient is called which one of the following?
    A. NCCN
    B. SWAT
    C. ECOG
    D. EQOL

11. K. L. has been placed on hospice care following treatment for metastatic lung cancer. Terminal secretions–also commonly referred to as a "death rattle"–occur when the dying patient is too weak to clear or swallow pharyngeal secretions. The oncology nurse instructs the family that which of the following is one of the least invasive ways to manage terminal secretions in dying patients?
    A. Giving anti-cholinergic drugs
    B. Position patient on their side
    C. Using suctioning
    D. Applying cool wash cloths

12. The oncology nurse does distress screening for every patient prior to chemotherapy. According to the National Comprehensive Cancer Network (NCCN) Distress Screening tool, a patient who scores less than a "4" should be referred to which one of the following services or members of the health care team?
    A. Psychiatrist
    B. Support group
    C. Primary oncologist
    D. Clergy person

13. M. S. is an 80-year-old male, who has been admitted into hospice care with an advanced form of cancer. He has been in hospice care for less than 24 hours, but his health is rapidly declining. After an evaluation from the hospice team, it is determined that M. S.'s death is eminent. Which one of the following signs should the hospice team have considered as a sign of eminent death?
    A. Rapid breathing
    B. Restless movements
    C. Cheyne-Stoke breathing
    D. Bounding pulse

14. An oncology nurse is providing education to a terminally ill patient about medical administration of nutrition and hydration (MANH). The nurse tells the patient and family that MANH is:
    A. unlikely to prolong life
    B. only provided at night so it is less disruptive to sleep
    C. likely to relieve thirst
    D. not associated with fluid overload because only small amounts are given

15. G.T. is a 48-year-old mother of two with metastatic breast cancer which has metastasized to her pancreas. She has recently begun palliative care. She has been suffering from periods of extreme pain, to the point of being debilitating. After consulting with the patient and the patient's family, her palliative care team has decided to initiate a regimen of pain medication. Which one of the following statements best illustrates a standard of palliative care? G.T.'s palliative care team:
    A. respected her autonomy as a patient, as well as her family's wishes, and developed a treatment plan to aggressively treat her cancer
    B. dealt with her psychosocial and spiritual distress
    C. began end-of-life care
    D. respected her autonomy as a patient, as well as her family's wishes, and initiated a plan to ease her pain

16. The social worker meets with a patient recently diagnosed with metastatic cancer. The patient is asked if they have any advance directives, which might include:
    A. last will and testament
    B. living trust
    C. durable power of attorney
    D. title on death documents

17. An example of specialty palliative care is:
    A. interdisciplinary team
    B. certified palliative care advance practice nurse
    C. acute inpatient consultative teams
    D. outpatient pain specialist

18. The diagnosis most commonly seen in hospice care is:
    A. cancer
    B. stroke
    C. dementia
    D. cardiopulmonary failure

19. M. T. is exhausted from providing home hospice care for her husband over the last 3 months. The hospice nurse recommends M. T. consider:
    A. taking scheduled rest breaks
    B. asking a neighbor for help
    C. sending a nurse to the home an extra time each week
    D. utilizing inpatient respite care

20. The hospice nurse has been providing bereavement care for nearly 12 months to the family of a patient who died from leukemia at age 16. The patient's mother is still having difficulty leaving her home, speaking to friends on the phone, or preparing basic meals for her family. The hospice nurse knows this might be a sign of:
    A. anticipatory grief
    B. complicated grief
    C. disenfranchised grief
    D. pathological grief

21. The oncology nurse is providing education to new nurses on the unit about death and dying. The nurse explains that medical aid in dying is also known as:
    A. euthanasia
    B. hospice care
    C. palliative care
    D. physician-assisted suicide

22. Regular assessment of symptoms is important in palliative care. The oncology nurse utilizes the Edmonton Symptom Assessment System–Revised (ESAS-r) to assess for which of the following symptoms?
    A. Pain, delirium, muscle aches
    B. Tiredness, anxiety, chest pain
    C. Shortness of breath, well-being, drowsiness
    D. Depression, nausea, delirium

23. P. T. has metastatic colon cancer and is experiencing delirium. The palliative care nurse recommends:
    A. considering a trial of antidepressants
    B. scheduling opioids for pain management
    C. ensuring the patient has eyeglasses and hearing aids
    D. assessing for changes in mental status every 2 hours

24. D. J. is close to death and has uncontrolled nausea. The hospice nurse explains to the family that palliative sedation:
    A. uses opioids around the clock
    B. can only be done in an inpatient facility
    C. requires placement of an intravenous line
    D. uses nonopioid medications

25. The oncology nurse administers the Palliative Performance Scale to P. L. who was recently diagnosed with metastatic breast cancer. This scale measures:
    A. activity level, orientation, pain
    B. self-care, oral intake, level of consciousness
    C. activity level, pain, hydration
    D. ambulation, orientation, pain

5 Nurse Navigation Across the Cancer Continuum

1. Harold Freeman, in 1990, developed the first patient navigation program for underserved patients in the Harlem neighborhood of New York City. The goal of the first patient navigation program was to reduce mortality in women with which one of the following types of cancer?
   A. Breast
   B. Cervical
   C. Colon
   D. Melanoma

2. Which one of the following is a goal of a patient navigation service?
   A. Identify and resolve barriers to care.
   B. Care for patients at end of life.
   C. Supply medical advice by phone.
   D. Provide telehealth services.

3. A trained nonprofessional or volunteer who provides individualized assistance to patients, families, and caregivers to help overcome health care system barriers and facilitate timely access to quality health and psychosocial care is which one of the following types of navigators?
   A. Lay
   B. Novice
   C. Expert
   D. Community clinic

4. The first navigation program in 1990 started by Harold Freeman in the Harlem neighborhood of New York City focusing on an underserved population of women with breast cancer demonstrated an increase in 5-year cancer survival rates from which one of the following ranges?
   A. 10% to 17%
   B. 25% to 49%
   C. 39% to 70%
   D. 75% to 92%

5. The Academy of Oncology Nurse and Patient Navigators (AONN+) was incorporated in which one of the following years?
   A. 1990
   B. 2000
   C. 2009
   D. 2018

6. Data compiled from the Patient Navigation Research Program (PNRP) revealed that a delay in diagnosis has been correlated with which one of the following conditions?
   A. Unemployment
   B. Coverage from disability insurance
   C. Adequate social support
   D. Higher education levels

7. Sue is collecting and organizing information for a report that she must compile to show the value of the new navigation program that her department is considering implementing. A key part of her report is to show the value of an individual oncology nurse navigator (ONN). As Sue is developing her report, which one of the following measures should be utilized to calculate the value of an ONN?
   A. Improved staffing ratios in inpatient oncology units
   B. Increased length of stay for patient comfort
   C. Provider, patient, and family satisfaction scores
   D. Improved drug costs

8. As part of their role, nurse navigators assess the level of psychosocial distress in patients with cancer as a barrier of care. Which one of the following represents the best time for a nurse navigator to access psychosocial distress in a patient?
   A. At each clinic visit
   B. During the end stage of disease
   C. When a psychologist is present during a clinic visit
   D. When patients have a remote psychiatric diagnosis

9. The most appropriate way to overcome the limitations that determine the effectiveness of nurse navigator programs would be to include data from which one of the following prospective studies?
   A. Gather data from lung cancer patients
   B. Provide navigation services focused on newly diagnosed patients
   C. Studies that use standardized instruments to gather data and measure outcomes
   D. Gather data from large metropolitan cities

10. Ms. J. is a 74-year-old woman who is currently receiving immunotherapy. She calls to report that her car has broken down and she is unable to attend the treatment appointment. She is unsure how long it will be until her car is repaired, and she is concerned about transportation to her future treatment appointments. Ms. J.'s car trouble is an example of which one of the following types of barriers to care that nurse navigators must try to mitigate for their patients with cancer?
    A. Transportation
    B. Cultural
    C. Language
    D. Family support

11. J.S. is a 42-year-old female, who has been diagnosed with breast cancer. She calls stating that she just lost her job and is now unemployed. With mounting medical bills and no income coming in, she'll have no choice but to file for bankruptcy and, from now on, she will no longer be able to afford her medications. After hearing her story, her nurse navigator knows that which one of the following resource(s) may be available for her?
    A. Transition to hospice care because of her financial barriers
    B. Charity care and medication assistance programs
    C. Receiving donated medications from other patients
    D. The treating facility's staff members will pay for her medications

12. Navigators can receive navigator-specific certification via which one of the following?
    A. ACOS
    B. ONS
    C. OCN
    D. AONN+

13. The ONN competency categories for nurse navigators lists four competency categories for navigation. Which one is part of the coordination category?
    A. Identifies potential and realized barriers to care (e.g., transportation, child care, elder care, housing, language, culture, literacy, role disparity, psychosocial, employment, financial, insurance) and facilitates referrals as appropriate to mitigate barriers
    B. Provides appropriate and timely education to patients, families, and caregivers to facilitate understanding and support informed decision making
    C. Develops quality improvement studies for the navigation program
    D. Facilitates timely scheduling of appointments, diagnostic testing, and procedures to expedite the plan of care and to promote continuity of care

6 Communication and Shared Decision-Making

1. An oncology nurse attends a staff development program on communication. The presenter explains that shared decision making (SDM) is described as:
   - A. a theoretical model of care delivery designed to lower health care costs
   - B. an *a priori* model lacking structural validation in actual practice
   - C. a theoretical care delivery model that involves collaboration of the patient and clinician
   - D. a model of local care delivery implemented within specific regions in a state

2. The Agency for Healthcare Research and Quality (AHRQ) developed five steps for SDM referred to as the SHARE approach. Which one of the following clinician's statements exemplifies the first of the five steps?
   - A. "Do you already know which treatment you want to choose?"
   - B. "Share with me what you are taking away from our discussion of treatment options."
   - C. "There are two treatments we should discuss, then I would like to explore your thoughts for treatment."
   - D. "When reviewing the treatment options, are there any worries that immediately come to mind?"

3. SDM has demonstrated short- and long-term benefit and has become a preferred model of care delivery. Which one of the following statements by the patient reflects an immediate, short-term benefit of SDM?
   - A. "I think my quality of life is good to very good on the treatment I was prescribed."
   - B. "I have been taking my oral chemotherapy regularly."
   - C. "My confidence in my provider really improved after receiving the information that I needed."
   - D. "I have been in remission for over 4 years now without any episode of cancer recurrence."

4. In a study among oncology nurses on their perceived barriers to SDM, which one of the following statements about SDM is correct?
   - A. Multiple reminders in the electronic medical record for SDM are utilized.
   - B. Oncology nurses have more than adequate time for SDM.
   - C. There is a lack of resources for education and training about SDM implementation.
   - D. Institutional mandate exists for SDM as a standard of care.

5. The oncology nurse meets G. R., an 80-year-old female newly diagnosed with early stage breast cancer. The nurse realizes that which of the following is a significant influence in an older adult's cancer treatment decisions?
   - A. Number of infusion nurses in clinic
   - B. Availability of educational videos
   - C. Provider recommendations
   - D. Access to patient decision aids

6. The oncology nurse would like to better understand a patient's preferences for making decisions. The most frequently used instrument to measure the degree of patient role preferences in the cancer setting is the:
   - A. OPTION tool
   - B. Pattern of Treatment Decision Making questionnaire (Control Preferences Scale)
   - C. Decisional Conflict Scale
   - D. Satisfaction with Decision Scale

7. During a performance review an oncology nurse is being evaluated on SDM processes. Which one of the following statements indicates the oncology nurse understands the complex role of variables within the context of uncertainty?
   - A. "I will reinforce to the patient that she should make her decision about treatment after a discussion of options with her oncologist."
   - B. "The patient has been given education based on National Comprehensive Cancer Network (NCCN) guidelines."
   - C. "The patient lives on her own and her support comes from her neighbor, who has a full-time job."
   - D. "I didn't tell the patient my concern regarding the possibility of her developing brain metastasis. I know that her mom is currently in hospice care and I didn't want to add even more stress to her life."

8. S. T., a 52-year-old single mother of three, who has been newly diagnosed with breast cancer, meets with her nurse to discuss the diagnosis and next steps. The nurse shares brochures and pamphlets with the patient about her type of cancer and the cancer treatments available. These materials describe some of the possible tests and treatments and outline what patients can expect to happen next. During their conversation, S.T. expresses her concern over, not only the diagnosis, but how she will be treated during the continuum of care, and shares her deep worries over caring for her teenage children. Which of the following best illustrates the nurse's role during SDM in this encounter? The nurse provides:
   A. patient education and psychosocial support
   B. psychosocial support and advocacy
   C. patient education and patient needs assessment
   D. patient education and outcome evaluation

7 Carcinogenesis

1. L.S. is a 49-year-old female with pancreatic cancer. During the course of her tumor work-up, L.S. asks the oncology nurse about the cause of her cancer. The oncology nurse responds to L.S. with the understanding that the genetic alteration frequently associated with her cancer is caused by which one of the following:
   A. an insertion variant
   B. a missense variant
   C. a chromosome translocation
   D. a proto-oncogene

2. The oncology nurse is aware that pathologic variants can develop in genes that normally function to control cell growth. The occurrence of pathologic variants in which one of the following growth-regulating gene types leads to uncontrolled cell proliferation?
   A. Caretaker genes
   B. Tumor suppressor genes
   C. Sex-linked genes
   D. Senescent genes

3. Deoxyribonucleic acid (DNA) contained within the genes located within the chromosomes in the cell nucleus provides the instructions for the cell's function. When a cell with pathologically altered DNA is inherited from an individual's parent, this is called which one of the following?
   A. Germline variant
   B. Somatic variant
   C. Microsatellite
   D. Carcinogen

4. Which one of the following is a definition of carcinogenesis?
   A. The creation of new blood vessels from existing ones to provide nutrients and remove waste products
   B. The transformation of a normal cell into a cancer cell is a complex and dynamic process that starts with pathogenic alterations in regulatory cells and is promoted by genomic instability, inflammation, and interactions within the tumor microenvironment
   C. The process by which epithelial cells lose cell polarity and cell-to-cell adhesion and gain invasive properties so that they can become mesenchymal cells
   D. Mechanism that may change the activity of a gene without changing the sequence of DNA

5. Changes in the normal activity of a gene may occur even when the sequence of DNA in the gene is unaltered. However, certain factors can cause the addition or subtraction of methyl groups within the DNA molecule. This type of acquired genetic reprogramming is caused by which one of the following?
   A. Epigenetic changes
   B. Polymorphic microbiomes
   C. Stimulation of angiogenesis
   D. Release of tumor necrosis factor

6. Tumor formation involves a step-wise process from a single precursor cell with genetic alterations that undergoes clonal expansion as it continues to replicate. Clonal evolution is the process of cells within a tumor accumulating genetic changes over time that are different from one cell to the next. Thus, a tumor may become heterogeneous and consist of cells that initially arose from the same mother cell but are genotypically different from one another. In this model, which is the <u>second</u> phase in the process of tumor formation?
   A. Initiating pathogenic variant
   B. Proliferation of additional driver variants
   C. Acquisition of cancer hallmarks
   D. Acquisition of genomic instability

7. Cancer cells acquire certain biologic capabilities that normal cells do not possess. Among the characteristics of cancer cells is the ability to do which one of the following?
   A. Inhibit angiogenesis
   B. Inactivate cell division
   C. Increase contact inhibition
   D. Resist programmed cell death

8. According to 2022 statistics from the American Cancer Society, colorectal cancer is the third leading cause of new cancer cases and cancer-related deaths in both men and in women. Mr. P., a 55-year-old man who has been diagnosed with metastatic colon cancer, comes to the oncology clinic. The nurse caring for him is aware that the signaling pathway that may be playing a role in the metastases of his colon cancer is which one of the following?
   A. Vascular endothelial growth factor
   B. Epidermal growth factor receptor
   C. Medial growth factor
   D. Nerve growth factor

9. A new oncology nurse is reviewing a patient's medical record and requests help in understanding the process of carcinogenesis. A seasoned nurse explains that the process is due to which one of the following?
   A. Clonal evolution
   B. Convergent evolution
   C. Coevolution
   D. Perseverance

10. R.J. is a 70-year-old male who has been diagnosed with metastatic lung cancer. At his clinic visit, R. J. asks the oncology nurse how the spread of his lung cancer has occurred. The nurse explains that the process of metastasis involves providing the distant tumor deposits with enough oxygen and nutrients so that they can continue to grow and enlarge. The part of the metastatic process that the nurse has described to R.J. is called which one of the following?
    A. Carcinogenesis
    B. Glycolysis
    C. Pathogenesis
    D. Angiogenesis

11. The oncology nurse caring for R. J. explains that the metastatic process begins when tumor cells break off from the primary tumor in the lung and spread through the bloodstream to distant tissues and organs in the body. The cancer cells may be able to avoid detection while circulating in the bloodstream because they are able to do which one of the following?
    A. Secrete proteases that break down solid tissues
    B. Combine with platelets and create emboli
    C. Enter nearby lymph nodes
    D. Become senescent

12. An oncology nurse is caring for a newly diagnosed patient with osteosarcoma who has "skip metastasis." The nurse is aware that this occurs when:
    A. cells bypass one organ and metastasize in another
    B. cells spread into nearby capillary beds or pulmonary arteriovenous shunts
    C. cells bypass the first lymph node and reach more distant sites
    D. tumor cells embed into distant arteries

13. The type of primary tumor that most frequently metastasizes to the brain is which one of the following?
    A. Non–small cell lung cancer
    B. Prostate cancer
    C. Liver cancer
    D. Colorectal cancer

14. Which one of the following is a key association and cause of cancer?
    A. Three servings of fresh fruits and vegetables weekly
    B. White meat in daily diet
    C. Too much fiber in daily diet
    D. Sun exposure and indoor tanning parlors

15. At the clinic, the oncology nurse meets P.J, a 62-year-old woman newly diagnosed with early stage breast cancer. The nurse is aware that the most frequent cause of cancer death is due to which one of the following?
    A. Primary disease in the breast
    B. Lymph node involvement with tumor cells
    C. Metastatic spread of cancer cells
    D. Comorbid disease conditions

8 Immunology

1. Recent surveillance imaging has revealed that an oncology patient, who is currently in remission, has developed new lesions. The phase of tumor suppression mechanism most likely to be implicated in this new development can be classified as which one of the following?
   A. Elimination
   B. Equilibrium
   C. Escape
   D. Progression

2. The concept of immune surveillance occurs:
   A. when innate and adaptive immunity destroy clinically unmeasurable tumors
   B. when a rare cancer clone requires resistance to innate immunity but is stabilized by the adaptive immune system
   C. when tumors enter the equilibrium phase of the proposed tumor suppression mechanism
   D. as a result of receiving multiple, sequential chemotherapeutic agents

3. Adaptive immunity differs from innate immunity in that adaptive immunity:
   A. creates memory cells for a longer-lived immune response
   B. uses humoral immunity through T-cell activation
   C. uses feedback inhibition mechanisms to control tissue damage due to inflammatory response
   D. uses nonspecific processes for immune defense

4. An example of how tumor cells can evade the adaptive immune system would include which one of the following?
   A. Becoming resistant to chemotherapy through drug activation
   B. Promoting T-cell exhaustion by upregulating checkpoint molecules
   C. Keeping the disease in check through actions of the innate immune system
   D. Increasing antigens that are recognized by the adaptive immune system

5. An example of humoral immunity is:
   A. antigen presentation to naïve T cells by antigen-producing cells (APCs)
   B. T lymphocyte activation
   C. the destruction of foreign particles by neutrophils
   D. the production of plasma cells

6. Cytokines function to do which one of the following?
   A. Assist with cell signaling during immune responses
   B. Recognize, ingest, and kill microbes
   C. Produce antibodies against antigens after exposure
   D. Supply tissue nourishment, improve oxygenation, and modulate blood viscosity

7. Organ and tissue components of the immune system include primary lymphoid organs and secondary lymphoid organs and tissues. Secondary lymphoid tissues are sites where antigens are captured and processed in the body. Which one of the following is an example of both primary and secondary lymphoid tissue?
   A. Spleen
   B. Lymph nodes
   C. Bone marrow
   D. Thymus

8. Lymphoid stem cell lineage has several types of lymphocytes that play a key role in immune responses. Which one of the following cells migrate to the thymus gland for maturation and are integral to immune surveillance and response?
   A. NK cells
   B. Dendritic cells
   C. T cells
   D. B cells

9. Which one of the following is the most abundant granulocyte?
   A. Neutrophils
   B. Basophils
   C. Eosinophils
   D. Macrophages

9 Precision Medicine

1. Which of the following information is most important in the application of precision medicine in a patient with a cholangiocarcinoma?
   A. 11.5 × 10.0 × 9.5 cm right hepatic lobe mass
   B. High positive expression of programmed death-ligand 1 (>50%)
   C. Tolerated adjuvant therapy with leucovorin, fluorouracil, and oxaliplatin (FOLFOX)
   D. Alanine aminotransferase 80 U/L, aspartate aminotransferase 123 U/L, total bilirubin 2.9 mg/dL

2. K.T. is a 29-year-old female patient, who has been newly diagnosed with breast cancer. K. T. has asked her oncology nurse why the oncologist would require the result of the biomarker test to determine the treatment plan. Which of the teach-back responses indicates that the patient did *not* fully understand her oncology nurse's explanation?
   A. "The results will tell us how long I have had the cancer."
   B. "The results can predict if the treatment will work for me."
   C. "My doctor will use the results to find out if I will need chemotherapy after surgery."
   D. "The results can be used to measure how aggressive my cancer is."

3. The use of ER/PR/Her-2/Neu status to guide decisions on the use of adjuvant systemic chemotherapy is an example of:
   A. use of a cancer-risk assessment tool to confirm suspected familial cancer syndromes
   B. dose determination based on genomics
   C. use of biomarkers to guide treatment decisions
   D. use of testing to determine eligibility for a clinical trial

4. The field of pharmacogenomics has revolutionized cancer care because it:
   A. increased rates of nonadherence to therapy
   B. lowered the cost of cancer treatment
   C. increased enrollment in clinical trials
   D. increased the safety and efficacy of cancer drugs

5. The use of targeted therapies is common within oncology practice and involves the use of genetic and genomic information of the cancer tissue to guide selection of an appropriate targeted drug therapy. One of the benefits of using targeted therapies is:
   A. less severe adverse reactions
   B. not classified as hazardous drugs
   C. spares normal cells
   D. only available in oral formulation

6. K.T., a 29-year-old female patient with breast cancer, has requested information on genetic and molecular testing. Her oncology nurse knows that her patient will need more information when she is heard saying:
   A. "Please expedite the results. I need them in 2 days for my second opinion."
   B. "I understand that my results may have implications to the rest of my family."
   C. "I will need to inquire if my health insurance will cover the costs related to genetic and molecular testing."
   D. "There are known risks to my privacy and confidentiality."

7. Which of the following is a definition of gene deletion?
   A. Heritable change that does not alter the DNA sequence but changes gene expression
   B. Loss of all or part of a gene found in cancer cells and other genetic diseases
   C. Increase in the copies of a protein made from a gene that may play a role in cancer development
   D. Increase in the number of copies of a gene that may cause cancer cell growth or resistance to anticancer drugs

8. When administering precision medicine treatments, the health care team must be aware of ethical considerations affecting the patient. Which one of the following is an ethical concern?
   A. After beginning treatment of a targeted therapy, the patient develops an unexpected adverse event, leading to life-threatening complications that neither the patient nor the patient's family had expected.
   B. Though the patient has been educated on the topic, the side effects of a particular treatment have severely comprised the patient's quality of life.
   C. The cost of the treatments is such that the patient experiences financial toxicity and must stop treatment while deciding how to pay the price of drugs.
   D. The patient is concerned about data security and fears government intrusion that may affect health care coverage.

10 Genetics and Cancer

1. Application of the Central Dogma of molecular biology to oncology nursing practice is important because:
   A. Canines have the same DNA nucleotides as humans.
   B. It explains the production of protein for all body functions.
   C. DNA and RNA contain identical nucleic acids for genetic information important in genetic testing in hereditary risk.
   D. The genetic make-up of humans is 95.5% similar and 4.5% different.

2. The experienced oncology nurse is explaining basic genetic concepts to new orientees. The nurse explains that humans have:
   A. 46 pairs of chromosomes comprised of 92 autosomes
   B. 23 pairs of chromosomes comprised of 46 autosomes
   C. 46 pairs of chromosomes with half from each parent
   D. 23 pairs of chromosomes with one copy from each parent

3. The oncology nurse is caring for a 29-year-old female patient newly diagnosed with bilateral breast cancer. Which of the following would raise suspicion for hereditary breast and ovarian cancer (HBOC) syndrome?
   A. Maternal aunt and paternal uncle with a history of brain cancer at unknown ages
   B. Mother was diagnosed with ovarian cancer at age 33 years
   C. Brother was diagnosed with testicular cancer at age 25 years after he served in the military during Vietnam
   D. 4-year-old nephew diagnosed with leukemia

4. A new oncology nurse asks how to determine if a cell is somatic or germline. You explain that:
   A. Germline cells will have single nucleotide variants (SNVs) associated with pathogenicity.
   B. A somatic cell acquires pathogenic changes during the monthly reproductive cycle of the body.
   C. Germline pathogenic variants occur in the egg or sperm of a person with an inherited cancer predisposition.
   D. Somatic cells accumulate pathogenic changes prior to conception while *in utero*.

5. Which of the following statements explains the derivation of a cancerous tumor?
   A. Genetic alterations in genes that control cell growth and proliferation are commonly associated with the development of cancer.
   B. Proto-oncogenes are frequently associated with the proliferation and development of malignancies.
   C. Passenger pathogenic variants are essential to cancers caused by driver variants.
   D. Pathogenic variants in a DNA repair gene are not associated with environmental carcinogens or inheritance.

6. A patient is being seen in the high-risk cancer clinic because they possess features suggestive of an inherited risk for developing malignancy. These features could include:
   A. same malignancy seen in both grandmothers
   B. no known germline pathogenic variants in a cancer susceptibility gene
   C. multiple close relatives with the same or related types of cancer in multiple generations
   D. a unique variety of cancer types on both sides of the family in multiple generations.

7. Pedigree construction that identifies a family at high risk for inherited cancer should include:
   A. at least four generations of cancer information for both lineages
   B. the use of squares to designate females and circles to designate males
   C. race, ethnicity, and age of individuals, but only if there is cancer in the generation
   D. history of treatments that may have reduced risk of cancer

8. A negative genetic testing result for a known germline pathogenic variant should include the following caveat:
   A. risk of malignancy is negligible
   B. the family may be affected by a somatic variant in another gene
   C. family history from the other parent influences the risk of developing cancer
   D. the cancer in the family may not be caused by a germline pathogenic variant

19

9. A "variant of unknown significance" (VUS) has which of the following characteristics?
   A. It is identified when a cancer risk has been established.
   B. It identifies a genetic change in which the association with cancer risk cannot be established.
   C. Once identified, a VUS maintains that label forever.
   D. A VUS is an uncommon genetic finding.

10. A patient with a family history of breast cancer has had genetic testing with "23 and Me" and reports her result was "negative." Which of the following information should be discussed with her?
    A. This tests for *BRCA1/2* genetic testing only and includes three pathogenic variants.
    B. Breast cancer predisposition testing from this test is not United States Food and Drug Administration approved.
    C. Direct-to-consumer testing is approved for use in diagnosis and treatment of breast cancer.
    D. All direct-to-consumer testing is the same.

11. Which testing strategy is used to identify chromosomal abnormalities?
    A. Cytogenetics
    B. Sanger sequencing
    C. Genome-wide association studies (GWAS)
    D. Transcriptome analysis

12. A germline pathogenic variant occurs in the gametes and:
    A. is present only in first generation
    B. is present in nonreproductive cells
    C. can include a *de novo* pathogenic variant
    D. occurs after conception

13. Which one of the following may be a psychological consequence to the patient who receives genetic testing results that reveal substantially increased risk for developing cancer?
    A. Depression, yet a sense of relief
    B. Transmitter guilt
    C. Heightened anxiety
    D. Survivor guilt

14. Which of the following groups are included in the Genetic Non-Discrimination Act (GINA)?
    A. Indian Health Service
    B. Active duty military
    C. Veterans Administration
    D. Adolescents

15. Which one of the following provisions of informed consent for genetic testing is not included when consented for testing?
    A. Purpose of the test
    B. Motivation for testing
    C. Impact of test result on health care decision-making
    D. Longevity of life after testing

16. Which one of the following diseases does not increase the risk for a primary brain tumor?
    A. Peutz-Jeghers syndrome
    B. Neurofibromatosis type 1
    C. Li-Fraumeni syndrome
    D. von Hippel-Lindau disease

17. The small arm of the chromosome is labeled as
    A. o
    B. p
    C. q
    D. s

18. The protein coding section of a gene is referred to as
    A. Exon
    B. Codon
    C. Intron
    D. Autosome

19. Which of the following hereditary cancer syndromes is inherited in an autosomal recessive fashion?
    A. Hereditary retinoblastoma
    B. MUYTH associated polyposis
    C. Hereditary diffuse gastric cancer
    D. Multiple endocrine neoplasia type 1

20. Pathogenic variants in the MSH2 gene are associated with cancers of the:
    A. lung
    B. ovary
    C. sarcoma
    D. thyroid

11 Research Protocols and Clinical Trials

1. A clinical trial study in which participants are not assigned to a specific intervention and health care outcomes are assessed is described as which one of the following?
   A. Experimental
   B. Interventional
   C. Expanded access
   D. Observational

2. Individuals from the general population who are enrolled in a clinical trial study to evaluate a new technique for early detection of skin cancer are in which type of the following clinical trials?
   A. Screening
   B. Diagnostic
   C. Quality of life
   D. Prevention

3. Which one of the following is a characteristic of an expanded access protocol?
   A. An investigational drug is used outside of a designated clinical trial
   B. Provides a means to use a therapy off label
   C. Patient must have early-stage cancer
   D. Designed to evaluate the safety and efficacy of an intervention

4. The individual with primary responsibility to ensure the ethical conduct of the research study is which one of the following?
   A. Study coordinator
   B. Principal investigator
   C. Statistician
   D. Data manager

5. The code of ethics and conduct that focuses primarily on beneficence, respect for persons, and justice is known as which one of the following?
   A. Nuremberg Code
   B. Declaration of Helsinki
   C. Common Rule
   D. Belmont Report

6. A common inclusion criteria for eligibility for enrollment into an oncology clinical trial is which of the following?
   A. Geographic area of residence
   B. Performance status
   C. No prior research participation
   D. Number of children

7. The approximate number of subjects needed to be enrolled in a Phase I study is which one of the following?
   A. 10 to 12
   B. 20 to 100
   C. 80 to 300
   D. 500 to 1000

8. The clinical trial endpoint of "time from randomization until death" is known as which one of the following terms?
   A. Disease-free survival
   B. Objective response rate
   C. Overall survival
   D. Time to progression

9. Which one of the following depicts a factorial design? Randomization to treatment:
   A. A or B
   B. A→outcome→B
   C. A, B, A and B
   D. A, B, A and B, placebo

10. A clinical trial study where subjects who have no reported outcomes or conditions are followed and compared, based on exposure, is described as which one of the following?
    A. Experimental
    B. Outcomes research
    C. Cohort studies
    D. Observational

11. A clinical trial study which explores the results of health care practices and interventions, includes patient-based outcomes, as well as the study of populations, databases, and the delivery of health care, is described as which one of the following?
    A. Interventional
    B. Outcomes research
    C. Cohort studies
    D. Experimental

12. J. L. is a 49-year-old male with lung cancer who has recently enrolled into a clinical trial. The clinical trial explores new interventions to minimize toxicities related to cancer and cancer treatments. The clinical trial is an example of which one of the following?
    A. Screening
    B. Prevention
    C. Quality of life
    D. Therapeutic

12 Bone and Soft Tissue Cancers

1. Primary tumors that have been known to spread to the bone include which one of the following?
   A. Prostate
   B. Brain
   C. Leukemia
   D. Ovary

2. T.K. is a 43-year-old male patient. During a physical assessment, the nurse notes a palpable mass in the area of a patient's tibia. A key part of physical assessment and documentation would be to include a(n):
   A. needle aspiration
   B. incision and drainage
   C. comparison to the unaffected side
   D. evaluation of complete blood count results

3. Nursing management post-reconstruction of a bone or soft tissue tumor includes a focus on assessing for which one of the following?
   A. Thrombocytopenia
   B. Pruritis
   C. Cytokine response
   D. Infection

4. Adjuvant radiotherapy can be a component of treatment in soft tissue tumors:
   A. only before surgery
   B. when the tumor has metastasized
   C. as the primary standard of care
   D. after the tumor has been debulked

5. After amputation, the patient may experience phantom limb pain:
   A. for 1 to 2 weeks after surgery
   B. postoperatively, starting 8 weeks or more after surgery
   C. chronically
   D. intermittently when standing

6. The oncology nurse is meeting with a patient who has been diagnosed with Kaposi sarcoma. The nurse is aware that Kaposi sarcoma more commonly occurs in which of these groups?
   A. Men younger than age 45
   B. People who have HIV or AIDS
   C. High socioeconomic populations
   D. Women who are postmenopausal

7. The treatment of choice for a patient diagnosed with chondrosarcoma is which of the following methods?
   A. chemotherapy
   B. surgery
   C. immunotherapy
   D. radiation therapy

8. According to the American Cancer Society and the National Cancer Institute, which one of the following is the most important risk factor for developing a soft tissue sarcoma?
   A. Prior radiation therapy
   B. Smoking history
   C. Food allergies
   D. Middle age

13 Breast Cancer

1. Which one of the following factors makes a patient more likely to have a germline pathogenic variant associated with an increased risk of developing breast cancer?
   A. History of multiple breast surgeries
   B. First-degree relative with breast cancer
   C. Age of menopause or menarche prior to diagnosis
   D. Nulliparity

2. Which one of the following patients should undergo genetic testing for the presence of a pathogenic variant associated with increased susceptibility for breast cancer?
   A. A 60-year-old male with breast cancer
   B. An 80-year-old female with grade 1, estrogen receptor (ER)-positive, progestogen receptor (PR)-positive breast cancer
   C. A 55-year-old female with ductal carcinoma *in situ* (DCIS)
   D. A 62-year-old female who is the first to be diagnosed in her family

3. An approved agent that could be utilized for the primary prevention of breast cancer in high-risk postmenopausal women with breast cancer is the use of which one of the following?
   A. Retinoids
   B. Metformin
   C. Raloxifene
   D. Cox-2 inhibitors

4. What type of breast cancer is suggestive of poor prognosis?
   A. ER-positive, PR-positive invasive ductal carcinoma
   B. ER-positive, PR-positive invasive lobular carcinoma
   C. ER-negative, PR-negative, Her-2/Neu-negative breast cancer
   D. T2 tumor between 2cm and 5cm with no lymph nodes positive.

5. W. J. is a 56-year-old woman who has just had a right-sided mastectomy and an axillary lymph node dissection. The nurse should provide instructions about which of these measures at the patient's first postoperative visit?
   A. Measure the circumference of the affected arm
   B. Avoid upper extremity exercise on the left arm.
   C. Take temperature and report a temperature of 99°F.
   D. Reduce sodium intake to less than 1800 mg daily.

6. S. L. is a 67-year-old women who has been diagnosed with stage I ER/PR-positive, HER2-negative breast cancer. During her extent of disease work-up, the patient has an Oncotype DX test that shows a recurrence score of 24. She asks her nurse what that means. The nurse should respond with which one of the following statements?
   A. "This recurrence score indicates that you will need additional chemotherapy."
   B. "This is a 70-gene assay test that shows you have a low risk of metastases."
   C. "Most likely you will not benefit from the addition of chemotherapy."
   D. "There is a high likelihood that your breast cancer will recur after therapy."

7. Which one of the following patients is most likely to develop breast cancer during their lifetime?
   A. J.L., who is a 30-year-old Hispanic woman
   B. D.C., who is a 44-year-old white male
   C. B.R., who is a 37-year-old African American woman
   D. T.K., who is a 27-year-old white woman

8. Breast milk is produced by which one of the following?
   A. Adipose tissue
   B. Sebaceous tissue
   C. Primary duct units
   D. Terminal duct lobular units

9. Which one of the following is true about luminal A tumors?
   A. Luminal A tumors have the highest levels of ER expression: ER positive and/or PR-positive
   B. Luminal A tumors tend to be high grade
   C. Luminal A tumors seldom respond to endocrine therapy
   D. Luminal A tumors have a poor prognosis

10. Histologic characteristics of breast cancer are often determined by the Bloom-Richardson system. Which statement correctly reflects this histologic classification?
    A. Grade 1 - low grade and poorly differentiated
    B. Grade 1 - low grade and well differentiated
    C. Grade 1 - high grade and well differentiated
    D. Grade 1 - high grade and poorly differentiated

14 Gastrointestinal Cancers

1. S.R. is experiencing difficulty swallowing. The oncology nurse knows that the diagnostic work-up for esophageal cancer includes:
   A. colonoscopy
   B. endoscopy
   C. brain MRI
   D. abdominal ultrasound

2. F.G. is concerned about his risk for gastrointestinal cancer. The oncology nurse explains to the patient that a modifiable risk factor for stomach cancer is:
   A. excessive alcohol use
   B. family history
   C. achalasia
   D. Lynch syndrome

3. The oncology nurse is providing a seminar on cancer prevention and detection. Which one of the following procedures is a screening technique for colorectal cancer?
   A. Abdominal CT
   B. Abdominal ultrasound
   C. Pelvic CT
   D. Immunochemical fecal occult blood test

4. J.L.'s pathology report from her colon cancer resection is available. The oncology nurse explains to the patient that molecular classification for metastatic colorectal cancer includes:
   A. programmed death ligand-1
   B. KRAS/NRAS
   C. estrogen receptor/progesterone receptors
   D. EGFR pathogenic variant

5. B. B. questions vaccination recommendations for the prevention of cancer. The oncology nurse provides education and tells B. B. that anal cancer risk is associated with infection with which of these viruses?
   A. Hepatitis B virus
   B. Epstein-Barr virus
   C. Human papillomavirus (HPV)
   D. Human T-lymphotrophic virus (HTLV-1)

6. The oncology nurse is performing a cancer risk assessment. The nurse knows which one of the following viruses is most commonly associated with hepatocellular cancer?
   A. Hepatitis C virus
   B. Influenza
   C. Human immunodeficiency virus (HIV)
   D. *H. pylori* infection

7. V.O., a 56-year-old African American female, was recently diagnosed with hepatocellular carcinoma. The oncology team discusses her treatment options. Which one of the following is a potential curative therapy for hepatocellular carcinoma?
   A. Transarterial chemoembolization
   B. Nivolumab
   C. Sorafenib
   D. Liver transplant

8. What percentage of pancreatic cancers are classified as adenocarcinomas?
   A. 5%
   B. 25%
   C. 75%
   D. 95%

9. Which one of the following is a systemic therapy for metastatic colon cancer?
   A. Trastuzumab
   B. Carboplatin/paclitaxel
   C. Regorafenib
   D. Gemcitabine

10. T.J. is a 41-year-old male, in good health, but whose family history of colon cancer has made him concerned about the possibility of developing colorectal cancer. Which one of the following should T.J.'s nurse recommend to him as a means of primary cancer prevention?
    A. Treat *H. pylori*, gastric ulcers
    B. Vaccinate against hepatitis B
    C. Begin testing with fecal immunochemistry test at age 45
    D. Exercise at least 150 minutes per week

11. The oncology nurse is providing a lecture on the epidemiology and screening for colorectal cancer. The nurse explains that there are multiple risk factors for developing colon cancer, some of which are modifiable and some which are not. The nurse discussed that although it is not modifiable, the following group is at highest risk for developing colon cancer:
    A. White males
    B. Asian females
    C. African American males
    D. Native American females

12. The oncology team is discussing treatment options for L. M. who was diagnosed with Stage I adenocarcinoma of the pancreas. The oncology nurse knows that the most likely treatment option to be recommended is:
    A. pancreatoduodenectomy
    B. palliative radiation
    C. pembrolizumab
    D. gemcitabine/nab-paclitaxel

15 Genitourinary Cancers

1. M.K. is a 59-year-old male patient who has been diagnosed with clear-cell carcinoma of the kidney. The oncology nurse caring for him is aware that which one of the following is true about M.K.'s cancer?
   A. This type of kidney cancer is unusual.
   B. This type of kidney cancer arises in the renal pelvis.
   C. This type of kidney cancer has the worst prognosis.
   D. This type of kidney cancer is the most common.

2. J.L. is a 63-year-old female who has recently been diagnosed with kidney cancer. She is concerned and confused because kidney cancer does not run in her family, and she asks her nurse for an explanation. Her nurse explains that two factors associated with increased risk include which one of the following?
   A. having a history of non-Hodgkin lymphoma and being overweight
   B. being of Asian descent and having a history of kidney stones
   C. consuming processed meats and sedentary occupation
   D. having a tall stature and being underweight

3. T.F. is a 54-year-old female patient who reports episodes of hematuria. The nurse anticipates which one of these diagnostic tests to determine etiology?
   A. Colonoscopy
   B. Kidney biopsy
   C. Intravenous pyelogram
   D. Blood chemistries

4. Diagnostic tests reveal that a patient with limited renal function has developed a primary tumor in the kidney. The nurse should anticipate an order to prepare the patient for which one of the following treatments?
   A. Partial nephrectomy
   B. Cytoreductive nephrectomy
   C. Radiation therapy
   D. Chemotherapy

5. H.R. is a 67-year-old male patient. He arrives at his local infusion center to receive treatment for kidney cancer. Treatment options that have been shown to improve response rates for this type of disease include use of which one of the following?
   A. Systemic radiation therapy
   B. Antibody-drug conjugates
   C. Cytotoxic chemotherapy
   D. Immunotherapy agents

6. C.M. is a 47-year-old female who has been diagnosed with urothelial carcinoma of the bladder. The nurse educating the patient and her family about this type of bladder cancer explains that urothelial carcinoma of the bladder is:
   A. the least common type of bladder cancer
   B. responsible for most cases of bladder cancer
   C. most likely to be invasive at diagnosis
   D. associated with changes to chromosome 9

7. T.C. is a 35-year-old son of a patient with bladder cancer. During a recent visit, he asks the oncology nurse for advice on which behaviors he should adopt to help him reduce the risk of developing bladder cancer, like his father. The nurse explains that factors associated with increased risk include which one of the following?
   A. Weight loss
   B. Tobacco use
   C. Excessive fluid intake
   D. Diet low in processed meats

8. J.C. is a 44-year-old man who presents for his annual well-visit examination and asks his nurse about prostate screening. The nurse informs him that guidelines for prostate-specific antigen (PSA) screening in men at average risk of prostate cancer recommend that screening:
   A. begins at age 45 years
   B. is not useful for men at any age
   C. should be done between ages 55 and 69 years
   D. once initiated, should be repeated every year

9. Grading for prostate cancer is based on the Gleason Score, which is determined by results from which one of the following?
   A. Imaging tests using MRI or CT
   B. Tissue specimen examination
   C. Blood tests for PSA levels
   D. Bone marrow aspiration

10. K.L. is a 47-year-old male who has been diagnosed with metastatic prostate cancer. At the physician's office he asks the oncology nurse about recommended treatment options. The nurse explains that the standard treatment option for K.L. is which one of the following?
    A. Radical prostatectomy
    B. Hormonal manipulation
    C. Insertion of radioactive seeds into the prostate
    D. Cryosurgery to freeze the involved prostatic tissue

11. Potential complications after treatment with radioactive seed placement into the prostate include which one of the following?
    A. Increased libido
    B. Constipation
    C. Impotence
    D. Anemia

12. Which one of the following is an essential nursing measure when trying to maximize and promote a patient's safety after surgery?
    A. Teaching a patient to manage and identify symptoms, including providing recommendations on when to report symptoms
    B. Monitoring vital signs, hemoglobin, hematocrit, kidney function tests, and urine output
    C. Teaching patients how to perform coping skills to control anxiety and fear
    D. Monitoring patients for signs of distress

13. A patient will be undergoing urologic diagnostic testing. Which one of the following nursing interventions should the nurse perform for a radiographic examination of the kidneys, ureter, and bladder (KUB)?
    A. Assess the patient for history of allergy to iodine dyes or contrast media before performing the test.
    B. Explain to the patient the need to lie flat on examination table.
    C. Observe the patient for a reaction to anesthetic or analgesic.
    D. Monitor the patient for bleeding, and symptoms of a urinary tract infection.

14. Mr. S. is a 70-year-old man who has been diagnosed with bladder cancer. At the clinic, the oncology nurse describes the treatment options for his bladder cancer. The nurse is aware that Mr. S. understands the difference between the treatments when he states that which one of the following options preserves the bladder?
    A. Radical cystectomy
    B. Continent ileal reservoir
    C. Ileal conduit
    D. External beam radiation therapy

15. Screening guidelines exist for which of these cancers of the urologic system?
    A. Prostate cancer
    B. Bladder cancer
    C. Kidney cancer
    D. Testicular cancer

16 Head and Neck Cancers

1. The oncology nurse is reviewing the chart of a patient who has been diagnosed with a head and neck cancer. Which one of the following cancers does the patient have that is considered a head and neck cancer?
   A. Esophagus
   B. Thyroid
   C. Brain
   D. Bone

2. The oncology nurse is aware that which one of the following is a risk factor for developing head and neck cancer?
   A. Human papillomavirus (HPV)
   B. Diabetes
   C. Menopause
   D. Dental implants

3. In order to develop a treatment plan for a patient with head and neck cancer, the results of which of the following procedures is needed initially?
   A. Hereditary genetic test
   B. Detailed family history
   C. Neutrophil count
   D. Biopsy of the tumor

4. For head and neck cancers, the disease work-up would most likely include which of the following imaging procedures?
   A. Chest radiograph and Gallium scan
   B. CT and/or MRI
   C. Neck ultrasound and intravenous pyelogram
   D. Positron emission tomography and barium enema

5. The oncology nurse caring for a patient being treated for a head and neck cancer should specifically focus on which one of the following measures?
   A. Monitoring swallowing ability
   B. Delivering skin care
   C. Assessing for lymphedema
   D. Evaluation of neutropenia

6. Before a patient's scheduled laryngectomy, the oncology nurse should provide patient teaching focused on which one of the following?
   A. Gait disturbance
   B. Lack of endurance
   C. Avoidance of opioid addiction
   D. Communication strategies

7. Immediate postoperative nursing care of patients with surgical grafting done during head and neck cancer surgery would include assessment of which one of the following?
   A. Perfusion of blood supply to the graft site
   B. Range of motion in the shoulders
   C. Need for debridement of necrotic tissue
   D. Presence of blood clots and need for lavage

8. Which one of the following outpatient referrals should the oncology nurse make for a patient who has had a neck dissection for treatment for head and neck cancer?
   A. Occupational therapy
   B. Physical therapy
   C. Pain management
   D. Gastroenterologist

9. A.P. is a male patient who is postoperative after a supraglottic laryngectomy. The oncology nurse caring for him understands that the primary nursing concern for A.P. following this surgery is the risk for which one of the following?
   A. Fall
   B. Dehydration
   C. Aspiration
   D. Somnolence

10. The oncology nurse should be aware that which of these signs or symptoms, if reported by a patient, would lead to a disease work-up for head and neck cancer?
    A. Bilateral ear pain with hearing loss
    B. A temperature >100°F accompanied by a sore throat
    C. Episodic hoarseness that resolves in 1 week
    D. A lump or sore in the mouth or lip that does not heal

11. The oncology nurse is caring for a patient who has been diagnosed with cancer of the oropharynx. The nurse is aware that which one of the following descriptions is accurate about the anatomy of the oropharynx?
    A. Extends from the lips to the hard palate above and the circumvallate papillae below, and structures include lips, buccal mucosa, floor of the mouth, and upper and lower alveoli
    B. Located below the base of the skull and behind the nasal cavity and continuous with the posterior pharyngeal wall
    C. Extends from the circumvallate papillae below and hard palate above to the level of the hyoid bone
    D. Extends from the epiglottis to the cricoid cartilage; protected by the thyroid cartilage, which encases it

29

12. The oncology nurse notes that a patient with head and neck cancer is on the surgery schedule for a hemilaryngectomy. The nurse understands that which of the following describes the physical alteration and nursing care implications for the patient undergoing a hemilaryngectomy procedure?
    A. Little to no physical alteration and minimal bleeding
    B. Vertical excision of one true and one false cord, hoarse voice, and minimal to no swallowing problems
    C. Partial or total en-bloc resection of the cavity that may include the ethmoid sinus and lateral nasal wall, and requires daily care to the surgical cavity and placement of obturator
    D. Surgical approach to inaccessible midfacial and extensive paranasal sinus and nasopharyngeal lesions that may create facial defect and cranial nerve (III, IV, V) deficits

13. Which one of the following is a definition for the hypopharynx?
    A. Located below the base of the tongue, and extending to but not including the true vocal cord
    B. Extends from the circumvallate papillae below and hard palate above to the level of the hyoid bone
    C. Extends from the hyoid bone to the lower border of the cricoid cartilage
    D. Includes the nasal vestibule; paired maxillary, ethmoid, and frontal sinuses

14. The nurse in the oncology clinic should be aware that cancers of the head and neck occur most often in which of the following groups?
    A. Women who never gave birth
    B. Men with HPV infections
    C. Those who use hair dye
    D. Those under age 40

15. The oncology clinical nurse specialist (CNS) is providing education to staff nurses on the oncology unit. The CNS should teach that screening strategies to detect cancers of the oral cavity include which of the following?
    A. Screening guidelines
    B. Mouth radiographs
    C. Sputum evaluation
    D. Dental inspection

16. An oncology nurse working in the head and neck cancer clinic needs to be up to date with statistics regarding disease prognosis and survival. After review, the nurse should be aware that which of these statements about head and neck cancers is accurate?
    A. Survival rates are higher in black patients compared to white patients.
    B. New cases of laryngeal cancer are increasing by 2% to 3% a year.
    C. Thyroid cancer has the highest 5-year relative survival rate.
    D. Patients with oral HPV infections do worse than those without.

17. A patient is admitted to the hospital for treatment of nasopharyngeal cancer. Which one of the following choices is accurate about cancers located in the nasopharynx? These cancers:
    A. involve the vocal cords
    B. arise from the floor of the mouth
    C. are in an area close to the brain
    D. originate in the soft palate

18. P.L., a 47-year-old male, is being worked up for cancer of the oropharynx. In taking his history, the oncology nurse questions him about his lifestyle habits. Which of these habits, if reported by P.L., is associated with increased risk of cancer of the oropharynx?
    A. Drinks alcohol at home each evening
    B. Likes fried foods and sugary beverages
    C. Works in a natural history museum
    D. Wears glasses for nearsightedness

17 Infection-Related Cancers

1. The average time from human immunodeficiency virus (HIV) infection to symptomatic disease is best described as which one of the following?
   A. Dependent on preexisting health
   B. Approximately 15 years
   C. Dependent on age at time of exposure
   D. Dependent on number of sexual partners

2. The oncology nurse knows that the three stages of HIV are described by which one of the following? (choose the correct progression of disease):
   A. Chronic/progressive disease, acquired immune deficiency syndrome (AIDS), acute infection
   B. Acute infection, AIDS, chronic/progressive infection
   C. Acute infection, chronic/progressive infection, AIDS
   D. Chronic/progressive disease/acute infection

3. Lifestyle factors such as nutritional status, overall health, and smoking may result in infection with other strains of HIV and:
   A. slow the disease progression
   B. influence the course of infection
   C. may hasten the disease progression
   D. are seen in approximately 37% of cases

4. The oncology nurse is providing an educational program on the epidemiology of HIV in the United States. In the nurse's discussion, which one of the following statements is TRUE regarding HIV in the United States?
   A. One-half of individuals with HIV will die from cancer.
   B. One in 10 persons infected with HIV does not realize it.
   C. Heterosexual contact with HIV-infected individuals accounts for about 34% of new HIV diagnoses.
   D. Those older than 50 years of age are the fastest growing HIV-positive population.

5. The nurse at the HIV clinic educates HIV-positive patients that they are at risk for which one of the following AIDs-defining malignancies?
   A. Oral and esophageal cancers
   B. Prostate and anal cancers
   C. Breast and ovarian cancers
   D. B-cell lymphoma and Burkitt lymphoma

6. A nurse is caring for a 29-year-old female patient who was recently diagnosed with AIDS. Her CD4 count is 293, and she is on active antiretroviral therapy. Based on the information provided, the nurse would educate the patient on the fact that she is at increased risk for developing which one of the following types of cancer?
   A. Lung cancer
   B. Acute myeloid leukemia
   C. Cervical cancer
   D. Kidney cancer

7. While a patient with AIDS-related diffuse large-cell B-cell lymphoma (DLBCL) is receiving R-CHOP immuno-chemotherapy, the oncology nurse should make every attempt to continue chimeric antigen receptor T-cell therapy (cART) throughout the course of antineoplastic therapy by doing which one of the following?
   A. Monitor for overlapping toxicities that may occur with combination therapy.
   B. Administer steroids to decrease the risk of inflammatory response.
   C. Administer Shingrix vaccine to decrease risk of varicella-zoster virus reactivation.
   D. Hold antineoplastic therapy in the setting of low CD4+ counts.

8. A characteristic of HIV-related lymphoma includes which one of the following?
   A. A CD4+ count of 400/mm^3
   B. An active EBV infection
   C. The presence of CD20+ marker
   D. An early manifestation of HIV infection

9. HIV-infected patients diagnosed with primary CNS lymphoma have which one of the following?
   A. Extensive bone marrow involvement
   B. A normal CD4+ count
   C. A 20% chance of ocular involvement
   D. Absent BCL6 pathogenic variant

10. J. J. is a 54-year-old HIV-infected male patient who has been admitted for treatment of PCP pneumonia with intravenous Bactrim. On day 2 of his admission, the patient develops altered mental status, fever, shortness of breath, and leukocytosis. His nurse anticipates the patient is experiencing signs and symptoms of which one of the following?
    A. Worsening PCP pneumonia
    B. Anaphylactic reaction to Bactrim
    C. Immune reconstitution syndrome
    D. Superimposing infection

11. Based on a nurse's current knowledge of survival factors in Kaposi sarcoma, the nurse understands that which of the following is true?
    A. There has been a dramatic decrease in survival despite the era of cART.
    B. The median survival is less than 6 months.
    C. Prior or comorbid major opportunistic infections have no impact on survival.
    D. Survival is shorter in patients with gastrointestinal lesions or B symptoms.

12. An oncology nurse has volunteered her time at a community health fair and is staffing a booth on the prevention of various cancers. Included in her materials are teaching materials on how to reduce the possibility of HIV transmission. Which one of the following would most likely be included in the educational materials she plans to hand out?
    A. Provide education about the use of latex condom with a water-based lubricant to reduce risk.
    B. Provide education about the use of latex condom with a petroleum-based lubricant to reduce risk.
    C. Provide education about the best way to share household toiletries such as razors and other personal items.
    D. Provide education about how to mix a solution of 1-part household bleach to 5 parts water to use with gloves in the clean up of emesis or other body fluid spills.

13. As part of any patient education program, an oncology nurse must assess the patient's health literacy and ability to comply with complex therapies and multiple appointments with medical specialists. Which one of the following is a factor that health literacy has on a patient's quality of care?
    A. Low health literacy in patients has little impact on maintaining regular medical care.
    B. Low health literacy is not associated with English not being the first language spoken by a patient since interpreters are readily available at most health care institutions.
    C. Only 50% of patients who score low on a health literacy assessment have been found to maintain regular medical care.
    D. Studies of antiretroviral adherence reflect low rates of medication adherence among individuals with low health literacy.

14. The oncology nurse is providing an inservice on cancer epidemiology. The nurse explains that schistosomiasis is associated with an increased risk of developing which one of the following cancers?
    A. Cholangiocarcinoma
    B. Bladder cancer
    C. Pancreatic cancer
    D. Leukemia

15. During the initial assessment of a patient, the oncology nurse notes the patient has a history of Epstein Barr virus (EBV) infection. The nurse knows that EBV infection is associated with an increased risk of developing which one of the following cancers?
    A. Leukemia
    B. Liver cancer
    C. Cholangiocarcinoma
    D. Lymphoma

16. An oncology nurse would like to develop a support program and other services for persons with a history of infection-related cancers. In making the proposal, the nurse should emphasize that infections are associated with what percentage of malignancies?
    A. 5%
    B. 15%
    C. 25%
    D. 30%

17. The oncology nurse is discussing how to reduce gastric cancer incidence due to *H. pylori* infection. Which one of these measures should the nurse include?
    A. Improved sanitation
    B. Annual colonoscopy beginning at age 45
    C. Treatment with zidovudine
    D. Upper endoscopy every 3 years beginning at age 45

18. Vaccination is one means to prevent infection-related cancers. The oncology nurse tells a patient that currently there are vaccines to prevent which of the following?
    A. HPV and HCV
    B. HBV and EBV
    C. HPV and HBV
    D. HCV and EBV

19. The oncology nurse is presenting a program in the community about viruses and their associated risks for developing cancer. The oncology nurse discusses screening recommendations, which include which one of the following?
    A. Screening for EBV at age 10
    B. Screening for HBV at age 15
    C. Screening for HCV at least once
    D. Screening for HIV at least once age 15 to 30 years

20. The oncology nurse is instructing a patient about possible mechanisms with which COVID-19 infection might lead to cancer occurrence, progression, or recurrence. These mechanisms include which one of the following?
    A. T-cells initiate a hyperactive response.
    B. Cytokines are suppressed.
    C. Growth factors are disabled.
    D. Tissue damage and chronic inflammation from "long-COVID-19."

18 Leukemia

1. The oncology nurse explains to a patient newly diagnosed with acute lymphoblastic leukemia (ALL) that a risk factor for this disease is which one of the following?
   A. Exposure to Epstein-Barr virus (EBV)
   B. Being of African descent
   C. Being of Asian descent
   D. Having had a diagnosis of measles as a child

2. A patient is being evaluated for possible ALL. The oncology nurse knows that a commonly reported constitutional symptom is:
   A. weight loss
   B. dizziness
   C. dyspnea
   D. easy bruising or bleeding

3. G.R. is an otherwise healthy 60-year-old patient who has been newly diagnosed with Philadelphia chromosome-positive acute lymphoblastic leukemia. Induction therapy has been ordered for this patient. Induction therapy would consist of which one of the following?
   A. Allogeneic hematopoietic cell transplantation
   B. A pediatric chemotherapy regimen
   C. A monoclonal antibody and corticosteroids
   D. A multi-agent chemotherapy regimen in combination with a tyrosine kinase inhibitor

4. S.T. is a 59-year-old female with newly diagnosed acute myeloid leukemia with a FLT3 pathogenic variant. In addition to standard-of-care induction therapy, the oncology nurse caring for her would anticipate that S.T. would receive which one of the following oral agents?
   A. Venetoclax
   B. Ibrutinib
   C. Rituximab
   D. Midostaurin

5. D.R. is a 44-year-old male who has a new diagnosis of high-risk acute promyelocytic leukemia. D.R. has no known comorbidities. His oncology nurse knows he will begin induction treatment with a regimen of all-trans-retinoic acid (ATRA) plus which one of the following?
   A. Arsenic trioxide
   B. Arsenic trioxide plus anthracycline
   C. Anthracycline alone
   D. Arsenic trioxide plus intrathecal chemotherapy

6. Chronic lymphocytic leukemia accounts for 25% of all diagnosed leukemias. The oncology nurse is aware that which one of the following statements is also true regarding chronic lymphocytic leukemia? It is:
   A. the second most frequent form of leukemia
   B. more frequently seen in women than men
   C. most commonly diagnosed at a median age of 60 years, with less than 15% diagnosed under age 50
   D. a leukemia that originates from immature B lymphocytes

7. S.W. is a 60-year-old female patient with a diagnosis of chronic lymphocytic leukemia (CLL). Upon review of her medication list, the oncology nurse notes that S.W. is taking ibrutinib for her diagnosis. The nurse would expect which one of the following biomarkers of CLL to be present?
   A. 17p deletion
   B. TP53 mutation
   C. CD20 antigen
   D. CD52 antigen

8. W.M. is a 67-year-old male patient who has been newly diagnosed with chronic myelocytic leukemia (CML). Upon review of his chart, the oncology nurse finds that he has been diagnosed with Rai stage III, high-risk disease based on his clinical findings. The nurse anticipates that W.M.'s laboratory results will show lymphocytosis and which one of the following?
   A. Adenopathy
   B. Leukopenia
   C. Splenomegaly
   D. Anemia

9. J.T. is a 68-year-old man who has recently been diagnosed with acute myeloid leukemia (AML). Which one of the following risk factors most likely contributed to his developing the disease?
   A. Prior history of radiation therapy
   B. Long-term exposure to benzene
   C. Heavy usage of alcohol
   D. A diet rich in red meats

10. Which statement is accurate regarding the epidemiology of leukemia?
    A. The most common type of leukemia in children is acute lymphocytic leukemia.
    B. The most common type of leukemia in children is chronic myelogenous leukemia.
    C. The most common type of leukemia in children is chronic lymphocytic leukemia.
    D. The most common type of leukemia in adults is acute lymphocytic leukemia.

11. M.L., a 59-year-old male, is being worked up for recent health changes. Laboratory test results reveal a lymphocyte count greater than 6000 B lymphocytes/μL and thrombocytopenia with a platelet count of 86,000. M.L. also reports he has noticed some swollen lymph nodes in the groin and the left axilla. He also reports he has early satiety. Using the Rai staging system for CLL, the oncology nurse determines that his extent of disease is which one of the following?
    A. Low
    B. Medium
    C. Intermediate
    D. High

12. CML is a clonal disorder that originates from which one of the following?
    A. Philadelphia chromosome
    B. Ataxia telangiectasia mutated (ATM) gene
    C. Germline tp53 mutated gene
    D. Trisomy 21

13. The oncology nurse is reviewing the labs from M.T., a 65-year-old male being evaluated for CML. He has more than 30% blasts on his peripheral blood smear. The nurse knows M.T. is most likely in what phase?
    A. Chronic
    B. Intermediate
    C. Accelerated
    D. Blast

14. The oncology nurse is teaching a newly diagnosed 42-year-old female about acute promyelocytic leukemia (APML). The nurse tells the patient that APML is due to:
    A. *RARA* (retinoic acid receptor [RAR] alpha) gene on chromosome 17
    B. Philadelphia chromosome translocation between chromosome 9 and 22
    C. intrachromosomal amplification of chromosome (iAMP21)
    D. trisomy 8

15. M.S. is a 59-year-old male with AML. The oncology nurse knows that AML that expresses CD33-positive antigens is treated with:
    A. ATRA plus arsenic trioxide (ATO)
    B. gemtuzumab ozogamicin
    C. alemtuzumab
    D. imatinib

19 Lung Cancer

1. An oncology nurse is caring for a patient with lung cancer who is exhibiting intrathoracic effects of his disease. The oncology nurse is aware that the signs and symptoms of this disease include which one of the following?
   A. Shoulder pain
   B. Neuropathy in bilateral lower extremities
   C. Hypomagnesia
   D. Darkening of the skin

2. F.R. is a 52-year-old male who arrives on the oncology unit with a diagnosis of extensive small-cell carcinoma (SCLC) of the lung. Which one of the following statements indicates that the oncology nurse assigned to the patient is knowledgeable about this type of lung cancer? Small-cell carcinoma of the lung:
   A. is slow growing and less likely to metastasize
   B. has a more aggressive course than non-small-cell lung cancer
   C. has a better prognosis than the other forms of lung cancer
   D. has multiple surgical options

3. An oncology nurse is staffing a cancer prevention booth at a local health fair. A man comes to the booth and questions whether or not he should have screening for lung cancer. The oncology nurse explains that the guidelines for screening for lung cancer include which one of the following?
   A. ≥30 pack-years history
   B. Age 75 years or older
   C. Use of inhaled marijuana for 15 years
   D. Current vaporized cigarette use

4. G.L. is a 70-year-old male patient with Stage I lung cancer. He is seen in the outpatient clinic to evaluate treatment options, including surgery. The oncology nurse caring for him knows that the type of treatment with the least risk for morbidity includes which one of the following?
   A. Pneumonectomy with wedge resection
   B. Sleeve resection
   C. Resuscitative thoracotomy
   D. Video-assisted thoracic surgery with wedge resection

5. H.M. is a 64-year-old female who has been newly diagnosed with Stage IIa non-small-cell lung cancer (NSCLC). After consultation with her oncology health care team, she has decided against having surgery. The oncology nurse caring for the patient knows that the next best treatment for this patient would be which one of the following?
   A. Stereotactic ablative radiotherapy (SABR)
   B. Oral chemotherapy
   C. Low-energy radiation
   D. Immunotherapy

6. An oncology nurse on the oncology unit is administering an immune checkpoint inhibitor drug to a patient with NSCLC. The oncology nurse understands that the family of immune checkpoint inhibitor drugs:
   A. acts to dampen the immune response stimulated by the presence of cancer cells
   B. is used only after other types of antineoplastic agents have not been effective
   C. can produce immune-related side effects that can harm normal tissues
   D. harbors molecules that break down cancer cells.

7. An oncology nurse caring for a patient with SCLC is aware that, with this type of lung cancer, which one of the following is correct?
   A. Brain radiation therapy is given to prevent metastasis.
   B. There is greater than 5-year survival with response to treatment.
   C. Alterations in the KRAS oncogene guides treatment choice.
   D. A lobectomy is often performed.

8. E.W. is a 59-year-old man who has worked in construction doing home remodeling, renovation, and demolition for the past 35 years. He was a smoker for a brief time as a teenager but has not touched a tobacco product in the intervening years. And, yet, despite being successful in his efforts for long-term smoking cessation, he has developed lung cancer. He is overweight and has been trying unsuccessfully to control his weight for the past few years. He is confused about how he developed lung cancer since he does not smoke. The oncology nurse reviews his chart and decides which one of the following could have contributed to his developing lung cancer?
   A. His gender and age
   B. His weight, which is above the average for his age
   C. His exposure to paint and paint thinners on the job
   D. His exposure to asbestos in his career in home construction

9. A.E., a 71-year-old man, arrives at the thoracic clinic complaining of cough and shortness of breath. Chest x-ray reveals the presence of a large left-sided pleural effusion. The oncology nurse is aware that A.E. will need to be prepared for which one of these procedures?
   A. Endoscopy
   B. Mediastinoscopy
   C. Thoracentesis
   D. Bronchoscopy

10. The oncology nurse is caring for a hospitalized patient being treated with radiation therapy for Stage III lung cancer. Which of these symptoms should the oncology nurse monitor for in order to help provide palliation?
   A. Fatigue and weakness
   B. Stomach cramps and diarrhea
   C. Constipation
   D. Night sweats

20 Lymphoma

1. An oncology nurse is caring for L.J., a 25-year-old male diagnosed with favorable Hodgkin's lymphoma (HL). After speaking with his health care provider, L.J. asks the nurse about his standard course of treatment. The nurse explains that he will receive which one of the following?
   A. Five cycles of chemotherapy followed by radiation therapy
   B. Two to three cycles chemotherapy, plus radiation therapy
   C. High-dose chemotherapy and autologous bone marrow transplant
   D. Palliative chemotherapy and radiation therapy

2. R.K. is a 46-year-old male with Stage II diffuse large B-cell lymphoma, who has been admitted for treatment. The oncology nurse caring for him knows that the standard treatment for a patient with this diagnosis is which one of the following?
   A. Autologous peripheral blood stem cell transplant
   B. Rituximab, cyclophosphamide, doxorubicin, vincristine, prednisone
   C. Salvage radiation therapy with 6000 cGy
   D. Ifosfamide, carboplatin, etoposide, prednisone

3. A 37-year-old female patient presents to the clinic with signs of HL. The patient undergoes testing and her oncology nurse should anticipate which one of these results that would confirm the diagnosis of HL? The presence of:
   A. Reed-Steenberg cells
   B. bone marrow involvement
   C. extranodal involvement in distal sites
   D. metastases to the long bones

4. An oncology nurse is caring for a 36-year-old patient who is newly diagnosed with HL. The staging system most commonly used for this type of lymphoma is which one of the following?
   A. The Tumor Nodes Metastasis staging system
   B. The Rai staging system of leukemia and lymphoma
   C. The Reed-Steenberg pathologic staging system
   D. The Lugano Classification modification of the Ann Arbor Staging system

5. S.D. is a 49-year-old man who has come to the clinic for treatment. An oncology nurse is assessing his past medical history and discovers that S.D. has a history of *Helicobacter pylori* bacterial infection. The nurse

reports this finding, as this is a significant risk factor for the development of which one of the following?
   A. Inflammatory breast cancer
   B. Cancer of the distal colon
   C. Mucosa-associated lymphoid tissue (MALT) lymphoma
   D. Burkitt lymphoma

6. A nurse is caring for G.F., a 37-year-old male patient, who has a high-grade non-Hodgkin lymphoma with localized disease. In a meeting with the physician, the patient asks about his prognosis. The nurse caring for G.F. would most likely expect the provider to respond that:
   A. "We could achieve a cure with combination chemotherapy and your overall survival at 5 years would be over 60%."
   B. "You will most likely relapse within 2 years, and, unfortunately, your overall cure rate is only 10%."
   C. "We have encouraging news. You have a greater than 80% cure rate and a survival time of more than 20 years."
   D. "This disease is completely curable, after you have undergone an autologous stem cell transplant."

7. T.J. is a 22-year-old male who comes to the oncology clinic after complaining of systemic symptoms that have gotten his clinician concerned that he could have a lymphoma. Reading over his chart, the oncology nurse would most likely be suspicious of which of the following systemic symptoms?
   A. Pain in the chest area
   B. Swelling of the limbs
   C. Extreme thirst and frequent urination
   D. Fever, weight loss, fatigue, and night sweats

8. J.B. is a 46-year-old male patient, whose chest radiography done in the emergency department reveals mediastinal widening. A chest CT is done, and a large mediastinal mass is detected. Upon axillary lymph node biopsy, a large cell follicular non-Hodgkin lymphoma is diagnosed. Which one of the following diagnostic tests is *not* necessary to determine disease staging?
   A. Obtain a 24-hour urine.
   B. Determine whether the lymph node biopsy is CD 20+.
   C. Obtain a CT scan of the abdomen and pelvis.
   D. Perform a bilateral bone marrow biopsy and aspirate.

37

21 Multiple Myeloma

1. L.M. is an oncology nurse who is studying for the oncology nursing certification exam. Which option should L.M. select as the correct answer to the question "Which one of the following risk factors have been found to be associated with the incidence of newly diagnosed multiple myeloma (MM)"?
   A. Employment status
   B. History of monoclonal gammopathy of undetermined significance (MGUS)
   C. Female gender
   D. Exposure to Epstein-Barr virus

2. L.M. learns that the incidence of multiple myeloma is highest in which of these groups?
   A. Blacks men
   B. White women
   C. Young adults
   D. Diabetic individuals

3. L.M. understands that three pathologic features of MM are listed in which one of the following set of examples?
   A. Renal dysfunction, polycythemia, hypercalcemia
   B. Anemia, hypocalcemia, immunodeficiency
   C. Hyperkalemia, osteolytic bone lesions, anemia
   D. Osteolytic bone lesions, renal disease, hypercalcemia

4. L.M. is aware that the diagnosis of multiple myeloma is confirmed by which one of these tests?
   A. Bone scan
   B. Complete blood count
   C. Bone marrow biopsy
   D. Renal ultrasound

5. L.M. learns that pain reported by a person with MM is most commonly due to which one of the following conditions?
   A. Anemia
   B. Neural infiltration of plasma cells
   C. Intestinal obstruction due to an abdominal mass
   D. Presence of lytic bone lesions

6. J.M. is a 67-year-old male patient who has been newly diagnosed with multiple myeloma. The oncology nurse caring for J.M. is aware that myeloma defining events are indicated by evidence of end organ damage attributable to the underlying plasma cell disorder (known as CRAB features). The presence of which one of the following diagnostic criteria for active or symptomatic multiple myeloma would require that MM therapy be initiated?
   A. 50% clonal bone marrow plasma cells
   B. Serum-free light chain ration Kappa: lambda <100
   C. Magnetic resonance imaging (MRI) studies with <1 focal lesion (>8 mm in size)
   D. Serum calcium elevated above 11.0 ng/L or above the upper limit of normal

7. A patient presents to the oncology clinic to discuss treatment for his new diagnosis of multiple myeloma and is ruled out as a candidate for stem cell transplant. The patient asks the nurse if he has a terminal disease. The nurse responds with the understanding that medication treatment in multiple myeloma:
   A. has a high likelihood of cure
   B. is curable in some trisomy translocations
   C. is used prior to surgery
   D. is aimed at controlling disease

8. The oncology nurse is teaching a class of adults about primary prevention strategies for multiple myeloma. Which of the following statements, if made by the nurse, would be accurate about MM prevention?
   A. Decrease alcohol consumption.
   B. Limit exposure to pesticides.
   C. Avoid using tobacco products.
   D. Increase physical activity.

22 Myelofibrosis

1. M.S. is a 66-year-old man who arrives at the oncology clinic with a new diagnosis of myelofibrosis. The oncology nurse who reads his chart is aware that myelofibrosis is often grouped together with which of the following conditions?
   A. Multiple myeloma
   B. Polycythemia vera
   C. Amyloidosis
   D. Lymphoma

2. The oncology nurse takes a history from M.S. and notes that which of the following factors increases his risk for developing myelofibrosis?
   A. Cigarette smoker for 40 years
   B. 50 pounds overweight
   C. Hispanic ethnicity
   D. 66 years of age

3. The oncology nurse understands that the occurrence of a pathologic variant of the JAK2 gene contributes to the development of primary myelofibrosis. Which of the following descriptions characterizes the pathophysiology of primary myelofibrosis?
   A. Alterations in myeloid stem cells, megakaryocyte hyperplasia, bone marrow scarring
   B. Thickening of the parietal pleura, shortness of breath, pneumonitis
   C. Paroxysmal nocturnal dyspnea, inflammation of the lungs, alveolar collapse
   D. Peripheral vascular disease, intermittent claudication, leg weakness

4. M.S. reports several changes in his usual health to the oncology nurse. Which of the following signs or symptoms could be a result of his myelofibrosis?
   A. Recent weight gain of 10 pounds
   B. Leg cramps during the night while in bed
   C. Heart palpitations on arising in the morning
   D. Pain localized to the left upper quadrant of the abdomen

5. The oncology nurse caring for M.S. reviews the results of his laboratory tests. Which of the following results would the nurse expect to see in a patient with myelofibrosis?
   A. Polycythemia
   B. Decreased lactate dehydrogenase
   C. Anemia and thrombocytopenia
   D. High neutrophils and low eosinophils

6. The oncology nurse in the hematology clinic reviews the chart of a patient with a history of essential thrombocythemia who has been diagnosed with secondary myelofibrosis. The nurse is aware that the median overall survival for a patient with secondary myelofibrosis is:
   A. 10 years
   B. 2 to 6 years
   C. 8 years
   D. 15 to 20 years

7. P.B. is a 73-year-old man with a history of adult-onset diabetes and cardiomyopathy. He has been newly diagnosed with intermediate-risk myelofibrosis. The oncology nurse expects that he would be treated with which of these therapies?
   A. Entered into a clinical trial
   B. Hematopoietic stem cell transplant
   C. A Janus kinase (JAK) inhibitor, such as ruxolitinib
   D. Radiation therapy

23 Neurologic System Cancers

1. An oncology nurse working with a pediatric patient population recognizes that which one of the following statements on pediatric brain and spinal cord tumors is true? Brain and spinal cord tumors are:
   A. the second most commonly diagnosed pediatric cancer
   B. a rare diagnostic occurrence
   C. the most frequently diagnosed pediatric cancer
   D. most often diagnosed as benign tumors

2. A patient with cancer who has undergone a craniotomy and tumor resection and the nurse caring for the patient understand that the best practice is for a new baseline MRI or CT to be completed postoperatively within which one of the following time frames?
   A. 12 hours
   B. 24 hours
   C. 48 hours
   D. 72 hours

3. The oncology nurse recognizes that the most important first-line treatment for a malignant primary brain tumor is which one of the following?
   A. Maximal surgical tumor resection
   B. Chemotherapy
   C. Antiepileptic medications
   D. Corticosteroids

4. The mother of a child diagnosed with a primary central nervous system tumor asks the nurse about her child's chances of survival. The nurse responds to the mother with an understanding that the 5-year survival rate for children and teens diagnosed with a primary central nervous system tumor is which one of the following?
   A. 25%
   B. 50%
   C. 75%
   D. 90%

5. A patient with a progressive malignant brain tumor reports to the oncology nurse that he has been diagnosed with hyperglycemia, myopathy, and osteoporosis. The nurse understands these are most likely related to which one of the following?
   A. Bone resorption inhibitors
   B. Anticonvulsants
   C. Corticosteroids
   D. Immunosuppressants

6. The tumor type with the highest predilection to metastasize to the brain is which one of the following?
   A. Colorectal
   B. Lung
   C. Breast
   D. Renal cell

7. The tumor type most frequently associated with leptomeningeal carcinomatosis originates from which one of the following?
   A. Breast
   B. Lung
   C. Hematologic malignancies
   D. Prostate

8. Which one of the following is a common sign or symptom experienced by a patient that led to a diagnosis of a brain tumor?
   A. Substernal pain
   B. Ringing in the ears
   C. Seizures
   D. Constipation

9. When caring for a patient with brain cancer, treatment with anti-epileptic medication is indicated:
   A. for driving
   B. with radiation
   C. perioperatively
   D. at diagnosis

10. Primary central nervous system tumors are staged according to which one of the following?
    A. World Health Organization (WHO) classifications
    B. Tumor Node Metastasis (TNM) criteria
    C. National Comprehensive Cancer Network (NCCN) criteria
    D. American Joint Committee on Cancer (AJCC) classifications

11. Which one of the following sections of the brain would the oncology nurse most likely identify as being responsible for a person's personality? The section of the brain responsible for personality is the:
    A. temporal lobe
    B. occipital lobe
    C. parietal lobe
    D. frontal lobe

40

12. Among the following types of primary spinal tumors, which one is the most common?
    A. Sarcomas
    B. Astrocytomas
    C. Chordomas
    D. Schwannomas

13. Which one of the following sections of the brain is responsible for a person's coordination and balance?
    A. Temporal lobe
    B. Pituitary gland
    C. Brain stem
    D. Cerebellum

14. Risk factors for central nervous system tumors can be known intrinsic, known situational, known extrinsic, and genetic/inherited risk. Of the following risk factors, which one is a known extrinsic risk factor?
    A. Immunocompromise, including HIV/AIDS, immunosuppressive medical therapies, and congenital immunodeficiency
    B. Exposure to pesticides, aspartame, and petrochemicals
    C. Ionizing radiation (IR) to the CNS with doses >2500 cGy
    D. Race/ethnicity, with Caucasian northern European most common and meningioma more common in African American populations

15. The most common type of primary brain tumor is:
    A. pituitary tumor
    B. low grade astrocytoma
    C. glioblastoma
    D. meningioma

16. Global effects of radiation therapy to the brain include:
    A. optic nerve toxicity
    B. diffuse white matter changes
    C. cerebral vascular accidents
    D. headache

17. A 42-year-old male recently diagnosed with a brain tumor is undergoing germline genetic testing for *VHl, BRCA1/2, TSC1.* and *NF1.* The nurse knows this is a consideration because brain tumors are associated with having a germline pathogenic variant that increases the risk of developing a brain tumor by which of the following percentages?
    A. 1% to 5%
    B. 5% to 17%
    C. 17% to 24%
    D. 24% to 31%

18. The oncology nurse meets with a patient with a history of renal cancer who has been diagnosed with metastatic spread to the brain. The nurse anticipates the need to educate the patient about which one of these treatment modalities for brain metastases?
    A. Whole brain radiation therapy
    B. Systemic chemotherapy
    C. Targeted therapy
    D. Immunotherapy

24 Reproductive System Cancers

1. The oncology nurse is presenting an in-service training about cervical cancer to staff nurses in the ambulatory clinic. The nurse should teach that which of the following interventions helps prevent deaths from cervical cancer?
   A. Papanicolaou testing and human immunodeficiency virus (HIV) screening in all females over age 21 years
   B. Being vaccinated against oncogenic (high-risk) hepatitis C virus subtypes
   C. Explaining that smoking is not associated with increased risk
   D. Encouraging vaccination for human papilloma virus, regular screening exams, and discussing risks of multiple partners

2. The oncology nurse understands that major risk factors for uterine (endometrial) cancer include increasing age, obesity, and which one of the following?
   A. Early menopause
   B. Having Lynch syndrome
   C. Aromatase inhibitor use
   D. Late menarche

3. G.T. is a 35-year-old patient who is a one-half pack-per-day smoker with a history of pelvic inflammatory disease (PID). She was recently diagnosed with advanced ovarian cancer. She states that "cancer always happens to us," in reference to her elder sister who is a breast cancer survivor. She is concerned that her 10-year-old daughter could be at future risk for ovarian cancer, and asks the oncology nurse for advice. Which one of the following statements by the nurse is accurate?
   A. "Women should have routine ovarian cancer screening for early detection."
   B. "Tobacco use and history of PID are known risk factors for ovarian cancer, but you should also have a genetic evaluation."
   C. "A new diagnosis of ovarian cancer is more common in premenopausal than in postmenopausal women."
   D. "Your daughter should start hormone-replacement therapy after menopause to decrease her ovarian cancer risk."

4. A patient with a history of gestational trophoblastic neoplasia asks the oncology nurse about when it would be safe to attempt to conceive. Which one of the following statements should the oncology nurse make to the patient? "It is safe to attempt to conceive:
   A. after the patient has passed at least 1 year after completion of therapy."
   B. as soon as the patient's human chorionic gonadotropin (hCG) levels have started to respond to chemotherapy."
   C. after the patient's hCG levels have normalized for 6 to 8 weeks and menses have become regular."
   D. as soon as the patient's menses are regular, however, the chemotherapy treatment may have had deleterious effects on fertility."

5. Oncogenic human papillomavirus (HPV) infection and smoking have been associated with an increased risk of developing cervical cancer, vaginal cancer, and vulvar cancer. The oncology nurse understands that which one of the following additional risk factors would apply to which of the patients described below?
   A. Diethylstilbestrol use by the mother of a patient diagnosed with vaginal cancer
   B. Breast cancer in a first-degree relative of a patient diagnosed with cervical cancer
   C. Asbestos exposure in the mother of a patient diagnosed with vulvar cancer
   D. Use of hormone replacement therapy by a patient diagnosed with vulvar cancer

6. The oncology nurse is giving a presentation to staff nurses about testicular cancer. At the conclusion, they should have learned that which one of the following males is statistically more likely to be diagnosed with testicular cancer?
   A. 65-year-old white male with a weak urinary stream and a history of well-controlled HIV infection
   B. 25-year-old male of Pacific Islander descent with a history of recurrent herpes simplex virus-2 infection.
   C. 50-year-old African American male with two first-degree relatives with a history of colorectal cancer
   D. 32-year-old Hispanic male with a history of painless unilateral testicular swelling

7. The oncology nurse is counseling the parents of two pre-teen boys about modifiable risk factors for penile cancer. These include which one of the following measures?
   A. Hepatitis B vaccination
   B. Vaccination for human papilloma virus
   C. Circumcision performed after puberty
   D. Avoid retracting the foreskin while cleaning the glans

8. A patient with a history of ovarian cancer comes to the oncology clinic for follow up. The oncology nurse is aware that typical signs and symptoms of recurrent ovarian cancer, if present, include which one of the following?
   A. Rising CA125 tumor marker
   B. Weight gain
   C. Increased appetite
   D. Vaginal discharge or bleeding

9. The standard treatment for most patients with newly diagnosed Stage II endometrial cancer is which one of the following?
   A. Fertility sparing therapies whenever possible
   B. Hysterectomy and bilateral salpingo-oophorectomy
   C. Oral hormonal therapy for 10 years for estrogen suppression
   D. Dilatation and curettage followed by close observation for endometrial thickening

10. Which one of the following is a treatment for early-stage (IA1–IA2) cervical cancer?
    A. Radical hysterectomy plus lymphadenectomy
    B. Definitive chemoradiation (with or without ovarian transposition if premenopausal)
    C. Fertility sparing procedures, including conization with cold knife or loop electrosurgical excision (LEEP), or radical trachelectomy
    D. Primary chemotherapy followed by close observation

11. L.J. is a 47-year-old female patient with newly diagnosed metastatic cervical cancer. Which one of the following therapy recommendations would her oncology nurse anticipate that L.J. will be offered?
    A. Simple or modified radical hysterectomy with or without lymph node evaluation
    B. External beam radiation therapy (EBRT) followed by neoadjuvant chemotherapy
    C. Radiation therapy, systemic therapy, and surgical resection
    D. Radiation therapy, with or without chemotherapy, plus palliative systemic agents

12. Which one of the following stages of testicular cancer has the best 5-year survival rate in the United States?
    A. Distant
    B. Un-staged
    C. Regional
    D. Localized

13. Mr. H. and his wife are distressed with his recent diagnosis of testicular cancer. During the course of the nursing assessment, it becomes clear that some of this distress is related to fertility concerns. The oncology nurse discusses sperm banking with the couple and explains that sperm banking should ideally be completed:
    A. before surgery
    B. before chemotherapy
    C. after surgery
    D. after chemotherapy

14. F.D. is a 45-year-old woman who is scheduled for a total abdominal hysterectomy and bilateral oophorectomy (TAH-BSO) after being diagnosed with ovarian cancer. She had been experiencing irregular menses prior to diagnosis. Possible complications F.D. might experience after the surgery include which one of the following?
    A. Alternating constipation and diarrhea
    B. Vaginal drying and pelvic tissue atrophy
    C. Decreased risk of cardiovascular disease
    D. Changes in urinary function

15. The oncology nurse is teaching a group of staff nurses about gynecologic cancers. Which information should be included in the discussion of vulvar cancer? It is:
    A. a common cancer in young women
    B. a major cause of female cancer deaths
    C. diagnosed at an average age of 68 years
    D. responsible for repeated miscarriages

16. In the discussion of vulvar cancer, the oncology nurse describes risk factors for vulvar cancer, which include which one of the following?
    A. Prior squamous cell carcinoma of the skin
    B. High number of sexual partners
    C. History of multiple childbirths
    D. Beginning menses at age 15

17. In the presentation to staff nurses about gynecologic cancers, the oncology nurse should explain that which of the following information about ovarian cancer is accurate?
    A. As many as 20% of all ovarian cancer cases are due to hereditary factors.
    B. Use of oral contraceptive agents increases risk of developing ovarian cancer.
    C. With each year of ovulation, the risk of ovarian cancer decreases.
    D. Rates of ovarian cancer are lowest in developing countries.

18. The oncology nurse is caring for O. L., a 48-year-old female patient with recurrent ovarian cancer. Which of the following signs and symptoms would be most appropriate for the oncology nurse to assess for the presence of?
    A. Neck pain
    B. Weight gain
    C. Abdominal bloating
    D. Skin dryness

19. The oncology nurse meets with D.S., a 22-year-old female who has been diagnosed with a hydatidiform mole. The nurse explains that D.S.'s condition has originated from the:
A. placenta
B. cervix
C. vagina
D. ovary

20. G.N. is a 52-year-old woman who has been diagnosed with clear cell adenocarcinoma of the vagina. The oncology nurse knows that the risk of developing this kind of cancer is associated with which of the following?
A. Excessive alcohol intake
B. Never becoming pregnant
C. Prolonged use of talcum powder
D. Diethylstilbestrol (DES) exposure in utero

25 Skin Cancer

1. An oncology nurse is caring for N.M., a 72-year-old female patient who has had several basal cell carcinomas (BCC) diagnosed on her face and arms over the years. The nurse knows that the predominant risk factor for developing BCC is which one of the following?
   A. Sunlight overexposure
   B. Tobacco smoking
   C. Family history
   D. Young age

2. An oncology nurse is assessing a patient in the clinic who has a history of nonmelanoma skin cancer. Which one of the following findings would be considered a precursor for squamous cell carcinoma?
   A. Atypical nevi
   B. Multiple moles
   C. Actinic keratoses
   D. Skin viral infection

3. A Mohs procedure is recommended to treat a patient with a nonmelanoma skin cancer on the face. In teaching the patient about what to expect during the procedure, the nurse explains that which one of the following will occur?
   A. Subzero temperature swabs will be applied to the area
   B. The area will be injected with a chemotherapy drug
   C. A curette will be used to scrape away tumor cells, then the area will be cauterized
   D. Thin layers will be removed from the area and examined under a microscope

4. J.R. is a 40-year-old female kidney transplant patient who is being treated for Merkel cell carcinoma. During an office visit, she begins showing signs of distress and asks the oncology nurse "Why me?" The nurse explains that which one of the following factors is associated with increased risk?
   A. Female gender
   B. Organ transplant
   C. African American descent
   D. Age between 35 and 50 years

5. The oncology nurse is teaching K.T., a 40-year-old female patient, how to recognize skin signs that could indicate a need for melanoma assessment by a specialist. The nurse should instruct the patient to report the sighting of a mole showing signs of which one of the following?
   A. Regular border
   B. Symmetrical shape
   C. Tendency to bleed
   D. Uniform brown color

6. F.R. is a 60-year-old male patient who has been diagnosed with metastatic melanoma. During an office visit, F.R. asks the nurse, "What are next steps in my treatment?" In answering his question, the oncology nurse anticipates that his standard treatment will include which one of the following treatments?
   A. Isolated limb perfusion
   B. Immunotherapy
   C. Cranial radiation therapy
   D. Photodynamic therapy

7. Which one of the following is a characteristic of Merkel cell carcinoma?
   A. Develops primarily on sun-exposed skin; rarely found on palmoplantar surfaces and never appears on the mucosa
   B. Presents as papules, plaques, and cyst-like structures or pruritic tumors on the lower extremities
   C. Often presents as a new or enlarging lesion that may bleed, weep, be tender, or be painful
   D. Can develop at sites of chemical exposure or chronic trauma

8. Which one of the following statements about basal cell carcinoma is true?
   A. Major risk factor is exposure to ultraviolet radiation (UVR), especially intermittent exposure early in life
   B. Most commonly presents as an erythematous or violaceous, tender, dome-shaped nodule on sun-exposed areas on the head or neck of an elderly white male
   C. Typically, these are slow growing; however those arising in non–sun-exposed sites (i.e., lips, genitalia, perianal areas) are more aggressive with a higher risk of metastases
   D. Most lesions are <2 cm in diameter at the time of diagnosis; rapid growth is common

45

9. The oncology nurse is giving a community lecture on cancer prevention and discusses the ABCDE rule for the early detection of melanoma. The nurse should explain that:
   A. B stands for Bigger than 3 cm
   B. C stands for Crevices in borders
   C. D stands for Diameter greater than 3 cm
   D. E stands for Evolving changes

10. The most common subtype of malignant melanoma is:
    A. superficial spreading
    B. nodular
    C. lentigo maligna
    D. acral lentiginous

11. The oncology nurse is reviewing a pathology report for a melanoma specimen. The nurse understands that there are recommended and optional components for reporting histopathology. The nurse knows that which of the following is considered an optional component:
    A. Clark's level
    B. Breslow's level
    C. specimen size
    D. ulceration

12. The nurse is providing a patient with postoperative care instructions after excision of a cutaneous squamous cell carcinoma (cSCC). It is a high-risk lesion. The nurse knows that the surgical margin for this type of squamous cell carcinoma should be at least:
    A. 2 mm
    B. 6 mm
    C. 10 mm
    D. 14 mm

13. The oncology nurse is preparing to give pembrolizumab to a patient with melanoma. The nurse knows this agent belongs to which type of immune checkpoint inhibitors?
    A. Anti-PD-L1 (anti-programmed death ligand-1) antibody
    B. Anti-CTLA-4 (anti-cytotoxic lymphocyte 4 [CTLA-4]) antibody
    C. Anti-PD-1 (anti-programmed death-1) antibody
    D. Anti-LAG-3 antibody

14. The nurse is reviewing the pathology report for a patient with melanoma. The nurse checks to see if there are abnormalities in the MAPK signaling pathway. The nurse knows that the most common pathogenic variant seen is in which one of these genes?
    A. NRAS
    B. EGFR
    C. BRAF
    D. HER2

15. The oncology nurse meets with a patient diagnosed with a basal cell skin cancer. The nurse is providing patient education about the use of imiquimod. The nurse should explain that imiquimod is a:
    A. MEK inhibitor
    B. topical therapy
    C. systemic therapy
    D. HH inhibitor

26 Surgery

1. D.J. is a 45-year-old male patient who is on a surgical oncology unit. He is scheduled for surgery the following day for removal of a malignant tumor. The nurse caring for D.J. understands that prior to surgery, it is most important to define whether which one of the following is happening?
   A. Is the organ being removed necessary for bodily function?
   B. Will there be placement of a jugular venous catheter during surgery?
   C. Will the physician involved be engaged in proper positioning of the patient?
   D. Will the wound be prepared and irrigated during the procedure?

2. T.G. is. a 40 year-old male who is scheduled for a wide excision of the left axilla. Before the procedure T.G. asks the oncology nurse to explain to him what a wide excision is. Which one of the following explanations should the nurse provide?
   A. "Your cancer will be removed along with a large margin of the surrounding tissue."
   B. "Your cancer will be removed, along with some adjacent tissue, and your regional lymph nodes."
   C. "A very small amount of cancerous tissue and many lymph nodes will be removed."
   D. "The planned procedure involves removal of the entire lesion along with your upper pectoral muscle."

3. H.R. is a 50-year-old male patient with cancer. He presents for presurgical evaluation and, during the assessment, he reports to the oncology nurse that he has been diagnosed with uncontrolled diabetes. The nurse is aware that the patient is at risk for developing which one of the following conditions?
   A. Kidney disease
   B. Hypertension postoperatively
   C. Electrolyte disturbances
   D. Hypoglycemia postoperatively

4. C.K. is a 45-year-old female patient with breast cancer. She has an appointment in the breast clinic to discuss the management of her breast cancer. The physician has recommended surgical treatment with a lumpectomy followed by adjuvant radiation therapy. The oncology nurse working with C.K. understands that the purpose of this type of disease management is to do which one of the following?
   A. Block the action of proteins to prevent the growth of cancer cells
   B. Treat microscopic disease potentially remaining after conservative breast surgery
   C. Fight cancer cells using the patient's own immune system
   D. Conserve the patient's breast tissue for later reconstruction

5. A nurse is preparing a patient for surgery in the perioperative suite. The nurse maintains standards of care through the World Health Organization, which ensure which one of the following?
   A. There is a "pause" completed, and that staff are in position for surgery
   B. Safety standards are met to decrease the length and cost of surgery
   C. Consent for treatment is completed, and there is team collaboration
   D. Hazardous drugs are properly used and disposed of

6. Which one of the following is a definition of a laparoscopic surgical approach? It is a procedure in which:
   A. surgical tools are passed through an existing orifice (mouth, nares, anus, urethra) without external incision/scar
   B. an extended, full-thickness incision is made to allow thorough exploration and manipulation of tissues
   C. multiple small incisions ("ports'") are made for surgical camera insertion and application of operative tools allowing less tissue manipulation
   D. remotely controlled instruments are used allowing less tissue invasion, improved optics, and finer control and ergonomics to lessen tissue manipulation

47

7. Which one of the following defines the characteristics of palliative cancer surgery? This type of surgery:
A. removes primary tumor, lymph nodes, adjacent affected organs with negative margins attained via the least invasive means available
B. improves function or appearance of a surgical defect improving the quality of life
C. improves comfort when curative resection is not possible; includes surgical debulking or decompression or diversion via stent or ostomy.
D. is performed for issues such hemorrhage, organ ischemia or perforation, drainage/washout for abscess or infection, and cord compression

8. The oncology nurse is caring for J.P., a patient who has just returned to his hospital room from the surgical recovery suite. The nurse knows that the number one cause of preventable death following surgery is:
A. venous thromboembolism
B. hyperglycemic coma
C. urinary infection
D. ischemic stroke

27 Hematopoietic Stem Cell Transplantation and CAR T-Cell Therapy

1. Which one of the following statements is true regarding allogeneic hematopoietic stem cell transplantation?
   A. The recipient receives his or her own procured stem cells after high-dose chemotherapy.
   B. Immunosuppression is not required to prevent graft-versus-host disease (GVHD).
   C. Human leukocyte antigen (HLA) matching is not required as part of pre-transplantation work-up.
   D. The recipient receives hematopoietic stem cells from a healthy related or unrelated donor.

2. The use of posttransplant immunosuppression in allogeneic hematopoietic stem cell transplantation (HSCT) is to prevent which one of the following:
   A. donor T lymphocytes mounting an immune response against the stem cell recipient
   B. relapse due to a low undetectable level of tumor cells persisting in the infusing cells
   C. damage to the small sinusoid of the liver from pretransplant conditioning regimen
   D. posttransplant infectious complications with viral, bacterial, or fungal organisms

3. Which one of the following factors significantly impacts determination in the type of transplant a patient is to undergo?
   A. Underlying malignancy or nonmalignant hematologic disease
   B. Availability of an ABO-matched donor
   C. Donor's disease status
   D. Donor's physical and psychosocial status

4. G.L. is a 47-year-old female patient with acute myeloid leukemia (AML), who underwent a HSCT a month ago. The patient now is presenting with new onset of erythematous skin on her face, palms of hands, and soles of feet. The oncology nurse caring for this patient is concerned about the development of which one of the following posttransplant complications?
   A. Hepatic sinusoidal obstruction syndrome
   B. Hand-foot-mouth disease
   C. Graft versus host disease
   D. Graft-versus-leukemia effect

5. The oncology nurse should assess which one of the following for hepatic sinusoidal obstruction syndrome?
   A. Tacrolimus levels
   B. Daily weights
   C. Characteristics of stool
   D. Skin conditions

6. Which one of the following medications is often used to treat cytomegalovirus (CMV) infection?
   A. Voriconazole
   B. Posaconazole
   C. Foscarnet
   D. Acyclovir

7. Reduced-intensity or nonmyeloablative regimens are used in the setting of HSCT when the patient presents which one of the following traits?
   A. The patient is less than 60 years old.
   B. The patient has no preexisting comorbidities.
   C. The patient has excellent organ function status.
   D. The patient will benefit from a graft-versus-tumor immunologic effect.

8. Which one of the following statements is true regarding autologous HSCT?
   A. Autografting is most frequently used for the treatment of AML and aplastic anemia.
   B. Autologous HSCT can be effective in treating some autoimmune diseases.
   C. Immunosuppressant agents are routinely used in autologous stem cell transplantation.
   D. A conditioning regimen is not required prior to stem cell transplantation.

9. Preventative measures for idiopathic pulmonary interstitial pneumonitis include the use of which one of the following?
   A. A filtered air system and high-dose steroid
   B. A filtered air system and CMV sero-negative blood products
   C. Mycophenolate and depletion of T cells from marrow
   D. Trimethoprim/sulfamethoxazole and tacrolimus

10. Which one of the following medications is used to prevent sinusoidal obstruction syndrome (SOS)?
    A. Ursodiol
    B. Lovenox
    C. Pantoprazole
    D. Bactrim DS

49

11. J.R. is a 56-year-old male patient with history of AML who has completed an allogeneic transplant. He is at day +48 and presented with total bilirubin of 4 mg/dl with more than 1000 ml of stool per day. The nurse grades his GVHD as:
    A. Acute GVHD, overall clinical Grade II
    B. Acute GVHD, overall clinical Grade III
    C. Chronic GVHD, overall clinical Grade II
    D. Chronic GVHD, overall clinical Grade III

12. One of the risk factors for the development of hepatic SOS is which one of the following?
    A. Karnofsky score > 90% before transplantation
    B. First transplantation
    C. Pretransplantation hepatotoxic drug therapy
    D. 10/10 HLA-matched unrelated allogeneic transplantation

13. Which one of the following medications requires frequent monitoring of drug blood levels?
    A. Acyclovir
    B. Ursodil
    C. Thalidomide
    D. Tacrolimus

14. Which one of the following statements is true regarding goals of a pretransplant conditioning regimen? The goal is to:
    A. boost the patient's immune system to allow for marrow engraftment
    B. eradicate remaining malignancy and to open spaces within marrow
    C. prevent GVHD and promote a graft-versus-tumor effect
    D. prevent posttransplant complications such as infections and SOS

15. The oncology nurse understands that which one of the following is a nursing intervention for the management of GVHD, both acute and chronic?
    A. Implement routine of coughing, and deep breathing
    B. Monitor reports on patient's hearing acuity
    C. Assess patients' weight gain
    D. Evaluate the patient's cyclosporine or tacrolimus levels

16. The oncology nurse should be aware that which one of the following is true regarding an infection in a patient with idiopathic pulmonary interstitial pneumonitis (infectious)?
    A. Occurs most frequently in patients >30 years old with a history of chest irradiation or previous bleomycin therapy
    B. Results from engraftment of immunocompetent donor T lymphocytes
    C. Occurs in 30% to 60% of all autologous bone marrow transplant recipients
    D. Occurs most commonly in women <30 years of age with a history of anthracycline therapy

17. Which one of the following is a fungal infection complication that can develop in HSCT recipients 1 to 4 months after transplantation?
    A. Gram-positive organisms
    B. Parainfluenza
    C. *Aspergillus* species
    D. *Pneumocystis jiroveci (carinii)*

18. Which one of the following is a bacterial infection complication that occurs in HSCT recipients 4 to 12 months after transplantation?
    A. Varicella-zoster
    B. *P. jiroveci (carinii)*
    C. *Streptococcus pneumoniae*
    D. Coccidioidomycosis

19. Which one of the following should be included in a social evaluation during assessment for a potential recipient of a HSCT?
    A. Number, type, effectiveness of coping mechanisms used in past stressful situations (before transplantation therapy) by patient and family members
    B. Perceptions of patient and family about isolation, prolonged hospitalization, living will, use of life-support technology, and potential death or survival
    C. Understanding of treatment aggressiveness, goals of therapy, chances of survival
    D. Type, number, and history of use of support systems in the family and community

20. CAR T-cells can identify the malignant cells that had previously:
    A. evaded B-cell destruction
    B. been destroyed by targeted chemotherapy
    C. evaded T-cell destruction
    D. been destroyed by an autologous stem cell transplant

21. The oncology nurse knows that the FDA requires individuals who prescribe, dispense, and administer CAR T-cell therapy to:
    A. consider performance status and comorbidities
    B. complete the risk evaluation and mitigation strategy program
    C. complete staff education and training program
    D. provide patient and caregiver education

22. The oncology nurse is caring for a patient who has received CAR T-cell therapy. The nurse is monitoring for complications, including cytokine release syndrome (CRS). The hallmark sign of CRS is:
    A. fever
    B. hypotension
    C. seizures
    D. hemorrhage

28 Radiation Therapy

1. The oncology nurse caring for the patient receiving external beam radiation understands the purpose of radiation safety measures, especially which one of the following?
   A. Wearing silicone ring to monitor radiation exposure
   B. Full knowledge of radiation effects, risk of exposure, and safety practices
   C. Adhering to principles of time, source, and distance
   D. Ensuring that radiation beams turn on when entering rooms

2. C.K. is a 60-year-old female patient with cervical cancer. She will be receiving external beam radiation as well as brachytherapy as part of her treatment. C.K. asks the oncology nurse caring for her why she would be required to have both types of radiation therapy. The nurse should tell C.K. which one of the following?
   A. "You are receiving combined therapy because this type of therapy treats bulky local disease and improves local control."
   B. "You are receiving brachytherapy because this type of therapy uses a lower dose, whereas the external uses higher doses in a small area."
   C. "Combining the two therapies will result in virtually no side effects for you."
   D. "Receiving both external and internal radiation will decrease the need for you to undergo surgery."

3. An oncology nurse is caring for a patient who has been diagnosed with lung cancer. This patient will be treated with stereotactic body radiation therapy (SBRT). The nurse knows that with this type of therapy which one of the following statements is true?
   A. Normal tissues and organs are not spared treatment-related toxicity.
   B. The patient will receive anywhere between 1 and 10 treatments.
   C. Immobilization is not required for this type of treatment.
   D. Doses are higher than conventional radiation treatments.

4. D.K. is a 56-year-old female patient who has had radiation therapy to the head and neck. In caring for this patient, the oncology nurse instructs the patient about the long-term side effects of radiation, which includes which one of the following?
   A. Xerostomia
   B. Secondary cancers such as acute myeloid leukemia
   C. Moist desquamation
   D. Neurologic effects

5. A multidisciplinary team meets to discuss radiation therapy treatment for a 60-year-old male patient with pancreatic cancer and decides to use three-dimensional conformal radiotherapy (3DCRT). The oncology nurse is aware that treatment with this type of radiation therapy includes which one of the following?
   A. It uses cobalt as the radioactive source.
   B. It shapes the distribution of the radiation dose to the volume of the target tumor.
   C. It is delivered in a single fraction of radiation.
   D. It allows the treatment to the target tumor to be synchronized with patient movement.

6. An experienced oncology nurse is educating a new nurse on an oncology unit regarding the guidelines for brachytherapy radiation safety while delivering care to a patient who is receiving brachytherapy to treat cancer of the cervix. The experienced nurse instructs the novice nurse that barriers to exposure include which one of the following?
   A. The use of gloves to protect against radioisotopes excreted through body fluids
   B. The use of shielding that is placed between the person with the radiation source and others who enter the room
   C. The use of fluid-resistant materials to prevent sweat from evaporating and igniting radioactive ions
   D. The use of respiratory equipment to protect from fumes emitted from radioactive isotopes

7. Radiation therapy dosing is based on medical physics and depends upon which one of the following?
   A. Density of the bone type to be penetrated
   B. Distance from the radiation source to the skin
   C. Energy and circumference of the beam
   D. Density and type of skin surface

8. Which one of the following statements correctly reflects the principles of the 5 R's of radiobiology?
   A. "Reassortment" refers to the tumor cell proliferation that occurs during radiation.
   B. "Radiosensitizing" refers to the concept that ionizing radiation therapy is dependent on differences in cell metabolism, maturity, and microenvironment
   C. "Repair" refers to radioresistant cells that synchronize into a more radiosensitive phase of the cell cycle after a fraction of radiation.
   D. "Reassortment" refers to the importance of oxygen in mediating the cytotoxic effects of radiation due to free radical production.

9. Which one of the following does *not* influence the biologic response to radiation?
   A. Level of DNA damage
   B. Oxygen effect
   C. Sensitivity of cells to radiation
   D. Ability of the body to clear toxins

10. Which of the following statements is true about the reasoning behind why the delivery of radiation is divided into small fractions?
   A. Delivering the same total dose of radiation at one time can only be done by use of brachytherapy technique.
   B. Fractionation allows for recovery of surrounding normal tissues and redistribution of cells into a radiosensitive phase of the cell cycle.
   C. Daily treatments over several weeks allow for the development of a therapeutic relationship between the health care providers and the individual undergoing treatment.
   D. Fractionation helps to deoxygenate the malignant cells in the radiation field, making them more sensitive to the radiation.

29 Chemotherapy, Hormonal Therapy, and Oral Adherence

1. Both normal and malignant cells pass through the five stages of the cell cycle in order to reproduce and proliferate. In the synthesis phase of the cell cycle, which one of the following is correct?
   A. Cellular DNA is replicated.
   B. Cells are ready for division or mitosis.
   C. Cells are resting and are not dividing.
   D. Cellular ribonucleic acid (RNA) is being produced.

2. Cells from different organs reproduce at different rates depending on the type of cell. The amount of time required for a cell to move from one mitosis to the next mitosis is termed as which one of the following?
   A. Tumor burden
   B. Cell cycle time
   C. Growth fraction
   D. Cell cycle phase

3. In combination chemotherapy, different agents are used simultaneously. The advantage of combination chemotherapy is which one of the following?
   A. Combination chemotherapy increases the number of cells exposed to cytotoxic effects.
   B. Combination chemotherapy increases the opportunity for drug resistance.
   C. Combination chemotherapy is limited to the recurrent setting.
   D. Combination chemotherapy is limited to the adjuvant setting.

4. All of the following are chemotherapy agents used as radiosensitizers, *except* for which one of the following?
   A. Cisplatin
   B. 5-Fluorouracil
   C. Mitomycin C
   D. Protein-bound paclitaxel

5. Chemotherapy can be administered to a patient in a variety of ways. The method of delivering doses of chemotherapy to the specific site of the tumor is called which one of the following?
   A. Systemic chemotherapy
   B. Regional chemotherapy
   C. High-dose chemotherapy
   D. Dose-dense chemotherapy

6. An example of a cell cycle–specific chemotherapy drug is which one of the following?
   A. Gemcitabine
   B. Cyclophosphamide
   C. Busulfan
   D. Cisplatin

7. Chemotherapy drugs that exert their cytotoxic effects on cells that are in any phase of the cell cycle, even those in the resting, nondividing phase, are called cell cycle–nonspecific agents. An example of this type of chemotherapy drug is which one of the following?
   A. Faslodex
   B. Carboplatin
   C. Goserelin
   D. Paclitaxel

8. Chemotherapy drugs are classified into five different groups based on their mechanism of action. Fluorouracil, which is used to treat many types of solid tumors, is an example of which one of the following classes of chemotherapy?
   A. Nitrogen mustards
   B. Nitrosoureas
   C. Antimetabolite
   D. Platinum compounds

9. Aromatase inhibitors are a type of:
   A. differentiating agent
   B. hormonal therapy
   C. alkylating agent
   D. immunotherapy

10. Side effects of hormonal therapy include all of the following *except* which one of the following?
    A. Vaginal discharge
    B. Increased libido
    C. Weight gain
    D. Hot flashes

11. Nurses need to be alert to the potential for hypersensitivity reactions in patients receiving infusions of certain chemotherapy agents. For patients receiving paclitaxel and docetaxel, nurses need to assess for anaphylaxis-type reactions that are known to occur most frequently during which one of the following time frames?
    A. First infusion
    B. Third infusion
    C. Fifth infusion
    D. Seventh infusion

12. Chemotherapy precautions for handling body fluids and soiled linens should remain in effect for what period of time after chemotherapy administration is complete?
    A. 24 hours
    B. 48 hours
    C. 2 weeks
    D. 4 weeks

13. Mesna is an agent that is administered in conjunction with some chemotherapy drugs to protect against which one of the following toxicities?
    A. Cardiotoxicity in patients who require more than 300 mg/m² of doxorubicin
    B. Renal toxicity from cisplatin therapy
    C. Bladder toxicity from ifosfamide
    D. Ototoxicity from carboplatin dosage greater than 60 to 75 mg/m²

14. Extravasation can cause serious injury to tissues in the arm in which it occurs. Recommendations to avoid the risk of extravasation include which one of the following?
    A. Use the biggest vein in the antecubital area.
    B. Use veins between the wrist and the elbow.
    C. Use veins on the dorsal side of the hand.
    D. Select IV sites that have been in place at least 24 hours.

15. Nurses may not administer chemotherapy via which one of the following routes?
    A. Intravenous
    B. Intraperitoneal
    C. Subcutaneous
    D. Intrapleural

16. Every precaution should be taken to avoid a drug extravasation during chemotherapy administration. If an extravasation of a vinca alkaloid occurs or is suspected, the infusion should be stopped immediately and the area treated with which one of the following?
    A. Cold compress
    B. Hyaluronidase
    C. Sodium thiosulfate
    D. Dexrazoxane

17. Side effects of cisplatin include all of the following *except*:
    A. cutaneous rash
    B. peripheral neuropathy
    C. ototoxicity
    D. renal toxicity

18. Which one of the following chemotherapy agents has the ability to cause "wasabi nose"?
    A. Etoposide
    B. Cyclophosphamide
    C. Carboplatin
    D. Doxorubicin

19. The nurse is caring for a patient with colon cancer who is receiving oxaliplatin. Patient education about potential side effects of this drug should focus on providing teaching about which one of the following complications?
    A. Heat sensitivity
    B. Cardiotoxicity
    C. Hypersensitivity reaction with the first dose
    D. Peripheral neuropathy

20. A patient has been diagnosed with HER2-positive breast cancer. Assessment of her cardiac function is essential prior to initiating therapy with which one of the following drugs?
    A. Cisplatin
    B. Trastuzumab
    C. Vincristine
    D. Irinotecan

21. Over time, as a tumor increases in size and volume, changes occur in the cells within the tumor mass. This property is taken into account when planning for the most effective type of anti-tumor therapy. The cellular changes in the cancer cells of an enlarging tumor include which one of the following?
    A. Decrease in the number of actively dividing cells
    B. Increase in the number of cells undergoing mitosis
    C. Decreased cellular heterogeneity
    D. Increased cellular growth rate

22. Ms. M., a 68-year-old female patient, has been diagnosed with a 4.5 cm tumor in the left upper quadrant of her left breast. Her surgeon consults with the medical oncologist about the feasibility of reducing the size of the tumor so that subsequent breast surgery can be limited to a lumpectomy. The type of chemotherapy treatment that is given prior to surgery to shrink the size of a tumor is called which one of the following?
    A. Adjuvant
    B. Neoadjuvant
    C. Consolidation
    D. Concurrent

23. Ms. M. is also scheduled to receive doxorubicin as part of her combination chemotherapy regimen. The nurse is aware that Ms. M. should be assessed for signs of which one of these adverse side effects most likely related to doxorubicin?
    A. Cardiotoxicity
    B. Hemorrhagic cystitis
    C. Ototoxicity
    D. Neurotoxicity

24. Hormonal therapy may be used in patients with breast cancers to inhibit the actions of hormones that stimulate malignant cell growth. A class of hormonal agents that is used to prevent estrogen production in the breast and other body tissues is which one of the following?
    A. Adrenocorticoids
    B. Aromatase inhibitors (AIs)
    C. Selective estrogen receptor modulators (SERMS)
    D. Gonadotropin-releasing hormone (GnRH) agonists

25. Hormonal therapy used in the treatment of patients with breast cancer or prostate cancer can lead to side effects that are most likely to include which one of the following?
    A. Increased libido
    B. Hypoglycemia
    C. Weight loss
    D. Hot flashes

26. Which one of the following is an advantage of oral administration of antineoplastic agents?
    A. Requires adequate muscle mass and tissue for absorption
    B. Provides ease of administration and gives patients a sense of control and independence
    C. Provides increased dose to the tumor with decreased systemic side effects
    D. Allows the patient ease of administration and promotes rapid absorption

27. Which one of the following is a disadvantage of intrapleural administration of antineoplastic agents?
    A. Requires placement of Tenckhoff catheter or intraperitoneal port
    B. Requires lumbar puncture or surgical placement of a reservoir or implanted pump
    C. Requires insertion of a thoracotomy tube, and the Nurse Practice Act may not allow the nurse to administer the drug via this method
    D. Requires the insertion of an indwelling catheter

28. Which one of the following is a nursing consideration for subcutaneous or intramuscular administration of antineoplastic agents?
    A. Evaluate the patient's platelet count before administration and use smallest gauge needle possible.
    B. Monitor for signs and symptoms of bleeding or occlusion.
    C. Use smallest catheter available and avoid areas of flection, lower extremities, and arms where lymph nodes have been removed.
    D. Administer at room temperature, and place patient in semi-Fowler's position.

29. Which one of the following is a nursing consideration for intraperitoneal administration of antineoplastic agents?
    A. Place patient in Trendelenburg position.
    B. Ensure that infusion is heated to body temperature.
    C. Assess catheter for blood return.
    D. Rotate patient side to side every 15 minutes for 1 hour post infusion.

30. The oncology nurse meets with a patient who will be receiving oral chemotherapy at home. The nurse is aware that the patient may face challenges to oral drug adherence. All of the following are likely patient factors to nonadherence with oral drug regimens *except* which one of the following? The patient may:
    A. Self-modify the dose to reduce distressing side effects
    B. Forget the medication schedule, especially if there are multiple daily doses
    C. Possess an advanced college degree and live in an affluent neighborhood
    D. Have high medication out-of-pocket expenses and inadequate health insurance

30 Biotherapies: Targeted Therapies and Immunotherapies

1. Before initiating treatment for a patient with colon cancer, the oncologist asks about the results of testing for *KRAS* and epidermal growth factor receptor (EGFR). The oncology nurse responds with the understanding that which one of the following is true about testing?
   A. KRAS and EGFR testing is necessary prior to beginning therapy for those most likely to benefit from treatment in some cancer types.
   B. KRAS and EGFR testing is a United States Food and Drug Administration (FDA)-approved test used prior to starting targeted treatment for all types of cancers.
   C. KRAS and EGFR testing is designed to be paired with a specific drug, but does not have to be FDA approved.
   D. KRAS and EGFR testing can only test one biomarker at a time and generally does not improve outcomes.

2. H.L. is a 60-year-old female patient with cancer. She expresses to her oncology nurse that she is concerned about beginning treatment with Crizotinib, worrying that the drug will not be effective. The oncology nurse explains which one of the following is true about Crizotinib?
   A. "Crizotinib is an oral chemotherapy medication that will directly kill your cancer cells."
   B. "Crizotinib acts to block defective genes that caused your cancer."
   C. "Crizotinib works by replacing the defective genes identified in your cancer with genes that are healthy."
   D. "Crizotinib works quickly and has fewer side effects than chemotherapy."

3. The oncology nurse understands that it is important to assess and monitor blood pressure levels in a patient being placed on bevacizumab because which one of the following statements is true about hypertension?
   A. Hypertension will result in seizures.
   B. Hypertension can be the first sign of cardiomyopathy.
   C. Hypertension is a common problem with this drug that can be managed.
   D. Hypertension is most likely to occur in patients without risk factors.

4. Targeted therapies work in several ways to stop cancer growth. Which one of the following is a way that targeted therapies work?
   A. Deregulating cell signaling pathways
   B. Activating oncogenes
   C. Inhibiting excessive growth factors
   D. Blocking apoptosis

5. J.R. is a 60-year-old male patient with cancer who is receiving a treatment of gemtuzumab ozogamicin. Which one of the following statements is true regarding this agent?
   A. Gemtuzumab ozogamicin is a conjugated monoclonal antibody that is chemically linked to a chemotherapy agent.
   B. Gemtuzumab ozogamicin is an unconjugated monoclonal antibody that is linked to a radioisotope.
   C. Gemtuzumab ozogamicin is a chimeric conjugated monoclonal antibody linked to a chemotherapy agent.
   D. Gemtuzumab ozogamicin is a conjugated monoclonal antibody that has several antigens as targets.

6. An oncology nurse's patient is being placed on a monoclonal antibody in addition to chemotherapy. The patient is wondering why she needs both types of treatment. The oncology nurse caring for her replies that the monoclonal antibody:
   A. results in immediate cell death while chemotherapy blocks intracellular signaling
   B. flags cancer cells for destruction by the immune system and chemotherapy initiates the complement cascade
   C. targets primarily the nucleus of the cancer cell to stop proliferation
   D. targets a specific protein that is driving the growth of the cancer

7. S.J. is a 44-year-old female patient with cancer with a known BRCA pathogenic variant. She is being treated with olaparib. The oncology nurse caring for her is teaching her about her disease. As part of the teaching, the nurse most likely explains which one of the following?
   A. Genetically pathogenically altered ovarian cancer cells are sensitive to poly-ADP ribose polymerase (PARP) inhibition.
   B. PARP inhibitors repair damaged DNA single-strand breaks.
   C. Cyclin-dependent kinase inhibitors are used in the treatment of estrogen receptor–negative breast cancers.
   D. Proteasome inhibitors are effective in the treatment of breast cancer with a pathogenic variant in BRCA.

8. H.K. is a 67-year-old patient with cancer who is about to start adjuvant treatment with chemotherapy, pertuzumab, and trastuzumab. His baseline blood pressure is 140/88. Which one of the following test results would be of concern and should be investigated prior to him starting treatment?
   A. Liver enzymes show an aspartate transaminase of 35 µ/L and alanine aminotransferase of 40 µ/L.
   B. A left ventricular ejection fraction (LVEF) of 45%.
   C. Hemoglobin A1c (HbA1c) is 5.0%.
   D. Creatinine clearance is 100 mL/min.

9. An oncology nurse is caring for a patient with cancer who is about to start treatment with rituximab. Which one of the following medical diagnoses would be a concern?
   A. Hypertension
   B. Type 2 diabetes
   C. Hepatitis B
   D. Basal cell carcinomas

10. G.K. is a 50-year-old female patient who will be started on an EGFR inhibitor for treatment of her cancer. Which one of the following statements indicates that the patient understands the oncology nurse's education regarding rash?
    A. "If I do develop an acne-like condition, I know that it is OK to use an over-the-counter product containing benzoyl peroxide."
    B. "I should apply a moisturizer once a day after taking a hot shower."
    C. "If I develop a rash, that means that the drug is working effectively."
    D. "I need to avoid sun exposure as much as possible and use sunscreens that contain zinc oxide."

11. J.L. is a 61-year-old male patient with cancer who is being treated with bevacizumab. It is most important for the oncology nurse to do which one of the following?
    A. Monitor for signs and symptoms of hypertension.
    B. Schedule treatment 1 week after surgery.
    C. Ensure that the patient takes one tablet daily with water.
    D. Take medication on an empty stomach.

12. L.T., a 48-year-old male patient who is being treated with an EGFR inhibitor, comes into the clinic complaining of diarrhea. He reports having six unformed, watery stools per day. Infection has been ruled out through testing. Which one of the following is an appropriate intervention to manage L.T.'s diarrhea?
    A. Administer loperamide and instruct the patient on a high-fat, high-fiber diet.
    B. Administer loperamide and monitor the patient for signs and symptoms of dehydration.
    C. Instruct the patient to take probiotics and modify his diet by increasing fiber and fats.
    D. Instruct the patient to increase hypotonic fluids to at least 1 liter per day and report any fever.

13. M.S. is a patient who is receiving everolimus. The oncology nurse knows that an appropriate pharmacologic intervention for M.S. would include which one of the following?
    A. A steroid-based mouthwash to reduce the incidence and severity of stomatitis
    B. An oral hypoglycemic agent to prevent hyperglycemia
    C. Prophylactic loperamide to prevent diarrhea
    D. Prophylaxis with trimethoprim-sulfamethoxazole to prevent pneumocystis pneumonia

14. Immunotherapy offers the potential for effectiveness after treatment has ended. This may best be explained by which one of the following statements?
    A. The use of antibodies to direct activity against tumors
    B. The ability of the immune system to distinguish between healthy tissue and tumor
    C. The immune system's unique memory abilities
    D. Immune-mediated cytotoxicity against cancer cells

15. D.W. is a 58-year-old male patient with cancer who will be starting treatment with a checkpoint inhibitor. His oncology nurse explains that this type of treatment works by:
    A. blocking links between proteins and receptors that cancer cells use to turn off the immune system
    B. tagging a protein produced by the tumor to allow the immune system to recognize the protein and destroy it, leading to tumor cell death
    C. using viruses to directly infect tumor cells
    D. binding with antibodies to directly attack tumors

16. Adverse events (AEs) with immunotherapy differ from those associated with cytotoxic therapy in that AEs associated with immunotherapy are which one of the following?
    A. AEs associated with immunotherapy are predictable and limited in duration.
    B. AEs associated with immunotherapy are unpredictable and prolonged.
    C. AEs associated with immunotherapy are treated with supportive care measures that target the AE.
    D. AEs associated with immunotherapy are prolonged in duration and "off-target."

17. S.K. is a 52-year-old female patient who has received chimeric antigen receptor T-cell (CAR-T) cell therapy 5 days ago. She now presents with a fever of 104°F, and complains of fatigue and headache. Her heart rate is 90 beats/min and blood pressure is 100/60 mmHg. The oncology nurse caring for her suspects that she has which one of the following?
    A. Capillary leak syndrome
    B. Pseudoprogression
    C. Central nervous system metastases
    D. Cytokine release syndrome

18. An oncology nurse is caring for a patient who is experiencing Grade 2 pneumonitis from treatment with a checkpoint inhibitor. The oncology nurse anticipates that the health care provider will order which one of the following?
    A. Hold the checkpoint inhibitor therapy and initiate corticosteroids.
    B. Keep the patient on the checkpoint inhibitor and initiate corticosteroids.
    C. Permanently discontinue the checkpoint inhibitor.
    D. Initiate empiric antibiotics keep the patient on the checkpoint inhibitor.

19. A patient with cancer who is receiving a programmed death-1 (PD-1) therapy tells her oncology nurse that she is experiencing some fatigue and flu-like symptoms. The oncology nurse recommends that the patient do which one of the following?
    A. Go to Urgent Care if her symptoms become worse.
    B. Report this symptom to her primary care physician at her upcoming appointment.
    C. Document her symptoms and only seek medical attention if a fever develops.
    D. Report this symptom to the health care team who prescribed the treatment.

20. Patients who have received immunotherapy should alert all of their health care providers because of which one of the following?
    A. Each provider should be aware of the potential for immune-related adverse events.
    B. Most providers know how to manage long-term effects of immunotherapy.
    C. Adverse events generally occur while patients are receiving immunotherapy.
    D. Most adverse events are short term and require management by a multidisciplinary team.

21. S.E. is a 47-year-old female patient with metastatic ovarian cancer. She has had genetic testing due to an extensive family history of breast and ovarian cancer and is found to have a pathogenic variant in the BRCA1 gene. The genetic testing results may also influence treatment decisions. Her treatment might include which one of the following?
    A. Olaparib or rucaparib
    B. Niraparib or ceritinib
    C. Erlotinib or olaparib
    D. Alectinib or ceritinib

22. Which one of the following statements is true about monoclonal antibodies?
    A. Monoclonal antibodies are intracellular enzymes that control DNA repair and cellular apoptosis.
    B. Monoclonal antibodies bind to only one specific target substance with exceptional specificity.
    C. Monoclonal antibodies are circulating growth factors in serum that stimulate growth.
    D. Monoclonal antibodies block the binding site of the intracellular portion of a receptor

23. Companion tests are ordered for which one of the following reasons?
    A. To evaluate for germline pathogenic variants
    B. To evaluate for somatic pathogenic variants
    C. To determine the appropriate dose of a targeted therapy
    D. To determine the stage of the tumor

24. An oncology patient is receiving a targeted therapy that ends with the suffix –ximab. The oncology nurse knows that this suffix refers to which one of the following?
    A. A monoclonal antibody that is fully human
    B. A monoclonal antibody that is mouse (murine)
    C. A monoclonal antibody that is chimeric human
    D. A monoclonal antibody that is humanized mouse

25. Infusion reactions most commonly occur with which one of the following?
    A. EGFR-targeted therapies
    B. Anti-VEGFR therapies
    C. mTOR therapies
    D. Monoclonal antibody therapies

26. The oncology nurse is teaching a group of staff nurses about cancer therapies. In describing the actions of antibody-drug conjugates (ADCs), which one of the following should be included in the teaching?
    A. The cytotoxic agent is delivered directly to the target of the monoclonal antibody in the cancer cell.
    B. The cytotoxic agent circulates throughout the bloodstream and affects all body cells.
    C. Only chemotherapy agents can be conjugated with monoclonal antibodies.
    D. Antibody-drug conjugates are used to suppress immune checkpoints.

27. In explaining adoptive T-cell therapies to the group of nurses, the oncology nurse should include which one of the following?
    A. T-cells are pooled from numerous individuals and infused into the patient with cancer.
    B. T-cells taken from the patient are modified so that a smaller quantity, when reinfused into the patient, has increased effectiveness.
    C. T-cells are extracted from the patient, enhanced in a laboratory, then reinfused back to the patient to destroy tumor.
    D. T-cells found in the patient cannot participate in the immune response unless they are activated by chemotherapy exposure.

28. Chimeric antigen receptor (CAR) is one form of adoptive T-cell therapy. The description of this therapy provided by the oncology nurse should include which one of the following?
    A. CAR T-cell therapy recognizes one specific antigen.
    B. CAR T-cell therapy is used to identify occult cancer cells.
    C. Side effects arising from CAR T-cell therapy are typically mild.
    D. Autoimmune endocrine disease is treated with CAR T-cell therapy.

29. The oncology nurse is educating her patient on a proposed treatment plan. The nurse explains that biotherapy is which one of the following?
    A. Biotherapy is always made from substances produced in a laboratory.
    B. Biotherapy is made from living organisms.
    C. Biotherapy reverses the deleterious effects of tumor genes.
    D. Biotherapy directly kills cells.

30. The oncology nurse is providing education for new staff nurses. The nurse defines targeted therapy as which one of the following?
    A. Synthetically produced cytotoxic agents that are aimed at specific tumor types
    B. Naturally occurring cytotoxic agents that are aimed at specific tumor types
    C. Agents that interfere with specific molecules or pathways involved with tumor growth and progression
    D. Agents that stimulate the release of cytokines

31. The oncology nurse continues the staff education and defines immunotherapy as which one of the following?
    A. Immunotherapy uses naturally occurring substances that interfere with the immune system.
    B. Immunotherapy uses synthetically produced agents that target specific tumor types.
    C. Immunotherapy uses agents that stimulate apoptosis in tumor cells.
    D. Immunotherapy uses agents that use, stimulate, augment, or suppress the immune system.

32. A patient being treated for breast cancer asks the oncology nurse about the use of biosimilar drugs in her treatment. The nurse should provide which one of the following explanations about biosimilars?
    A. Biosimilars do not need FDA approval.
    B. Biosimilars are known to increase the risk of side effects.
    C. Biosimilars have minor differences in clinically active components.
    D. Biosimilars are small molecule drugs that are naturally occurring.

33. The oncology nurse is preparing to administer a targeted therapy to C.L., a male patient being treated for advanced kidney cancer. C.L. asks the nurse how targeted therapy differs from chemotherapy. The nurse's explanation should include which one of the following?
    A. Targeted therapies act on rapidly dividing cells.
    B. Targeted therapies act on specific molecules in cancer cells.
    C. Targeted therapies have cytotoxic effects on tumor cells.
    D. Targeted therapies are used to augment tumor cell metabolism.

34. The oncology nurse is teaching about targeted therapies that use engineered MoAbs. Which one of these explanations by the nurse is correct about MoAbs?
    A. MoAbs target molecules inside the cell.
    B. MoAbs are relatively small.
    C. MoAbs target molecules on the cell surface.
    D. MoAbs are not considered an immunotherapy.

59

35. The oncology nurse also explains that small molecule inhibitors:
    A. have similar molecular size and weight to MoAbs
    B. have a lower rate of cell entry relative to MoAbs
    C. are designed to interfere with intracellular signaling molecules
    D. stimulate an immune response

36. Immunotherapy capitalizes on the immune system's unique specificity and memory abilities. Specificity refers to ability to do which one of the following?
    A. Orchestrate immune-mediated cytotoxicity against the tumor
    B. Distinguish between molecules that characterize "self" and "nonself" tissues
    C. Recall previous encounters with an antigen
    D. Engage the immune system to fight cancer

37. The oncology nurse is teaching staff nurses about concepts of immunotherapy. The nurse explains that tumor escape occurs:
    A. in unsuppressed tumor microenvironments
    B. when there is sufficient host immunity
    C. when B-cell exhaustion occurs
    D. when there is failure to recognize an in situ tumor

38. The nurse is reviewing small molecule nomenclature. These molecules are named with Prefix + substem(s) + Stem. The prefix rafe + substem rafenib represents an RAF tyrosine kinase RAF/RAS/MEK pathway small molecule. An example would be which one of the following?
    A. Bortezomib
    B. Dabrafenib
    C. Olaparib
    D. Erlotinib

39. The oncology nurse understands that monoclonal antibodies are named for the species from which they are derived. A monoclonal antibody that ends with -zumab is derived from which one of the following?
    A. Chimeric human-mouse
    B. Fully human
    C. Mouse
    D. Humanized mouse

40. The oncology nurse is aware that there have been recent changes to the nomenclature for monoclonal antibodies. The new naming system eliminates the stem "mAb" and replaces it with one of four stems classifying the construction of the immunoglobulin. Which one of the following stems indicate that the agent is an engineered monospecific immunoglobulin?
    A. -bart
    B. -mig
    C. -tug
    D. -ment

41. The oncology nurse is providing teaching to a patient who is scheduled to receive immunotherapy treatments for his cancer. Which one of the following statements is *not* accurate about immunotherapy side effects?
    A. Multiple organ systems can be affected simultaneously by the immunotherapy.
    B. Autoimmune disorders can result from immune system activation from immunotherapy.
    C. Organs that share the same antigen as the target may be affected by immunotherapy.
    D. The risk for side effects peaks during the period that immunotherapy treatments are given.

42. The oncology nurse is monitoring for the development of immune-related adverse events (irAEs) in a patient receiving immunotherapy treatments. The nurse assesses the patient's symptoms and grade severity according to the Common Terminology Criteria for Adverse Events and determines that the patient has Moderate or Grade 2 AEs. The nurse should anticipate which one of the following?
    A. The patient will continue to be carefully monitored as treatment continues.
    B. There will be a dose interruption or treatment delay until symptoms resolve.
    C. The treatment will be discontinued and intensive long-term management instituted.
    D. The symptoms will be ascribed to the disease state unless proven otherwise.

43. The oncology nurse understands that the frequency and type of irAEs depends on the agents used, the length of exposure, the dose, and the patients' preexisting risk factors. Although almost any organ can be affected by immunotherapies, the most common ones are which of the following?
    A. Kidney and gastrointestinal tract
    B. Thyroid and adrenal glands
    C. Brain and pancreas
    D. Skin and lungs

44. B.F., a male patient who has completed treatment for non–small-cell lung cancer with erlotinib, an epidermal growth factor receptor (EGFR), comes to the oncology clinic for a follow-up visit. The oncology nurse should assess B.F. for which one of the following drug reactions?
    A. Rash
    B. Bruising
    C. Cognitive changes
    D. Peripheral neuropathy

45. J.L., a 77-year-old male, is being worked up for B-cell lymphoma. The oncology nurse caring for him anticipates that he will be treated with which one of these B-cell lymphoma 2 (BCL-2) inhibitor drugs that acts to regulate the intrinsic apoptosis pathway?
A. Olaparib
B. Palbociclib
C. Venetoclax
D. Bevacizumab

46. E.N., a female patient with breast cancer, is scheduled to receive therapy with trastuzumab. The oncology nurse is aware that "on-target, off-tumor" adverse events result from drug activity against normal tissue that displays similar or identical molecules as the primary target tissue. Because E.N. will be taking trastuzumab, the nurse should monitor her for the function of which one of the following normal organs?
A. Ovaries
B. Heart
C. Kidney
D. Liver

47. The oncology nurse is caring for A.F., a 66-year-old male patient with metastatic colorectal cancer, who is being treated with chemotherapy in combination with bevacizumab. The nurse is aware that which one of the following AEs, if experienced by A.F., may be a biomarker of bevacizumab efficacy?
A. Acneiform rash
B. Shortness of breath
C. Hypertension
D. Diarrhea

48. The oncology nurse meets with L.T., a male patient newly diagnosed with prostate cancer who is considering several treatment options. Among them is a prostate cancer vaccine. The oncology nurse understands that which one of the following descriptions of prostate cancer vaccine therapy is accurate?
A. It is a personalized therapy based on a patient's own extracted antigen-presenting cells (dendritic cells) engineered to recognize tumor-associated antigens.
B. It is the injection of an attenuated virus into the tumor, resulting in tumor lysis and presentation of tumor-associated antigen to immune cells.
C. It orchestrates the actions of host immune cells communicating inflammatory, stimulatory, or suppressive chemical signals.
D. It interrupts the binding between tumor-related growth factors in the serum and receptors on the cell surface, thereby restoring apoptosis and halting growth signaling pathways.

49. Bispecific antibody drugs differ from monoclonal antibody drugs because of which one of the following?
A. They have both a female and a male gender.
B. They target regulatory checkpoint molecules.
C. They can bind with either chemotherapy agents or radionuclide molecules.
D. They have two distinct antigen binding regions allowing them to bind to different target molecules simultaneously.

31 Support Therapies and Access Devices

1. A patient with acute leukemia had a previous febrile reaction to platelets and is scheduled for another platelet transfusion. The oncology nurse knows that which one of the following platelet products should be used?
   A. Human leukocyte antigen (HLA)-matched platelets
   B. Single-donor platelets
   C. Pooled platelets
   D. Leukocyte-reduced platelets

2. W.K. is a 56-year-old female patient with colon cancer who is undergoing surgical resection of her mass and may need red blood cells (RBCs) during her surgery. The oncology nurse understands that which one of the following methods of RBC collection is used to ensure that the correct blood component will be available?
   A. Whole blood
   B. Homologous blood
   C. Autologous blood
   D. Directly donated blood

3. After a patient has received a transfusion of platelets, the oncology nurse should expect correction of which one of the following conditions?
   A. Anemia
   B. Thrombocytopenia
   C. Hypogammaglobulinemia
   D. Clotting factors

4. An oncology nurse has administered an RBC transfusion to a patient with cancer. During the follow-up assessment, the nurse notes that the patient has an oral temperature of 102°F degrees, along with chills, and is complaining of nausea. Which type of reaction is this patient exhibiting?
   A. Febrile nonhemolytic reaction
   B. Hemolytic reaction
   C. Transfusion-related acute lung injury
   D. Iron overload

5. S.L. is a 65-year-old male patient with lung cancer who is undergoing chemotherapy. Ten days after a treatment he presents to the clinic for lab work. Results of his complete blood count reveals that his absolute neutrophil count is 1000/mm³, hemoglobin 6.8 g/dl, and platelets 30,000/mm³. The oncology nurse should anticipate that which one of the following blood products will be ordered for S.L.?
   A. Platelets
   B. Neutrophils
   C. Red blood cells
   D. Immunoglobulin

6. G.R. is a 49-year-old female patient who presents to the oncology clinic with a report that, during her last platelet transfusion, G.R. exhibited a mild case of hives with itching. The oncology nurse expects that which one of the following premedications will be ordered for G.R. prior to future platelet transfusions?
   A. Diphenhydramine
   B. Meperidine
   C. Hydrocortisone
   D. Diuretic

7. The nurse on the oncology unit has received an order to transfuse one of the inpatients. The nurse is aware that to decrease the incidence and severity of a transfusion reaction, which one of the following is the best nursing intervention to follow?
   A. Use of normal saline as a diluent during the transfusion
   B. Use the maximum number of units according to the lab value
   C. Attach an appropriate filter to the blood product
   D. Monitor patients for 4 hours after transfusion

8. A husband asks the oncology nurse about which blood product is the safest should his wife require a blood product transfusion for an upcoming elective surgery. The nurse should explain that blood received from which one of the following is safest?
   A. HLA matched
   B. Collected during a blood drive
   C. Collected from the intended recipient
   D. Directly donated blood

9. V.K. is a 59-year-old female patient who presents to the oncology clinic 7 days after receiving a chemotherapy treatment, and states that her gums have been bleeding. Complete blood count reveals a platelet count of 38,000/mm³ and hemoglobin of 8.5 g/dL. Which one of the following blood component therapies would the oncology nurse anticipate being ordered for this patient?
   A. Red blood cells
   B. Plasma
   C. No blood product
   D. Platelets

10. Which one of the following techniques can be used to minimize blood loss in a patient who refuses blood component therapy while undergoing cancer treatment?
    A. Routinely check complete blood counts
    B. Administer iron and vitamin supplementation
    C. Use of histamine-2 antagonist
    D. Use of regular blood collection tubes

11. A patient receiving red blood cells begins to demonstrate uncontrolled shaking chills, shortness of breath, and wheezing. Which one of the following would be the appropriate initial nursing intervention?
    A. Notify the provider and blood bank of potential reaction.
    B. Administer diphenhydramine intravenously.
    C. Administer meperidine intravenously.
    D. Stop the infusion immediately and start intravenous normal saline.

12. An oncology nurse is teaching a patient and the patient's family about a peripherally inserted central catheter (PICC). The nurse knows the patient needs more teaching when the patient describes the PICC as:
    A. inserted into a central vein
    B. inserted with single, double, or triple lumen
    C. inserted at the antecubital fossa
    D. inserted for 6 months and removed

13. J.D. is a 62-year-old male patient who returns from having surgical insertion of a tunneled venous catheter. The nurse caring for him can begin chemotherapy treatments when which one of the following is performed?
    A. Computed tomography scan
    B. Blood return on aspiration
    C. Chest x-ray
    D. Fluids infuse without difficulty

14. Bundled care is incorporated upon insertion of venous catheters to decrease risk of which one of the following?
    A. Bleeding
    B. Infection
    C. Catheter dislodgement
    D. Catheter migration

15. A patient presents to the oncology clinic for a chemotherapy infusion. The nurse caring for the patient accesses the implantable port and attempts to flush. The port flushes easily; however, a blood return is unobtainable. Which one of the following is the most common cause for no blood return?
    A. Precipitation
    B. Deep vein thrombosis
    C. Fibrin sheath
    D. Intraluminal blood clot

16. T.S. is a 57-year-old male patient who will be discharged from the hospital to receive intravenous antibiotics at home for the next 10 days. Which of the following pumps is not equipped with audible alarms?
    A. Peristaltic
    B. Syringe
    C. Smart pump
    D. Elastomeric

17. A patient has been diagnosed with leptomeningeal disease requiring frequent administration of chemotherapy into the cerebral spinal fluid. Which one of the following devices would be implanted?
    A. Intraventricular catheter
    B. Peritoneal catheter
    C. Epidural long-term catheter
    D. Intrapleural catheter

18. Which one of the following is an example of an intervention to prevent a mechanical complication of an access device?
    A. Maintain flushing routine and flush with pulsatile (push-pause) method to cause swirling action in device
    B. Change intrathoracic pressures: have the patient inhale fully and hold breath or exhale fully and hold breath
    C. Surgical removal, as indicated, to avoid fracture
    D. Remove needle, and re-access port using a non-coring needle

19. Which one of the following is the best management strategy for catheter migration?
    A. Monitor the length of the catheter (tunnel, midline, PICC) to ensure placement is intact.
    B. Refer to the physician for repositioning the catheter using fluoroscopy.
    C. Avoid placing the port at the sites of actual or potential tissue damage (in radiation field).
    D. Use high-pressure infusions or flush catheter with 1 or 3 mL.

20. Which one of the following is a characteristic of a short-term or intermediate-term peripheral catheter?
    A. Insertion is done centrally into the jugular vein, subclavian vein, superior vena cava (SVC), or inferior vena cava
    B. Available with a pressure-activated safety valve (PASV) located in the catheter hub and designed to permit fluid infusion and decrease risk of blood reflux
    C. Catheter tip must be confirmed before initial use by ultrasound (during placement if used), fluoroscopy, or chest x-ray
    D. Infuses fluids, medications, blood products, and peripheral total parenteral nutrition (TPN) and to obtain blood specimens

63

21. In addition to monitoring for febrile complications of blood component therapy (BCT), an oncology nurse should monitor the recipient's response for which one of the following?
    A. Allergic reactions, hypothermia, and hemolytic reactions
    B. Fluid volume overload and deep vein thrombosis (DVT) caused by the platelet increase
    C. DVT and other coagulation problems
    D. Bone marrow reaction to the unrelated presence of unrelated stem cells

22. The oncology nurse is preparing a BCT infusion. The nurse knows that which one of the following guidelines maximizes patient safety?
    A. Using a gravity-flow infusion line
    B. Adding medications slowly through the Y-port
    C. Using the smallest gauge intravenous (IV) catheter available
    D. Together with a second registered nurse, checking BCT product with the patient's ID

23. An oncology nurse is evaluating the potential for a patient with cancer to receive an implanted venous access device. Which one of the following best supports the decision for the patient to have this type of device inserted?
    A. The patient demonstrates the ability to care for the device.
    B. The patient needs chemotherapy infusions and blood samples.
    C. The patient expresses concerns about implantation of the device.
    D. The patient and the patient's family are reluctant to care for an external device.

24. K.R. is a 69-year-old male who is being discharged from the ambulatory infusion center with an infusion system for continuous chemotherapy infusion. Which one of the following would indicate that the patient and his family are adequately prepared for use of the infusion system?
    A. They acknowledge understanding of how to flush the line with sterile water every 12 hours.
    B. They acknowledge understanding of how to monitor the infusion system for proper functioning.
    C. They acknowledge understanding of how to attach a second line to the infusion system for pain control.
    D. They acknowledge understanding of how to change the dose of the drug whenever the patient is sleeping.

25. E.L. has come to the oncology clinic for a blood transfusion. The oncology nurse caring for E.L. is aware that the use of blood component therapy in the oncology setting has increased because of which one of these reasons?
    A. Increased use of erythropoietin
    B. Delay in initiating antineoplastic therapies
    C. Use of more aggressive therapies resulting in bone marrow suppression
    D. Difficulty in providing timely hematopoietic stem cell transplantation therapies

26. A patient who is anemic after cytotoxic cancer therapy is scheduled to receive a blood transfusion of packed red cells (pRBCs). The oncology nurse caring for the patient anticipates that each unit of RBCs should have which one of the following effects?
    A. Hemoglobin should increase 1 g/dL or hematocrit by 3% with each unit.
    B. Hemoglobin should increase 3 g/dL or hematocrit by 1% with each unit.
    C. A single unit of pRBCs is unlikely to elevate hemoglobin or hematocrit.
    D. One unit of pRBCs will elevate the platelet count 35 to 40 μL.

27. The oncology nurse is preparing to give P.W., a male patient on the oncology unit, a transfusion of fresh frozen plasma. The nurse understands that the purpose of this transfusion is to achieve which one of the following?
    A. Maintain antibody levels to prevent infection
    B. Provide passive immunity protection against cytomegalovirus
    C. Increase WBC count, prevent and/or treat infections in neutropenic patients
    D. Correct clotting factor deficiencies, expand blood volume, provide osmotic diuresis

28. The nurse caring for P.W. should monitor him closely during his plasma transfusion for which one of these possible acute events?
    A. Hemolysis
    B. Hemorrhage
    C. Iron overload
    D. Allergic reaction

29. The oncology nurse caring for P.W. reviews his hospital chart and notes that he experienced posttransfusion purpura in the past. The nurse understands that this indicates which one of the following?
    A. This is a delayed reaction in which transfused antibodies destroy platelets in the transfused blood and the patient's own platelets.
    B. This is an acute reaction caused by WBC antibodies in the transfused product reacting with the patient's own WBCs.
    C. This is an acute hemolytic reaction causing immune destruction of transfused RBCs, which are attacked by the recipient's antibodies.
    D. This is a delayed reaction after blood component transfusion in which the recipient develops alloantibodies against the donor's antigens.

30. The oncology nurse is reviewing laboratory test results for L.G., a male patient being treated for bladder cancer. The nurse anticipates that the physician will order a blood component transfusion for L.G. when which one of these laboratory results is present?
    A. Platelet count > 60,000/mm³
    B. Hemoglobin < 7 g/dL
    C. Neutrophils > 1000/mm³
    D. International normalized ratio (INR) < 1.50

31. During the administration of blood component therapy, the oncology nurse should monitor the patient for the presence of which one of the following signs or symptoms indicating a transfusion complication?
    A. Diarrhea
    B. Flatulence
    C. Pale urine
    D. Flank/back pain

32. L.S. is a female patient who has experienced heavy bleeding from endometrial cancer. She may need a blood transfusion but is opposed to receiving blood products. The oncology nurse suggests which one of the following methods to diminish further blood loss?
    A. Minimize routine blood testing.
    B. Use large blood collection tubes.
    C. Add vitamin C supplementation.
    D. Increase frequency of heparin flushes.

33. The oncology nurse on the inpatient unit will be receiving a patient scheduled to be treated for pancreatic cancer with intraarterial chemotherapy. The nurse understands that the type of catheter used to deliver this type of therapy is which one of the following?
    A. A nontunneled catheter centrally inserted into the jugular vein, subclavian vein, or superior vena cava
    B. A midline catheter inserted into a peripheral vein and terminating in the axillary vein in the upper arm
    C. An arterial catheter directly threaded into the artery that feeds the tumor
    D. An intrathecal catheter inserted below the dura where cerebrospinal fluid circulates

34. The oncology nurse is explaining to a staff nurse the advantages of using arterial catheters for short- or long-term chemotherapy administration. The oncology nurse should include all of the following reasons *except* which one?
    A. They have smaller internal diameters and thicker walls because of higher vascular arterial pressures.
    B. They can be nontunneled for short-term use or tunneled for long-term use.
    C. They deliver high concentrations of drug directly to the tumor with decreased systemic exposure.
    D. They have a one-way valve to prevent retrograde blood flow.

35. The oncology nurse is providing orientation to new nurses to the unit about blood component therapy. The nurse explains that an allogeneic blood component is:
    A. blood collected from the intended recipient before surgery
    B. blood component collected from a donor designated by the intended recipient
    C. blood collected from screened donors for transfusion to another individual
    D. blood collected during surgery by the use of automated "cell saver" device

36. The nurse is caring for a patient who has experienced a dilution of clotting factors due to hemorrhage. The nurse anticipates the patient will be transfused with:
    A. HLA platelets
    B. fresh frozen plasma
    C. packed red blood cells
    D. cryoprecipitate

37. The nurse is caring for a 26-year-old male who was in an motor vehicle accident and has a large laceration on his arm. He has a known diagnosis of hemophilia A. The nurse anticipates that he will be transfused with:
    A. platelets
    B. plasma
    C. factor VIII
    D. factor IX

38. The nurse is caring for a patient who is experiencing thrombocytopenia (platelet count 19,000/mm³). The patient has never had a blood component transfusion. The nurse anticipates the patient will be transfused with:
    A. pooled platelets
    B. single donor platelets
    C. leukocyte reduced platelets
    D. HLA matched platelets

39. The oncology nurse is caring for a patient with a suspected access device infection. The nurse anticipates an order for which one of the following?
    A. acetaminophen for fever reduction
    B. institute a broad-spectrum antibiotic
    C. vancomycin for empiric therapy until organism identified
    D. remove access device

32 Pharmacologic Interventions

1. A patient who received chemotherapy 7 days ago presents to the emergency department (ED) with a fever of 102°F and chills. His absolute neutrophil count is 500 cells/µL. His spouse asks the nurse why he is being admitted to the hospital since he "doesn't look that sick." The oncology nurse explains that which one of the following is true?
   A. The patient's fever might be an early sign of infection.
   B. The patient is dehydrated and requires IV hydration.
   C. The patient needs a platelet transfusion.
   D. Fever might be a sign of an allergic drug reaction.

2. The oncology nurse understands that which one of the following antimicrobial agents is appropriate for the treatment of cytomegalovirus (CMV)?
   A. Levofloxacin
   B. Acyclovir
   C. Ganciclovir
   D. Fluconazole

3. Patients who are considered high risk for febrile neutropenia should avoid which one of the following medications?
   A. Antipyretics
   B. Antibiotics
   C. Antivirals
   D. Antifungals

4. Which one of the following statements regarding vancomycin as an empiric therapy is true?
   A. Dose adjustments per pharmacy are not required prior to initiation.
   B. Vancomycin provides appropriate empiric coverage of gram-negative bacteria.
   C. Empiric vancomycin is recommended for low-risk patients.
   D. Routine use of empiric vancomycin should be avoided.

5. The oncology nurse has an order to administer amphotericin B (deoxycholate) to a patient. Which one of the following adverse reactions associated with amphotericin B should the nurse monitor for?
   A. Nephrotoxicity and electrolyte wasting
   B. Myelosuppression and central nervous system (CNS) toxicity
   C. Ocular toxicity and prolonged QTc
   D. Serotonin syndrome and ototoxicity

6. A patient with cancer complains of burning on urination. Microbiology results show the urinalysis with leuko-esterase, white blood cell (WBC), and nitrate positivity, and it is positive for *Escherichia coli*. Which one of the following nursing actions would be indicated?
   A. Encourage patient to drink fluids in order to prevent antibiotic use.
   B. Ensure the patient has an order for prophylactic antibiotics upon discharge to prevent future urinary tract infections (UTIs).
   C. Report culture results to provider and anticipate orders for antibiotics.
   D. No further action is needed.

7. G.T. is a 58-year-old male who is in the clinic receiving chemotherapy for lung cancer and is inquiring about whether he can receive the flu vaccine before he leaves clinic today. The oncology nurse caring for him should respond with which one of the following statements?
   A. Influenza vaccines contain live virus and should be avoided.
   B. The influenza vaccine can be administered between chemotherapy cycles.
   C. Receiving the influenza vaccine may increase the risk for infection.
   D. The vaccination schedule is dependent on his CD34 counts.

8. Antiinflammatory agents are effective in treating pain and inflammation because they do which one of the following?
   A. Block major nerve pathways and conduction
   B. Inhibit cyclooxygenase and prostaglandin production
   C. Decrease platelet function and bleeding risk
   D. Lower temperature threshold and signs of infection

9. A patient has returned to clinic for a follow-up appointment and reports that she has been taking an over-the-counter NSAID for mild bone pain. Which other medication reported by the patient should prompt the oncology nurse to notify the medical team?
   A. Metoprolol
   B. Clopidogrel
   C. Multivitamin
   D. Ciprofloxacin

10. A patient is prescribed corticosteroids for the treatment of multiple myeloma. The oncology nurse caring for the patient knows to monitor for which one of the following?
    A. Signs of bleeding
    B. Renal and hepatic failure
    C. Nausea and vomiting
    D. Muscle weakness

11. The oncology nurse is caring for a female patient who will receive an antiemetic agent prior to the start of her infusion of highly emetic chemotherapy agents. The nurse understands that the antiemetic drugs ondansetron and granisetron disrupt signaling pathways by targeting which one of the following neurotransmitters?
    A. Serotonin
    B. Dopamine
    C. Histamine
    D. Neurokinin

12. During a follow-up visit, a patient reports that she is experiencing breakthrough chemotherapy-induced nausea and vomiting despite receiving palonosetron 0.25 mg PO prior to her chemotherapy infusion. The oncology nurse should anticipate administering which one of the following antiemetics?
    A. Ondansetron 8 mg IV
    B. Dexamethasone 12 mg IV
    C. Granisetron 2 mg PO
    D. Repeat dose of palonosetron

13. Metoclopramide has a black box warning for which adverse reaction?
    A. Drug-drug interactions
    B. Prolongation of QT interval
    C. Extrapyramidal symptoms
    D. Orthostatic hypotension

14. The oncology nurse understands that which one of the following is an essential principle of analgesic medication management?
    A. For chronic pain, patients should have long-acting and breakthrough options available.
    B. Patients with acute pain should avoid opioids to prevent physical dependence.
    C. Opioid tolerance means the patient has developed a psychological addiction to the drug.
    D. Stool softeners should only be administered once the patient reports changes in bowel movements.

15. S.L. is a 48-year-old male patient who arrives at the clinic with complaints of nausea, sweating, and insomnia. During the medication reconciliation, he states that he recently stopped taking his prescribed morphine sulfate. The oncology nurse suspects he is experiencing which one of the following?
    A. Poor pain control
    B. Constipation
    C. Addiction
    D. Withdrawal

16. The oncology nurse knows that which one of the following medications would be appropriate for a patient experiencing somnolence from opioid use?
    A. Methylphenidate
    B. Metoclopramide
    C. Micafungin
    D. Mithramycin

17. A patient with cancer has just been prescribed oral oxycodone. The oncology nurse caring for the patient knows that instructing the patient will include which one of the following?
    A. Avoid grapefruit juice.
    B. Take medication with food.
    C. Take medication on an empty stomach.
    D. Medication should be taken in combination with acetaminophen.

18. Anxiolytics can be used as supportive treatment for patients with cancer to do which one of the following?
    A. Prevent or manage anticipatory nausea.
    B. Replace the need for narcotic pain control.
    C. Prevent opportunistic infection.
    D. Treat clinical depression.

19. A patient has just been prescribed Lexapro 10 mg to manage depression. The oncology nurse is aware that which one of the following statements would most likely indicate that the patient needs additional teaching?
    A. "I should take this medication with food."
    B. "If I experience any side effects, I will notify my doctor."
    C. "I will carry a bottle of water with me to help relieve dry mouth."
    D. "My mood should be better by the end of the week."

20. Which one of the following medications is an appropriate option for managing sleeping disorders?
    A. Linezolid
    B. Posaconazole
    C. Zolpidem
    D. Temozolomide

21. A patient with cancer has been diagnosed with a major depressive disorder and has recently been prescribed an antidepressant. The oncology nurse understands that which one of the following is the most important question to ask during the patient's initial follow up appointment?
    A. "Is your pain being well controlled?"
    B. "Are you having any thoughts of harming yourself?"
    C. "How would you describe your sleep pattern over the last few nights?"
    D. "Did you drive yourself to clinic today?"

22. Which one of the following antidepressants is associated with a higher risk of anticholinergic effects (blurred vision, dry mouth, and constipation)?
    A. Fluoxetine
    B. Sertraline
    C. Citalopram
    D. Amitriptyline

23. Which one of the following chemotherapy drugs has the potential to lower the seizure threshold?
    A. Cytarabine
    B. Melphalan
    C. Carmustine
    D. Mitoxantrone

24. Levetiracetam is associated with which one of the following side effects?
    A. Somnolence
    B. Hepatotoxicity
    C. Nausea
    D. Hallucinations

25. Anticonvulsants have the potential to change drug metabolism and drug–drug interactions because they are categorized as which one of the following types of enzymes?
    A. Inducers
    B. Substrates
    C. Inhibitors
    D. Receptors

26. T.W. is a 60-year-old male patient who has received an autologous stem cell transplant 5 days ago and has an order for filgrastim. The oncology nurse caring for him understands this medication is used to do which one of the following?
    A. Filgrastim is used to prevent veno-occlusive disease.
    B. Filgrastim is used to support neutrophil engraftment.
    C. Filgrastim is used to reduce the need for red blood cell transfusions.
    D. Filgrastim is used to prevent delayed nausea and vomiting.

27. A patient with cancer being treated with chemotherapy is scheduled to receive a myeloid growth factor. The oncology nurse knows that myeloid growth factors are used to stimulate production of which one of the following?
    A. Neutrophils and macrophages
    B. Natural killer cells
    C. B lymphocytes
    D. Plasma cells

28. A patient with cancer is receiving erythropoietin growth factor. The oncology nurse should monitor the patient for which one of the following adverse events associated with erythropoietin?
    A. Bone pain
    B. Deep vein thrombosis
    C. Splenic rupture
    D. Peripheral neuropathy

29. In the neutropenic patient with cancer, which one of the following surgeries may impact the treatment of active infections?
    A. Lobectomy
    B. Appendectomy
    C. Splenectomy
    D. Cholecystectomy

30. S.R. is a 62-year-old male patient with cancer who is experiencing anxiety. The oncology nurse caring for him relays the patient assessment to the physician. The physician orders a serotonin selective reuptake inhibitor (SSRI) to begin while the patient remains hospitalized. Which one of the following should the nurse understand about SSRIs?
    A. SSRIs relieve anxiety symptoms early in therapy.
    B. SSRIs have an optimal effect when started at the maximum dose and then tapered down.
    C. SSRI effect will be seen in first 7 days of treatment.
    D. SSRI abrupt discontinuation may precipitate withdrawal syndrome.

31. A patient with cancer is diagnosed with major depressive disorder, which is characterized by which one of the following?
    A. Sad, empty, and irritable mood occurring late in the day
    B. Recurrent thoughts of dying
    C. Occurs in about 75% of patients with cancer
    D. Depressive symptoms occur daily for at least 5 days

32. The oncology nurse should counsel a patient with cancer to make dietary modifications to avoid foods containing tyramine when the patient is receiving which one of the following types of antidepressants?
    A. Serotonin selective reuptake inhibitors (SSRIs)
    B. Serotonin and norepinephrine reuptake inhibitors (SNRIs)
    C. Tricyclic antidepressants (TCA)
    D. Monoamine oxidase inhibitors (MAOIs)

33. S.R. is the 62-year-old male patient with cancer who was diagnosed with depression. He was recently started on an antidepressant. If improvement in symptoms occur, which one of the following is true about the therapy?
    A. The therapy should be continued for 6 months.
    B. The therapy should be continued for 6 weeks.
    C. The therapy should be discontinued.
    D. The patient should begin gradual tapering until off medication.

34. When applying the principles of medical management with myeloid growth factors (MGFs), the risk of neutropenia is increased in which one of the following patient populations?
    A. Patients with endocrine dysfunction
    B. Patients with recent surgery or open wounds
    C. Pediatric patients
    D. Patients with pulmonary hypertension

35. When evaluating the iron stores of a patient with cancer prior to use of erythropoiesis-stimulating agents (ESA) or erythropoietin (EPO) agents, such as epoetin alfa, epoetin alfa-epbx, and darbepoetin, the oncology nurse should consider which one of the following statements?
   A. Patients who are iron deficient will respond best to EPO stimulation.
   B. This medication is warranted in patients with hemoglobin greater than 16 g/dL.
   C. This patient will have an increased risk of venous thromboembolism.
   D. The patient will need an increased number of RBC transfusions to treat anemia.

36. When performing the medication reconciliation for the neutropenic patient, the oncology nurse would expect the cell nadir to occur during which one of the following?
   A. The cell nadir would occur the day after the last chemotherapy dose.
   B. The cell nadir would occur at the beginning of the third chemotherapy cycle.
   C. The cell nadir would occur when the absolute neutrophil count is greater than 500/mm^3.
   D. The cell nadir would occur in 7 to 14 days after chemotherapy treatment.

37. The potential for "Disturbed Body Image" would be important for the oncology nurse to assess and document with which one of the following drug classification?
   A. Corticosteroids
   B. NSAIDS: Cox-2 selective agent
   C. Salicylates
   D. Aminoglycosides

38. When requesting a prescription from the healthcare provider for Morphine to control pain, the oncology nurse should consider which one of the following?
   A. Morphine 30 mg IV has equivalent potency as morphine 10 mg oral
   B. Onset of effect for oral morphine is 30 minutes
   C. Peak effect is 60 minutes with morphine IV
   D. Morphine IV and oral have a duration of effect of 4 to 8 hours

39. Temperature threshold for neutropenic patients is defined as which one of the following?
   A. Multiple axillary temperatures over 37.5°C (99.5°F)
   B. Two consecutive rectal temps over 36.8°C (98.2°F)
   C. Single oral temperature of 38.3°C (101°F)
   D. Sustained temperature of 38°C (100.4°F) over 3 hours

40. A patient with lymphoma, who is currently receiving chemotherapy, presents to the urgent clinic complaining of fever and aching for past 36 hours. The patient has a central line with no redness, tenderness, or edema at the insertion site. Skin is warm and intact. The patient is tolerating oral fluids without nausea or vomiting. The physician orders blood cultures. When obtaining the blood cultures, the gold standard for diagnosis is to draw which one of the following?
   A. Two peripheral cultures
   B. Two central line cultures
   C. No cultures until 48 hours duration of symptoms
   D. One peripheral and one from the central line

41. In a low-risk patient with febrile neutropenia, the provider may prescribe viral prophylaxis in patients with which one of the following prior conditions?
   A. Herpes simplex virus (HSV)
   B. Human immunodeficiency virus (HIV)
   C. Pseudomonas
   D. Respiratory syncytial virus (RSV)

42. During which one of the following time frames would the oncology nurse anticipate discontinuation of antimicrobial therapy for the resolution of a fever in a low-risk patient who is clinically stable with negative cultures but has an ANC remaining less than 500?
   A. After a total of 14 days
   B. After a total of 5 to 7 days
   C. After a total of 17 to 21 days
   D. After the ANC is above 500 for 7 consecutive days

43. Stevens-Johnson syndrome is an adverse effect of antimicrobial therapy impacting which one of the following systems?
   A. Hepatic
   B. Cardiovascular
   C. Gastrointestinal
   D. Dermatologic

44. A patient who is on a chemotherapy regimen is requesting the measles, mumps, and rubella (MMR) vaccine since her grandchildren have been exposed to measles in school. If the health care provider warrants this as necessary, the nurse should administer the vaccine at which one of the following time periods?
   A. More than 2 weeks prior to chemotherapy
   B. 1 month after the chemotherapy regimen is completed
   C. Greater that 4 weeks prior to chemotherapy
   D. At the next chemotherapy appointment since it is not a live virus

45. Which one of the following results may be used as a means of timing vaccine administration in a patient that is post transplant?
    A. Human leukocyte antigen-DR
    B. CD34
    C. Vascular endothelial growth factor receptor (VEGFR)
    D. Complete blood count (CBC)

46. F.L. is a 75-year-old patient who presents at the cancer center with a history of renal insufficiency and cardiovascular disease and is complaining of musculoskeletal pain. The medication list also reveals the patient is prescribed coumadin. When prescribing a medication for the patient's pain, which one of the following would put the patient at high risk for toxicity?
    A. NSAIDs
    B. Anticonvulsants
    C. Acetaminophen
    D. Corticosteroids

47. Which one of the following describes the use of cannabis for chemotherapy-induced nausea and vomiting?
    A. Cannabis is used as an agent for highly emetogenic intravenous chemotherapy.
    B. Cannabis is legal in every state for medical use only with chemotherapy.
    C. Cannabis is not prescribed due to prolonged, irreversible side effects.
    D. Cannabis is used as an agent for breakthrough nausea and vomiting.

48. Fat-to-lean body ratio is important to assess when prescribing pain medication to be given by which one of the following routes?
    A. Buccal
    B. Transdermal
    C. Subcutaneous
    D. Rectal

49. G.H. is a 50-year-old male patient with cancer who has just been diagnosed as having a *Candida* infection. Which one of the following medications does his oncology nurse expect the primary practitioner to order?
    A. Amphotericin B or fluconazole (Diflucan)
    B. Caspofungin (Cancidas) or ciprofloxacin (Cipro)
    C. Voriconazole (Vfend) or fluconazole (Diflucan)
    D. Imipenem or cidofovir

50. Administration of acyclovir should take which one of the following into account?
    A. Dosing should be based on the patient's actual body weight to ensure adequate blood levels.
    B. It is an effective preemptive therapy for CMV in high-risk patients with cancer.
    C. Probenecid is given to patients to prevent renal reabsorption and related toxicities.
    D. Fluid hydration is necessary if therapeutic IV doses are used.

51. Antiemetics that belong to the same class as ondansetron (Zofran) affect nausea and vomiting by acting as which one of the following?
    A. 5 HT3 agonists
    B. D2 antagonists
    C. NK-1 antagonists
    D. 5 HT3 antagonists

52. Which one of the following statements places antiemetics with the appropriate neurotransmitter agent?
    A. Serotonin – aprepitant
    B. Cannabinoid agonist – dronabinol
    C. Histamine H1 antagonist – prochlorperazine
    D. Dopamine D2 antagonist – promethazine

53. The oncology nurse is aware that which one of the following is a common side effect of concern for patients receiving serotonin reuptake inhibitors?
    A. Hot flashes
    B. Neuropathy
    C. Sexual dysfunction
    D. Increased appetite

54. The oncology nurse meets with a patient who is receiving growth factor support with filgrastim. The nurse should explain to the patient that which one of the following is a common side effect of filgrastim (G-CSF)?
    A. Sedation
    B. Liver dysfunction
    C. Constipation
    D. Bone pain

55. A health care provider has ordered ciprofloxacin, a fluoroquinolone antibiotic, to treat an infection in an immunocompromised patient with cancer. Which one of the following side effects should the nurse be aware of when providing instructions to the patient?
    A. Risk of glaucoma
    B. Risk of permanent tendon damage
    C. Risk of chronic constipation
    D. Risk of developing hypertension

56. Per orders, the oncology nurse is giving acetaminophen to a patient with cancer who has a temperature of 101.8°F. The nurse understands that acetaminophen does *not* have which one of the following effects?
    A. Analgesic
    B. Antipyretic
    C. Antiinflammatory
    D. Fever reducing

33 Complementary and Integrative Modalities

1. Which one of the following classes describes the entire domain of therapies that are independent of conventional medicine?
   A. Integrative
   B. Complementary and alternative
   C. Allopathic
   D. Mind body

2. The two broad subgroups of complementary health approaches defined by National Center for Complementary and Integrative Health (NCCIH) are which of the following?
   A. Massage and acupuncture
   B. Tai chi and healing touch
   C. Chiropractic and osteopathic manipulation
   D. Natural products and mind and body practices

3. When an oncology nurse is discussing safety and risks with a patient, which one of the following factors is true regarding herbal and botanical medicine?
   A. United States Food and Drug Administration (FDA) approved
   B. Tightly regulated in the United States
   C. Efficacy ensured
   D. Interacts with prescribed medication

4. Art and music therapy are modalities labeled as which one of the following?
   A. Mind body
   B. Whole medicine
   C. Biologically based
   D. Manipulative

5. Which one of the following is an appropriate response by the oncology nurse when assessing the patient's use of complementary and alternative medicine at the patient's initial appointment?
   A. "We only need to know the medicines prescribed by your primary physician for your medical record."
   B. "Complementary therapy will be assessed at the end of your treatment visit."
   C. "If there are cultural or religious practices that you incorporate for your health, it should be noted for your oncology team."
   D. "Biologically based therapies are not part of your cancer care so they do not need be addressed at this time."

6. Which one of the following chemotherapy agents is commonly impacted by natural products and would warrant a review of the patient's medication and complementary and alternative medicine (CAM) list in their electronic medical record (EMR) to ensure safety?
   A. Adriamycin
   B. Docetaxel
   C. Lupron
   D. Bleomycin

7. Massage therapy is therapeutic to decrease emotional and physical tension, and is appropriate if which one of the following conditions is met?
   A. Platelets <50,000
   B. Applied directly at the bone metastatic site
   C. Peripheral neuropathy grade 3 or less
   D. White blood cell (WBC) count <1500

8. Which one of the following descriptions defines the mind-body modality of neurolinguistic programming (NLP)?
   A. This modality has a meditative component that brings harmony to body, mind, and spirit.
   B. With this modality, the patient focuses on positive aspects of his or her life to promote a positive outlook over time.
   C. Practices within this modality share characteristics and often involve focused breathing and a relaxed yet alert state that promotes control over thoughts and feelings.
   D. This is a modality with a structured process that uses live or recorded readings describing different scenarios or detailed images to guide the patient through a certain process.

9. Which one of the following descriptions defines the mind-body modality of guided imagery?
   A. A technique within this modality trains patients to develop awareness of experiences moment by moment and in the context of all senses
   B. Enhances coordination and balance and promotes physical, emotional, and spiritual well-being
   C. May lead the patient through progressive muscle relaxation or visualization of a treatment process (e.g., visualization of chemotherapy entering the body and seeking out cancer cells to remove them from the body)
   D. A psychotherapy technique based on the concept that distressing events are associated with specific rapid eye movements

71

10. Which one of the following descriptions defines the manipulative and body-based practice of acupressure?
    A. The use of vigorous massage to stimulate flow of lymphatic fluid
    B. The use of manual pressure and strokes on muscle tissue
    C. An ancient Oriental technique associated with traditional Chinese medicine (TCM), used to restore or promote health and well-being using fine-gauge needles inserted into specific points on the body to stimulate or disperse the flow of energy
    D. The use of finger or hand pressure over specific points on the body to relieve symptoms or to influence specific organ function

11. Which one of the following is a safety issue when using aromatherapy?
    A. Standardization is lacking in the preparation and clinical use of essential oils.
    B. Use of aromatherapy can trigger depression, and these agents can target psychological well-being.
    C. Agents have a narrow range of safe applicability.
    D. Patients frequently develop an allergy to the transporter.

12. The term Feldenkrais refers to which one of the following?
    A. Gentle manipulation of the skull to reestablish natural configuration and movement
    B. The use of vigorous massage to stimulate the flow of lymphatic fluid out of an area of the body
    C. A somatic education system that teaches movement and gentle manipulation to increase body awareness and function
    D. A technique that uses movement and touch to restore balance to the body

13. Which one of the following terms defines reiki?
    A. A technique for balancing the flow of energy in the body through the transfer of human energy
    B. An energy healing technique that uses nursing process and specific protocols
    C. The use of magnetic fields to positively impact the body to stimulate healing
    D. An energy healing modality in which the practitioner directs the flow of energy to various parts of the body to facilitate healing and relaxation

14. Acupuncture is often successful in alleviating pain because of which one of the following?
    A. The placebo effect in which patients expect pain relief and therefore feel less pain
    B. The introduction of pain at the insertion site allows the patient to refocus his or her perception of the original site of pain
    C. The stimulation of the nerve fibers entering the dorsal horn of the spinal cord, which mediates the impulses of the other parts of the body, and allows the patient to experience less pain the original site
    D. The pressure applied by exerting a finger and thumb on the specific point on the surface of the skin acts as an entrance and an exit for an internal healing force, thereby eliminating the overall sensation of pain

15. Following assessment the nurse learns that the patient is practicing qi gong. The nurse knows that this is which one of the following?
    A. Japanese form of body work like acupressure
    B. Chinese meditative practice that combines physical postures with focused intention and breathing techniques to release, cleanse, strengthen, and circulate energy
    C. Eastern homeopathy
    D. Movement and touch to restore balance in the body and neuromuscular function, thus allowing the body to regain a relaxed, healthy posture

34 Cardiovascular Symptoms

1. Which one of the following is a treatment-related risk factor for lymphedema?
   A. Lowered body mass index (BMI)
   B. Tumor invasion
   C. Prolonged immobilization
   D. Lymph node dissection

2. Which one of the following interventions would be an urgent priority for medical management of lymphedema?
   A. Treatment of suspected infection
   B. Weight management
   C. Exercise program
   D. Axillary reverse mapping (ARM)

3. When caring for the patient with lymphedema, the oncology nurse would expect to see which one of the following interventions in the plan of care?
   A. Restrict exercise
   B. Dangle extremities
   C. Apply extreme heat
   D. Wear a compression garment

4. H.K. is a 50-year-old female treated for breast cancer who has developed lymphedema in the arm on the affected side. When the oncology nurse is educating H.K. about lymphedema management at home, which one of the following is an appropriate point to convey?
   A. Wear tight-fitting clothes.
   B. Consume diet high in sodium and low in fiber.
   C. Maintain healthy weight.
   D. Follow up with health care team for 1 month.

5. Movement of fluid from the vascular space into the interstitial space causing edema would occur by which one of the following?
   A. Decreased capillary pressure
   B. Increased capillary permeability
   C. Increased plasma oncotic pressure
   D. Lowered hydrostatic pressure

6. B.L. is a 62-year-old patient who experiences edema after receiving plasma expanders. This condition would be documented as being caused by which one of the following?
   A. Medication related
   B. Allergic
   C. Systemic
   D. Iatrogenic

7. Which one of the following is a risk factor for edema?
   A. Increase in mobility
   B. Absent history of edema
   C. Long distance travel
   D. Hypotension

8. The primary medical management of edema is to do which one of the following?
   A. treat the underlying cause
   B. restrict beta blockers
   C. increase sodium in diet
   D. force fluids

9. A primary diagnosis that commonly results in malignant pericardial effusion is which one of the following?
   A. Basal cell skin cancer
   B. Mesothelioma
   C. Brain tumor
   D. Amyloidosis

10. A risk factor for malignant pericardial effusion is which one of the following?
    A. A fractionated radiation dose of 30 cGy/day to the iliac crest
    B. Simultaneous cancer treatment with hormones
    C. Coexisting renal infection
    D. Radiation targeted to more than 33% of the heart

11. The most common characteristic or symptom of malignancy-related pericardial disease is which one of the following?
    A. Hypertension
    B. Dyspnea
    C. Productive cough
    D. Abdominal distention

73

12. Normal pericardial fluid volume is which one of the following measurements?
    A. 15 to 50 ml
    B. 50 to 80 ml
    C. 900 to 1000 ml
    D. 1 to 5 ml

13. A patient's blood pressure (BP) is 120/80, pulse 60, and respirations 12. Thirty minutes later, the BP is 106/76, pulse 64, respirations 14. This difference in BP demonstrates which one of the following?
    A. Imminent stroke
    B. Narrowing pulse pressure
    C. Widening pulse pressure
    D. Pulsus paradoxus

14. Which one of the following drug classifications is associated with the cardiovascular toxicity that can cause coronary artery spasm?
    A. Alkylating agents
    B. Anthracyclines
    C. Antimetabolites
    D. Angiogenesis inhibitors

15. Which of the following is a characteristic of an acute cardiovascular toxicity from chemotherapy?
    A. Frequently occurs
    B. Occurs within 7 days of drug administration
    C. Is usually reversible
    D. Requires discontinuation of the drug

16. Prevention of cardiotoxicity would include which one of the following nursing interventions for a patient receiving doxorubicin?
    A. Ensure patient treated for hyperlipidemia.
    B. Prescribe a beta blocker.
    C. Prescribe a calcium channel blocker.
    D. Document total cumulative dose of chemotherapy.

17. A 70-year-old patient with advanced stomach cancer presents to the clinic with an infection. The oncology nurse's assessment reveals poor performance status, presence of a venous access device, and lymphadenopathy. The nurse would recognize that the patient is at high risk for which one of the following conditions?
    A. A thrombotic event
    B. Lymphedema
    C. Malignant pericardial effusion
    D. Cardiovascular toxicity

18. A 61-year-old patient with cancer presents to the clinic. A physical examination reveals severe pain in the patient's right leg. The right leg is also cool with a decreased pulse. This exam describes which one of the following conditions?
    A. Venous occlusion
    B. Arterial embolus
    C. Pulmonary embolus
    D. Valvular abnormality

19. A patient presents with mild, spontaneously reversible pitting edema of the extremity that feels slightly heavy. The skin has a smooth texture. Pain and erythema are present. These characteristics of lymphedema describe which one of the following stages?
    A. 0
    B. 1
    C. 2
    D. 3

20. When the limb starts to look disfigured with over 30% difference in size at the greatest point of the limb and interferes with activities of daily living, which of the following grades of lymphedema would this be?
    A. 1
    B. 2
    C. 3
    D. 4

21. Which of the following descriptions of cardiovascular toxicities is associated with the drug class of anthracyclines?
    A. Associated with toxicity from injury of free radicals that result in myocardial cell loss, fibrosis, and loss of contractility resulting in left ventricular dysfunction, heart failure, myopericarditis
    B. Associated with acute myopericarditis, pericardial effusions, arrhythmias, HTN, thromboembolism, and heart failure
    C. Associated with bradycardia, thromboembolism, and HTN
    D. Associated with coronary artery spasm resulting in angina, arrhythmia, myocardial infarction, cardiac arrest, and sudden death; coronary artery thrombosis and apoptosis of myocardial cells

22. Which one of the following techniques should oncology nurses use for the prevention of thrombotic events in high risk patients?
    A. Elevate the patient's foot with their knee extended.
    B. Elevate the patient's knee with their foot extended.
    C. Employ constant pneumatic compression device.
    D. Ambulate frequently, and implement leg exercises if the patient is bedridden.

23. Nursing management for treatment and prevention of issues related to lymphedema includes which one of the following?
    A. Implementing sterile technique before the administration of antineoplastic agents in the limb
    B. Using an electronic or automated, rather than a manual, blood pressure cuff
    C. Using massage therapy on and vigorous weightlifting with the affected limb
    D. Recording regular measurement of extremities and elevating the affected limb

24. If a patient with breast cancer has not developed lymphedema in the first 3 years after surgery, which one of the following statements is true?
    A. She will probably not develop lymphedema in the arm.
    B. She must be instructed that the potential for lymphedema exists and she should report any issues.
    C. She probably had sentinel node mapping at the time of her initial surgery.
    D. She most likely benefited from breast conservation and radiation therapy.

25. Findings related to edema of cancer include which one of the following?
    A. The presence of S2 heart sound
    B. Decreased levels of serum albumin and protein
    C. Increased peripheral pulses
    D. Decreased blood pressure and heart rate

35 Cognitive Symptoms

1. S.L. is a 45-year-old breast cancer survivor who has undergone treatment with multimodal therapies. She is reporting having difficulty juggling multiple tasks at work. She is likely experiencing which one of the following?
   A. Cognitive impairment
   B. Decreased self-confidence
   C. Delirium
   D. Posttraumatic stress

2. B.H. is a 71-year-old male patient with metastatic prostate cancer. He reports bilateral decreased strength in his lower extremities. The oncology nurse caring for him would anticipate receiving an order for which one of the following procedures?
   A. Bone scan
   B. Electrolytes, including calcium
   C. Liver function tests
   D. Magnetic resonance imaging

3. J.L. is a 43-year-old colon cancer survivor who has completed treatment but is concerned about "chemo brain" affecting his work performance. Which one of the following interventions could be recommended for management of chemotherapy-induced impairment?
   A. Cognitive training
   B. Mindfulness stress reduction
   C. Donepezil
   D. Methylphenidate

4. An oncology nurse recognizes that one of the hallmark symptoms in a patient with delirium when compared with other cognitive impairment is the presence of:
   A. decreased motor function
   B. hypervigilance
   C. impaired concentration
   D. memory changes

5. Which one of the following is a risk factor for delirium in the cancer patient?
   A. Multimodality therapy
   B. Sensory impairments
   C. Metabolic abnormalities
   D. Genetic polymorphism

6. The oncology nurse recognizes that the most appropriate initial step in assessing a patient with delirium would be to do which one of the following?
   A. Review current medications.
   B. Obtain an MRI of the brain.
   C. Consider CBC with differential.
   D. Perform a lumbar puncture.

7. In the patient with delirium, low-dose antipsychotics may be useful to do which one of the following?
   A. Treat metabolic imbalances
   B. Minimize sensory deficits
   C. Promote uninterrupted sleep
   D. Manage severe agitation

8. Which one of the following is a nursing management technique for cancer- and cancer treatment–related cognitive impairment?
   A. Avoid excessive sensory stimulation and/or restraints.
   B. Incorporate environmental strategies such as having a visible clock or calendar available.
   C. Provide frequent reorientation and reassurance.
   D. Reinforce cognitive and exercise training plans.

9. Ms. B. is an 87-year-old patient with breast cancer who has been diagnosed with delirium. In planning her care, the oncology nurse would do which one of the following?
   A. Remove calendars from the patient's environment because they increase confusion.
   B. Allow family photos only if the patient can identify the people depicted in the photos.
   C. Encourage the patient to consistently use assistive devices such as eyeglasses and hearing aids.
   D. Maximize the patient's exposure to environmental sounds, such as alarms, to remind her that she is in a hospital room and not in her own home.

36 Endocrine Symptoms

1. The adrenal gland produces which one of the following hormones?
   A. Antidiuretic hormone
   B. Luteinizing hormone
   C. Thyroxine
   D. Cortisol

2. F.H. is a 70-year-old female patient with cancer who arrives at the infusion center with reports of weakness, depression, and feeling cold most of the time. The oncology nurse caring for her is aware that these symptoms most likely represent the presence of which one of the following?
   A. Hypothyroidism
   B. Hyperthyroidism
   C. Hypoparathyroidism
   D. Adrenal insufficiency

3. A patient with a history of coronary artery disease has a new diagnosis of treatment-related hyperthyroidism secondary to an immune checkpoint inhibitor. He is admitted to the oncology unit. The oncology nurse caring for him should anticipate receiving an order for which one of the following?
   A. Methylprednisolone
   B. Dexamethasone
   C. Levothyroxine
   D. Cinacalcet

4. The oncology nurse is caring for a patient who is to begin levothyroxine therapy after being treated with radioactive iodine for a malignant thyroid nodule. The nurse should expect that levels of thyroid stimulating hormone (TSH) and thyroxine (T4) will be monitored on which one of the following schedules?
   A. Every week for a month
   B. Every 4–6 weeks until stable
   C. On an annual basis
   D. Daily for 6 months

5. An oncology nurse provides teaching to a patient diagnosed with asymptomatic primary hyperparathyroidism. Education should include instructions on which one of the following?
   A. Initiating thiazide diuretics
   B. How to take phosphate binders
   C. A low calcium, high phosphate diet
   D. A diet rich in calcium-containing foods

6. An oncology nurse is caring for a 54-year-old male patient following surgical removal of the parathyroid glands. The nurse anticipates that medication management of resulting hypoparathyroidism will be based on the level of which serum electrolyte?
   A. Potassium
   B. Chloride
   C. Sodium
   D. Calcium

7. S.L. is a 60-year-old male patient who is undergoing radiation for brain metastases. He presents to the clinic with reports of feeling thirsty much of the time and having to urinate frequently during the day and night. The oncology nurse suspects that the patient is demonstrating signs of which one of the following?
   A. Hypothyroidism
   B. Diabetes insipidus
   C. Adrenal insufficiency
   D. Hyperparathyroidism

8. An oncology nurse is caring for a 62-year-old patient who is being treated for adrenal insufficiency. Patient education should include which one of the following?
   A. Wear an alert bracelet indicating steroid stress doses.
   B. Decrease steroid doses prior to surgical procedures.
   C. Increase steroid doses five-fold for a head cold.
   D. Adjust the steroid doses on a weekly basis.

9. Which one of the following scenarios most likely describes a patient who would be diagnosed with hyperthyroidism/thyrotoxicosis?
   A. The patient presents with symptoms of anxiety, agitation, weakness, and heat intolerance. A physical examination shows the patient has lost weight and is hyperactive.
   B. The patient complains of bone pain, and is fatigued, weak, and is presenting with signs of anorexia. A physical examination reveals hypertension and bradycardia.
   C. The patient presents with fatigue, anxiety, depression, and irritability. The patient's physical examination reveals chronic skeletal abnormalities.
   D. The patient presents with visual changes, headache, and myalgias. A physical examination shows the patient has experienced weight loss and is showing signs of hypotension.

10. The oncology nurse is caring for a patient receiving levothyroxine. The nurse knows that some drugs alter the metabolism of this medication. Which one of the following drug classes might decrease absorption of levothyroxine?
A. H2 receptor antagonists
B. Potassium supplements
C. PARP inhibitors
D. Insulin

37 Fatigue

1. Which one of the following factors is an underlying physiologic mechanism of fatigue?
   A. Low levels of pro-inflammatory cytokines, interleukins, tumor necrosis factor
   B. 5-Hydroxytryptophan autoregulation
   C. Hypothalamic-pituitary-adrenal axis dysfunction
   D. Circadian rhythms that reflect a desire to stay up late in the evening

2. J.L. is a 65-year-old women being treated for endometrial cancer who is undergoing radiation therapy. She presents in a wheelchair due to increased weakness and a complaint of severe fatigue. The oncology nurse understands that which one of the following factors can significantly increase the risk of this patient's fatigue?
   A. Older age
   B. Female sex
   C. Low performance status
   D. High doses of ondansetron

3. The oncology nurse meets with a patient being treated for pancreatic cancer. In assessing the patient's condition, which one of the following should the nurse use as the best measurement strategy for a patient experiencing fatigue?
   A. Provider assessment
   B. Patient-reported questionnaire
   C. An Eastern Cooperative Oncology Group (ECOG) score
   D. Nurse-reported distress screening tool

4. The oncology nurse understands that which one of the following laboratory analyses should be considered initially to evaluate potential underlying causes of fatigue?
   A. Thyroid function
   B. Serum protein electrophoresis (SPEP)
   C. Tumor markers
   D. Platelet count

5. A 59-year-old female patient with Stage II breast cancer reports significant fatigue, and laboratory results during treatment have shown pancytopenia. Medical management of her fatigue should include which one of the following?
   A. Blood transfusions for severe anemia
   B. Routine use of erythropoiesis-stimulating agents
   C. High-dose dexamethasone for severe fatigue
   D. Benzodiazepines for fatigue

6. Which one of the following interventions show the greatest benefit for the management of cancer-related fatigue?
   A. Blood transfusions
   B. Dexamethasone
   C. Patient education on priority setting
   D. Exercise

7. An oncology nurse is meeting with T.K., a young adult patient who has just completed treatment for acute myelogenous leukemia. He is feeling better, but his primary complaint is fatigue. Which one of the following educational information statements should the nurse include for management of this patient's fatigue?
   A. Because of the patient's age, high-intensity exercise is recommended.
   B. Depression can mimic fatigue, and referral to psychosocial resources can be important.
   C. Increasing environmental stimuli can help alleviate fatigue.
   D. Fatigue is likely to resolve within 2 months.

8. Fatigue is often seen with other symptoms related to cancer. Which one of the following have been found to cluster with fatigue?
   A. Anxiety
   B. Dietary changes
   C. Cognitive changes
   D. Sleep disturbances

38 Gastrointestinal Symptoms

1. J.R. is 50-year-old male patient with head and neck cancer who is undergoing radiation therapy after surgery. The oncology nurse is aware that during the initiation phase of the pathogenesis of mucositis which one of the following statements is true?
   A. Cytokines and modulators produced are associated with mucositis production.
   B. Signs and symptoms are already present within the oral mucosa.
   C. Angiogenesis is absent, leading to the development of small nodules.
   D. Interferons and tumor necrosis factor (TNF) cells proliferate, leading to the development of mucositis.

2. M.K. is a 46-year-old male patient with cancer who arrives in the clinic for evaluation prior to the start of chemotherapy. Upon reviewing the patient's medical record, the oncology nurse finds that the patient is most at risk for developing mucositis due to which one of the following?
   A. A body mass index (BMI) of 19.0
   B. Past history of alcohol use
   C. A serum creatinine level of 2.7
   D. Use of nonalcohol-based mouthwash

3. An oncology nurse on the hematopoietic stem cell transplant unit is caring for T.L., a 45-year-old female patient with acute myelocytic leukemia. T.L. will soon be undergoing chemotherapy, along with total body irradiation (TBI) for an autologous hematopoietic stem cell transplantation (HSCT). The physician has ordered palifermin. The nurse instructs T.L. that this drug has been ordered to do which one of the following?
   A. Decrease nausea and vomiting during treatment
   B. Elevate blood counts after transplant
   C. Alleviate painful cramping during treatment
   D. Reduce the incidence and severity of mucositis

4. A male patient is admitted to the hospital for his course of chemotherapy. The treatment includes cisplatin. The oncology nurse caring for him is aware that when acute chemotherapy-induced nausea and vomiting (CINV) occurs which one of the following is true?
   A. The vagus nerve is stimulated by 5-HT3 agonists, and CINV occurs within 24 hours.
   B. Receptors in the brain send an intense emetic message, and CINV occurs within 48 hours.
   C. The small intestine is stimulated, and CINV persists from a few to many days.
   D. Abdominal muscle contraction leads to CINV within hours to days.

5. An oncology nurse is caring for S.K., a 56-year-old female patient on an oncology unit who is due to receive her first dose of chemotherapy. Which one of the following findings in S.K.'s history puts her at risk for CINV?
   A. Use of NSAIDs
   B. History of smoking
   C. History of gastroesophageal reflux disease (GERD)
   D. No previous alcohol use

6. T.J. is a 42-year-old male patient who arrives in the clinic for his first infusion of chemotherapy. The patient inquires what treatment he will receive for nausea and vomiting. The oncology nurse is aware that the standard-of-care antiemetic the patient would receive includes which one of the following?
   A. 5-HT3 antagonist
   B. Dopamine
   C. Benzodiazepine
   D. Antisecretory drugs

7. An oncology nurse on a gynecology unit is caring for a patient with ovarian cancer who has malignant ascites. The nurse understands that this is due to which one of the following?
   A. Increased drainage from malignant tumor, leading to accumulation of fluid
   B. Lymphatic cells draining fluid into the peritoneum
   C. Seeding by malignant cells within the peritoneal cavity
   D. Fluid moving from the intravascular space into the interstitial space

8. K.M. is a 58-year-old female patient on an oncology unit who has malignant ascites. The patient has been scheduled for a paracentesis. The oncology nurse should provide K.M. with which one of the following instructions?
   A. "With your procedure, there is the potential for cardiac effects."
   B. "Your procedure comes with a high risk for bowel obstruction."
   C. "The procedure requires deep sedation."
   D. "With this procedure, you will feel decreased abdominal distension discomfort."

80

9. G.L., a 62-year-old male patient who has diabetes, arrives in the oncology clinic with complaints of constipation. G.L. states that he has not been drinking much, and a urine sample shows indication of uremia. The etiology of his constipation is most likely due to which one of the following?
   A. Metabolic causes
   B. Dietary causes
   C. Kidney stones
   D. A urinary fistula

10. An oncology nurse is caring for M.R., a 70-year-old male patient on an oncology unit who is suffering from fecal impaction. An enema has been ordered for him. M.R. asks why he can't have an oral agent. His nurse should provide which one of the following explanations?
    A. The liquid in the enema has a fiber-forming agent that softens the stool.
    B. An enema is the preferred method and is more predictable for the discharge of stool.
    C. Oral stool softeners will cause further constipation without removing the stool.
    D. Water taken along with the oral medications will cause cramping and bloating.

11. A patient arrives in the clinic with complaints of diarrhea after receiving a course of chemotherapy. After reviewing the patient's medical record, the oncology nurse believes the diarrhea may be caused by which one of the following?
    A. A bacterial infection such as *Escherichia coli*
    B. Malabsorption due to chemicals in etoposide
    C. Recent treatment with methotrexate
    D. Recent constipation

12. The oncology nurse caring for a patient on an oncology unit is discharging a patient home who has been admitted for diarrhea. The patient inquires as to what he should eat and drink at home. The nurse responds by explaining to the patient which one of the following?
    A. Drink plenty of apple juice for rehydration.
    B. Eat high-fiber foods such as cereals to bulk up stool.
    C. Eat plenty of fruits, such as peaches and nectarines.
    D. Eat a low-fat, high-potassium diet, with small frequent meals.

13. A patient with asthma is receiving radiation therapy with concurrent chemotherapy for head and neck cancer. The radiation field includes the salivary glands. The physical assessment reveals the patient's complaints of dry mouth, difficulty chewing and wearing their dentures, difficulty swallowing, and altered taste. Medical management of this patient could include an agent to increase saliva secretion. With this patient's history and physical assessment, which one of the following drugs would be avoided in the plan of care for xerostomia?
    A. Cevimeline (Evoxac)
    B. Pilocarpine (Salagen)
    C. Aquoral
    D. Xero-Lube

14. A patient with cancer arrives at the urgent care clinic with complaints of nausea, frequent vomiting, and inadequate fluid and food intake. A feeding tube had been placed 2 days prior. The physician determines the patient should be admitted to the hospital and begin total parenteral nutrition (TPN). Using the National Cancer Institute's Common Terminology Criteria for Adverse Events (NCI-CTCAE) for gastrointestinal symptoms, the patient's vomiting would be rated as which one of the following?
    A. Grade 1
    B. Grade 2
    C. Grade 3
    D. Grade 4

15. A patient with cancer presents to the oncology nurse with symptoms of dysphagia. Symptoms reported include cough, a sense of choking with swallowing, voice change, frequent throat clearing, and earache. Which one of the following types of dysphagia is the patient most likely experiencing?
    A. Oropharyngeal dysphagia (OD)
    B. Mechanical dysphagia
    C. Esophageal dysphagia (ED)
    D. Radiation dysphagia

16. Which one of the following would be considered a lifestyle factor that could cause xerostomia?
    A. Use of an antihistamine
    B. Caffeinated beverage consumption
    C. Secondary Sjögren syndrome
    D. Use of anticholinergic agents

17. The patient with head and neck cancer is scheduled for a sialometry, and the oncology nurse is to instruct the patient before the procedure. Which one of the following would be an accurate explanation about this test?
    A. The evaluation of the patient is done at normal bedtime.
    B. The test is performed after a full meal.
    C. This test is a measure of regurgitation.
    D. The procedure is done with the patient upright.

18. Which one of the following is a preventative nursing management measure for oral mucositis?
    A. Have the patient apply a topical protective or coating agent to the affected area.
    B. Remind the patient to avoid spicy food or hot drinks.
    C. Have the patient use a solution of normal saline, salt, and baking soda.
    D. Remind the patient to have a pretreatment dental examination and provide instructions for an oral hygiene regimen.

19. S.L. is a 50-year-old male patient who complains of dry mouth after treatment. Within several weeks, he develops thick, ropy saliva. He also has trouble chewing his food. His oncology nurse suspects he has developed which one of the following?
    A. Dysphagia
    B. Xerostomia
    C. Mucositis
    D. Trismus

20. Which one of the following interventions is appropriate for patients with xerostomia?
    A. Encourage the patient to decrease intake of liquids.
    B. Encourage the patient to suck ice cubes or sugarless popsicles.
    C. Encourage the patient to eat dry and spicy foods.
    D. Encourage the patient to rinse with commercial mouthwashes frequently to increase moisture.

21. Ascites is most likely linked to which one of the following cancer types?
    A. Cervical cancer
    B. Ovarian cancer
    C. Malignant melanoma
    D. Head and neck cancer

22. T.H. is a 53-year-old female patient with cancer who is complaining of abdominal bloating and cramping with no bowel movement for the past 3 days. She has reported that she normally has a bowel movement daily. Bowel sounds are present. T.H. completed her last dose of chemotherapy (doxorubicin and cyclophosphamide) approximately 10 days ago. Which one of the following actions should be recommended to alleviate her constipation?
    A. An immediate glycerin suppository
    B. Use a Fleet enema to stimulate peristalsis
    C. A stimulate laxative until a bowel movement occurs, then evaluation, as needed, for daily stool softeners or lubricant laxatives
    D. Begin bulk-forming laxatives for constipation, and a mild narcotic for her pain

23. A patient is receiving radiation therapy to her abdomen and asks for dietary instructions to decrease her diarrhea. Which one of the following instructions should the oncology nurse include in the patient's dietary teaching?
    A. Eat a high-fiber diet that is high in protein.
    B. Begin a low-residue diet that is high in protein.
    C. Add fruit juices to the diet to increase fluid intake.
    D. Include stone fruits in the diet, such as apricots and cherries.

24. M.L., a 69-year-old male patient with pancreatic cancer, returns to the oncology clinic with recurrent ascites. The oncology nurse anticipates that the ascites will be drained using which one of the following methods?
    A. Paracentesis
    B. Nontunneled catheter
    C. Peritoneovenous shunts
    D. Intraperitoneal surgery

25. H.M., a 58-year-old female patient with a history of breast cancer, comes to the oncology clinic for a follow-up visit and reports recent onset constipation. Aside from assessing environmental factors that might contribute to H.M.'s constipation, the nurse anticipates monitoring H.M.'s laboratory reports for which one of the following electrolytes that might explain the onset of constipation?
    A. Bicarbonate
    B. Sodium
    C. Calcium
    D. Chloride

39 Genitourinary Symptoms

1. The nurse on the oncology unit notes that a patient in her care has a history of urinary stress incontinence. The nurse is aware that this type of incontinence is caused by which one of the following?
   A. Intensified psychological concerns
   B. Intrinsic urinary sphincter dysfunction
   C. Impaired reflexes controlling bladder emptying
   D. Physical activities that increase abdominal pressure

2. P.R. is a male patient who is receiving radiation therapy to the bladder. He reports frequent involuntary loss of urine. The oncology nurse caring for him is aware that this condition is most likely due to which one of the following?
   A. Treatment-induced bladder inflammation
   B. Reduced size of the bladder tumor
   C. Advanced age of the patient
   D. Presence of kidney stones

3. F.R. is a 60-year-old female patient with cancer. The patient has been experiencing recent onset urinary incontinence. The oncology nurse caring for her explains that the best diagnostic testing for this condition would include which one of the following?
   A. Determination of amount of residual urine after voiding
   B. Review of the patient's bladder diary of the past 2 weeks
   C. Colonoscopy if not performed in the previous 5 years
   D. Gathering information about usual voiding habits

4. J.T. is a 55-year-old female patient with cancer who is experiencing urinary incontinence. She asks the nurse in the outpatient oncology clinic about management of uncontrolled loss of urine. Appropriate nursing education might include which one of the following?
   A. Minimizing trips outside the house as much as possible
   B. Scheduled voiding at the same time daily
   C. Increase in fluid intake during the day
   D. Learning bladder self-catheterization

5. An oncology nurse is caring for a 57-year-old male patient who is scheduled for surgery to remove his bladder and create a continent urinary diversion with a stoma in the skin. In teaching the patient about what to expect after the procedure, the nurse should explain which one of the following?
   A. An external urine collection device will be required.
   B. It is possible that some urine will dribble continuously.
   C. Catheterization of urine will need to be done every 4 to 6 hours.
   D. The pouch will need to emptied before each chemotherapy treatment.

6. The oncology nurse is caring for a patient who has a newly created ileal conduit after removal of a malignant bladder. Patient teaching should include instructions to do which one of the following?
   A. Avoid eating cruciferous vegetables.
   B. Use alcohol to clean the peristomal skin.
   C. Catheterize the stoma several times per day.
   D. Empty the collection pouch when it is half full.

7. S.H. is a 44-year-old female patient with breast cancer who has widespread bone metastasis. She is now receiving radiation therapy to the bone lesions. Since radiation therapy has started, she reports a recent change in output of large amounts of urine. The nurse caring for her suspects that this change may be caused by which one of the following?
   A. Decreased renal blood flow
   B. Pelvic lymph nodes obstructed by tumor
   C. Hypercalcemia of malignancy
   D. Nephrotoxicity associated with radiation therapy

8. L.R. is a 58-year-old female patient being treated for cancer. The patient comes to the infusion center and reports that she has been experiencing the involuntary loss of urine with an abrupt and strong desire to void her bladder. The nurse is aware that this type of incontinence is most likely which one of the following?
   A. Stress incontinence
   B. Reflex incontinence
   C. Functional incontinence
   D. Urge incontinence

9. Which one of the following is an example of a pharmacologic intervention for a patient with cancer diagnosed with renal dysfunction?
   A. Anticholinergics
   B. Amifostine and sodium thiosulfate for cisplatin nephrotoxicity
   C. Tricyclic antidepressants
   D. Potassium channel openers

10. Which one of the following is an example of medical management of urinary incontinence?
    A. Saline hydration with appropriate diuretic
    B. Oral or intravenous (IV) sodium bicarbonate to maintain alkaline urine
    C. Replacement of electrolytes
    D. Electrostimulation

11. Which one of the following types of patients would be suitable candidates for neobladder surgery?
    A. A patient with a history of benign prostatic hypertrophy (BPH)
    B. A patient with inflammatory bowel disease
    C. A patient who has received radiation therapy
    D. A patient with urethral cancer

40 Hematologic and Immune Symptoms

1. Granulocyte cell counts include which one of the following types of cells?
   A. Red blood cells
   B. Platelets
   C. Monocytes
   D. Lymphocytes

2. When reviewing a patient's lab work, the oncology nurse knows that the patient's risk of infection is increased when which one of the following is true?
   A. Absolute neutrophil count rises above 2500/mm^3
   B. Absolute neutrophil count falls below 1500/mm^3
   C. White blood cell count decreases to 4.3×10^9/L
   D. Absolute basophil count increases above normal limits

3. A patient who received chemotherapy last week calls the infusion unit to report a temperature of 100.9°F. The oncology nurse is concerned that the patient is at risk for which one of the following?
   A. Febrile neutropenia
   B. Thrombocytopenia
   C. Hypercalcemia
   D. Hemolytic anemia

4. A patient at high risk for chemotherapy-induced neutropenia has an order for prophylactic injections of a granulocyte colony-stimulating factor (G-CSF) agent. The oncology nurse anticipates monitoring the patient for G-CSF-related adverse events, which include which one of the following?
   A. Eye inflammation
   B. Acne-like rash
   C. Lung fibrosis
   D. Bone pain

5. The oncology nurse meets with a patient with metastatic prostate cancer who is receiving radiation therapy to the pelvis, ischium, and left femur. The nurse is aware that the patient is at increased risk for which one of the following?
   A. Bone marrow suppression
   B. Peripheral neuropathy
   C. Wet desquamation
   D. Urinary retention

6. The oncology nurse is caring for an immunosuppressed patient who is being treated with concomitant chemotherapy and radiation therapy. Nursing interventions to minimize infection risk in this patient might include which one of the following?
   A. Avoid frequent bathing as it is drying to the skin.
   B. Change water in pitchers every 4 hours.
   C. Prohibit visits from family members.
   D. Restrict delivery of fresh flowers.

7. Patient education to minimize infection risk should include instructions to call the healthcare provider to report which one of the following?
   A. Dry mouth
   B. Sore throat
   C. Temperature of 99.8°F
   D. Urinary hesitancy

8. Results of a complete blood count in a patient being treated for esophageal cancer reveal anemia. The oncology nurse anticipates that further work-up might include tests to determine which one of the following?
   A. Iron overload
   B. Platelet function
   C. Gastrointestinal blood loss
   D. Estrogen level

9. A patient arrives at the chemotherapy infusion unit complaining of fatigue and dyspnea. A rapid heart rate is noted. The oncology nurse is aware that the patient is most likely exhibiting signs of which one of the following?
   A. Anemia
   B. Neutropenia
   C. Lymphocytopenia
   D. Thrombocytopenia

10. When receiving a transfusion of packed red blood cells, the optimal goal for a patient with symptomatic anemia would be to maintain a:
    A. Hemoglobin level that is greater than 10 g/dL
    B. Red blood cell count that is greater than 6.2 mcL
    C. Heart rate lower than 90 beats/min
    D. Glomerular filtration rate of 90 mL/min/1.73 m^2

11. A patient being treated for prostate cancer develops disseminated intravascular coagulation. The oncology nurse anticipates an order to monitor which one of the following laboratory results?
    A. The patient's red blood cell count
    B. The patient's hemoglobin level
    C. The patient's platelet count
    D. The patient's ferritin level

12. The oncology nurse provides teaching about bleeding precautions to a patient who is newly diagnosed with myelodysplastic syndrome. Education should include which one of the following?
    A. Prevention of falls
    B. Use of enemas for constipation
    C. Shave with a straight-edge razor
    D. Apply warm packs to cuts in the skin

13. A patient who is being treated with cytotoxic chemotherapy develops a urinary tract infection. Which one of the following findings, if recorded by the oncology nurse, indicates high risk for clinical deterioration?
    A. Blood pressure of 86/50 mmHg and respiratory rate of 26
    B. Blood pressure of 155/90 mmHg and respiratory rate of 20
    C. Temperature of 100.1°F and depression
    D. Heart rate of 80 beats/min and sleepiness

14. The oncology nurse is caring for a patient who underwent biopsy for suspected kidney cancer. During rounds, the oncology nurse notices that the patient has become pale, has a weak, irregular pulse, and has moist skin. The patient is exhibiting signs of which one of the following?
    A. Anemia
    B. Neutropenia
    C. Hemorrhage
    D. Thrombocytopenia

15. A patient on the oncology unit has developed fever and chills following completion of chemotherapy administration. Appropriate nursing interventions to promote comfort for this patient include which one of the following?
    A. Provide heating blankets
    B. Give tepid sponge baths
    C. Limit warm fluids by mouth
    D. Immerse in ice bath

16. Which one of the following factors is a disease and treatment-related risk factor associated with chemotherapy-induced myeloid toxicity?
    A. Decreased immune function
    B. Recently completed surgery
    C. Drug–drug interactions
    D. Dose intensity

17. The oncology nurse is caring for a patient with lung cancer receiving chemotherapy. The nurse anticipates that colony-stimulating growth factor (CSF) administration is initiated when which one of the following occurs?
    A. A chemotherapy dose has been reduced.
    B. A patient has experienced a previous anemia with chemotherapy administration.
    C. A patient is undergoing radiation therapy for cancer treatment.
    D. A patient is at risk of grade 3/4 chemotherapy-induced neutropenia or is febrile.

18. The oncology nurse is caring for a patient receiving immunotherapy and chemotherapy for pancreatic cancer. The nurse knows which one of the following places the patient with cancer at risk for opportunistic infection?
    A. Myalgia
    B. Lymphopenia
    C. Thrombocytopenia
    D. Anemia

19. The oncology nurse is orienting a new graduate to the unit and asks the orientee "how an ANC is calculated." Which of the following best represents the correct calculation?
    A. % neutrophils (segmented neutrophils + bands) divided by total WBC
    B. Total WBC divided by % neutrophils (segmented neutrophils + bands)
    C. % neutrophils (segmented neutrophils + bands) multiplied by WBC
    D. Actual number of neutrophils (segmented neutrophils + bands) multiplied by WBC

20. The oncology nurse is providing education to a patient and family about leukemia and its treatment. The nurse discusses the origin of various blood components. The nurse teaches the family that platelets arise from which type of stem cells:
    A. Lymphoid stem cells
    B. Megakaryocyte cells
    C. Myeloid stem cells
    D. Epithelial stem cells

21. As the oncology nurse provides education about types of blood cells to the family, the nurse explains that granulocytes collectively include which one of the following?
    A. Basophils, eosinophils, and neutrophils
    B. Basophils, lymphocytes, and neutrophils
    C. Eosinophils, lymphocytes, and monocytes
    D. Basophils, lymphocytes, and monocytes

22. The oncology nurse is providing patient education about thrombocytopenia. The nurse explains that patients with cancer are at a severe risk for bleeding when which one of the following occurs?
    A. Neutrophils are at 50%
    B. Lymphocytes are at 30%
    C. Platelets are less than 20,000 mm^3
    D. Erythrocytes are at 20%

23. The oncology nurse is caring for a patient who recently completed chemotherapy. The nurse knows which one of the following statements is true about nadir?
    A. Nadir is the highest point the WBCs reach after cancer treatment and occurs 7 to 14 days after treatment.
    B. Nadir is WBC lysis related to chemotherapy administration.
    C. Nadir is the lowest point blood cells reach after a cancer treatment and occurs 7 to 14 days after treatment.
    D. Nadir regularly occurs after biotherapy administration.

24. The oncology nurse is reviewing the laboratory report of a patient newly diagnosed with leukemia. The nurse knows that thrombocytopenia describes a decrease in the circulating:
    A. Platelets below 100,000/mm^3
    B. WBCs below 1500/mm^3
    C. Neutrophils below 1000/mm^3
    D. RBCs below 1000/mm^3

25. The oncology nurse is caring for a patient who recently had CAR T-cell therapy and is experiencing cytokine release syndrome. The patient has a fever of 38.3°C, and is receiving a vasoactive agent and high flow nasal cannula oxygen. The grade of cytokine release syndrome is:
    A. Grade 1
    B. Grade 2
    C. Grade 3
    D. Grade 4

26. The oncology nurse is caring for a 58-year-old woman with breast cancer who had a course of chemotherapy 7 days earlier. Her ANC is 625/mm^3. The nurse knows that this is which one of the following grades of neutropenia?
    A. Grade 1
    B. Grade 2
    C. Grade 3
    D. Grade 4

27. The oncology nurse is caring for a patient with febrile neutropenia following high-dose chemotherapy. Which of the following factors are associated with poor prognosis febrile neutropenia?
    A. Hypertension, hypoalbunemia, low procalcitonin level
    B. Hypotension, hypoalbunemia, low serum bicarbonate level
    C. Hypertension, hyperalbuminemia, high procalcitonin level
    D. Hypotension, hyperalbuminemia, high serum bicarbonate level

28. The oncology nurse is caring for a 28-year-old man who had chemotherapy for leukemia cancer 10 days earlier. His Hgb is 8.3 g/dL The nurse knows this is what grade of anemia?
    A. Grade 1
    B. Grade 2
    C. Grade 3
    D. Grade 4

41 Integumentary Symptoms

1. Which one of the following layers of skin serves as an insulator to temperature changes?
   A. The dermis
   B. The subcutaneous tissue
   C. The epidermis
   D. The inner connective tissue

2. R.K. is a 50-year-old patient who presents to the clinic with disease-related pruritus on the upper extremities. The oncology nurse caring for R.K. knows that his condition will require pharmacologic management. Which one of the following drugs utilized to treat R.K.'s pruritus is most likely to cause drowsiness?
   A. Corticosteroids
   B. Antihistamines
   C. Capsaicin
   D. Calamine lotion

3. F.M. is a 60-year-old man who has been diagnosed with colon cancer. He is receiving irinotecan and reports to the oncology nurse that he is experiencing frequent diarrhea on Day 2 after receiving treatment. When providing education for F.M., which one of the following measures related to perineal hygiene should be avoided?
   A. Use alcohol wipes to cleanse the affected area
   B. Frequent hand washing
   C. Mild soap, rinsing thoroughly, pat dry
   D. Apply a skin barrier after each stool

4. Graft-versus-host disease is most often related to which one of the following?
   A. A skin graft
   B. A bone marrow transplant
   C. Melanoma
   D. Malnutrition

5. H.W. is a 57-year-old male patient who has just completed radiation therapy. He was diagnosed with acute radiation dermatitis, and the oncology nurse caring for him recognizes that symptoms for his condition include which one of the following?
   A. Circular red scaly rash
   B. Rash involving extremities, including palms and soles
   C. Thinning of skin, scarring and contractures, and telangiectasias
   D. Erythema, pain, dermal swelling, itching, and necrosis

6. A skin reaction commonly seen in a patient who is receiving an epidermal growth factor receptor (EGFR) inhibitor is which one of the following?
   A. Onycholysis
   B. Acneiform rash without comedones
   C. Erythema of hands and feet
   D. Permanent hyperpigmentation of gums

7. The nurse is teaching a patient who is receiving chemotherapy about the importance of reducing ultraviolet light exposure during chemotherapy because many agents are photosensitizing. Photosensitivity associated with chemotherapy agents often manifests as which one of the following?
   A. Several days after sunburn, causing the sunburn to reappear
   B. Transverse lines in nails with bands corresponding to when drug was given
   C. A moderate-to-severe sunburn in sun-exposed areas
   D. Paronychia

8. Which one of the following is a description of symptoms related to chronic radiation dermatitis?
   A. Thinning of skin, scarring and contractures, telangiectasias, and long-term skin sensitivity to irritants and environmental agents
   B. Occurs in previously irradiated skin within 1 to 2 weeks after chemotherapy with erythema, edema, superficial ulcerations, and superficial skin sloughing
   C. Immediate dermatitis that occurs in irradiated areas with erythema, pain, dermal swelling, itching, and necrosis
   D. Allergic response where drug touches skin manifested by erythema, local swelling, desquamation, and blistering, and possible necrosis

9. Which one of the following is a description of symptoms related to erythema multiforme (antigen–antibody complexes) skin reaction?
   A. Itching, redness, and swelling within 1 hour after infusion has begun
   B. Outbreak of rash with typical target lesions involving extremities, including palms of the hands and soles of the feet, can progress to a generalized rash
   C. Occurs in previously irradiated skin within 1 to 2 weeks after chemotherapy and symptoms include erythema, edema, and superficial ulcerations
   D. Involves generalized vascular inflammation with end organ damage

10. Which one of the following skin reactions is known to be caused by treatment with platinum derivatives (e.g., cisplatin, carboplatin)?
   A. Contact allergy
   B. Acute radiation dermatitis
   C. Immunoglobulin E (IgE) mediated
   D. Vasculitis

11. After receiving radiation therapy treatment, J.T., a 47-year-old male patient with cancer, experiences a skin reaction involving blistering, local swelling, and erythema outside of the radiation field. The nurse caring for him suspects that a contact allergy could be to blame for his symptoms. Which one of the following could have been responsible?
   A. Reaction to his premedication
   B. Reaction to something he had eaten earlier in the day
   C. Reaction to the radiation therapy
   D. Latex found in gloves or rubberized protective clothing

12. Which one of the following is a description of symptoms related to radiation recall dermatitis?
   A. Reaction occurs in previously irradiated skin within 1 to 2 weeks after chemotherapy, and is associated with erythema, edema, superficial ulcerations, and superficial skin sloughing
   B. Rash with typical target lesions involving extremities, including palms and soles; can progress to generalized
   C. Thinning of skin, scarring and contractures, telangiectasias, and long-term skin sensitivity to irritants and environmental agents
   D. Flulike symptoms, which may progress to life threatening

1. When assessing a patient with sarcopenia, the oncology nurse would expect to see which one of the following?
   A. Loss of skeletal muscle mass
   B. Bone marrow suppression
   C. Joint contractures
   D. Muscle spasticity

2. W.R. is a 61-year-old female patient with a history of lymphoma. She arrives at the oncology clinic and reports difficulty standing after using the toilet. The oncology nurse is aware that which one of the following factors is most likely to increase risk for musculoskeletal alterations?
   A. Medical marijuana use
   B. Enteral tube feedings
   C. Vegetarian diet
   D. Increased bed rest

3. The oncology nurse is caring for a 58-year-old male patient on the oncology unit who has a Karnofsky performance status (KPS) of 50. The nurse caring for him anticipates which one of the following to be true?
   A. The patient will be able to participate in self-care independently.
   B. The patient will need considerable assistance with daily activities.
   C. The patient will show minor signs and symptoms of disease.
   D. The patient will be disabled and require complete care.

4. During a clinic visit the oncology nurse assesses a patient's musculoskeletal status by observing which of the following traits of the patient?
   A. Cleanliness
   B. Gait
   C. Body language
   D. Habitus

5. G.K. is a 47-year-old female patient who completed a course of cisplatin 2 weeks ago. She arrives at the oncology clinic complaining of muscle weakness in her legs. The oncology nurse anticipates that blood tests will be ordered to assess for which one of the following?
   A. Metabolic alkalosis
   B. Hypochloremia
   C. Hypokalemia
   D. Hyperphosphatemia

6. The oncology nurse is caring for a patient on the oncology unit who has impaired mobility. Appropriate nursing measures for this patient include which one of the following?
   A. Changing the patient's position every shift
   B. Instituting soft lighting during the day
   C. Placing a soft restraint vest while in bed to prevent falls
   D. Encouraging active range of motion exercises every 4 hours

7. J.B. is a 49-year-old male patient with cancer on the oncology unit who has an Eastern Cooperative Oncology Group (ECOG) Performance Status score of 3. The oncology nurse caring for him anticipates which one of the following to be true?
   A. The patient is disabled and unable to carry out any activities related to self-care.
   B. The patient is fully active and able to carry on all normal activities as he would have before his diagnosis.
   C. The patient is restricted in strenuous activity such as heavy lifting or vigorous aerobic workouts.
   D. The patient is capable of limited self-care and is restricted to a bed or chair during half of his waking hours.

8. H.R. is a 69-year-old female patient with cancer on the oncology unit who has an ECOG Performance Status score of 1. The nurse caring for her anticipates which one of the following to be true?
   A. The patient is capable of performing light activities such as housework.
   B. The patient is restricted to a bed or chair during half of her waking hours and capable of limited self-care.
   C. The patient is fully disabled with no capability for self-care.
   D. The patient has died.

9. An oncology nurse is caring for a 62-year-old male patient with cancer who reports to the clinic with complaints of a fast or irregular heartbeat and some pain in his legs. The oncology nurse caring for him knows she will be getting orders for a laboratory work-up. Which one of the following electrolyte abnormalities might the nurse expect to find in the results?
   A. An abnormality in his chloride level
   B. An abnormality in his calcium level
   C. An abnormality in his potassium level
   D. An abnormality in his phosphate level

43 Neurological Symptoms

1. The oncology nurse is orienting new staff nurses on the oncology unit and explains that factors that may put patients at increased risk for neuropathies include which one of the following?
   A. A diagnosis of cancer under the age of 60 years
   B. A diagnosis of anxiety and depression
   C. A history of vitamin B complex deficiency
   D. A history of a lumpectomy for breast cancer

2. During the staff nurse orientation, the oncology nurse further explains that seizures, encephalopathy, and cerebellar dysfunction in a patient with cancer are symptoms most likely to be attributed to which one of the following?
   A. Neuropathies of the central nervous system (CNS)
   B. Anxiety and depression
   C. A past medical history of childhood epilepsy
   D. Damage to the peripheral nervous system (PNS)

3. Medical management for cancer-related neuropathies include which one of the following?
   A. Fentanyl patch
   B. Solumedrol
   C. Pregabalin
   D. Alprazolam

4. Nursing management for cancer-related neuropathies includes instructing the patient on which one of the following?
   A. Use massage and lotions on hands and feet.
   B. Refrain from exercise.
   C. Avoid using assistive devices so muscle strength can be restored.
   D. Stimulate the skin of affected area often.

5. F.N. is a 51-year-old female patient with cancer, who has been receiving chemotherapy, and is complaining of decreased sensation in her hands. The oncology nurse understands that an appropriate intervention would include which one of the following?
   A. Engage in a hand-strengthening program.
   B. Wear gloves to protect from cold.
   C. Apply hand sanitizer at least hourly.
   D. Use a three point cane for ambulation.

6. S.W. is a 52-year-old female patient with cancer who is receiving a chemotherapy agent known to increase the risk of neuropathy. To assess proprioception, the oncology nurse would do which one of the following?
   A. Check vibration using a tuning fork.
   B. Assess for discrimination between sharp and dull sensations.
   C. Check for clonus in the extremities.
   D. Evaluate balance using a Romberg test.

7. When assessing for neuropathy, the patient will be evaluated for cerebellar function and proprioception, sensory function, and deep tendon reflexes. The oncology nurse knows that which one of the following would be the procedure for assessing sensory function related to neuropathy?
   A. Observe for accurate movement of extremities.
   B. Assess for discrimination between sharp and dull sensations.
   C. Have patient stand with feet together, arms at side with eyes closed. A slight sway is normal.
   D. Evaluate rapid alternating movement of hands.

8. G.R. is a 64-year-old male patient with cancer who has been experiencing a decline in mobility and ability to care for himself. The oncology nurse caring for G.R. knows that to improve his mobility and self-care ability, which one of the following interventions would be appropriate?
   A. Develop an exercise and muscle-strengthening program.
   B. Offer the patient access to acupressure and acupuncture services.
   C. Encourage the patient to implement relaxation techniques.
   D. Refer the patient for biofeedback teaching sessions.

9. R.H. is a 61-year-old female with cancer. She presents to the clinic with increased pain and signs of depression and anxiety. R.H. is not interested in any medications to alleviate pain or other symptoms and is seeking alternative solutions. The oncology nurse caring for R.H. understands that which one of the following would be an appropriate nonpharmacologic intervention for this patient?
   A. Teach the patient about the side effects of treatments.
   B. Provide assistive services for the patient in performing daily activities, as needed.
   C. Empower the patient to communicate with her physician and caregivers regarding the severity of her symptoms.
   D. Encourage the patient to enroll in a yoga class.

44 Nutritional Issues

1. M.J., a 75-year-old male patient, is currently undergoing treatment for tonsillar cancer and has a gastrostomy tube for tube feedings. Which one of the following symptoms might develop from the patient's enteral therapy?
   A. Confusion
   B. Constipation
   C. Bradycardia
   D. Bradypnea

2. E.N. is a 51-year-old female patient with Stage IV cancer. She is currently undergoing chemotherapy and reports no appetite, significant muscle weakness, and fatigue. The oncology nurse caring for her determines that she has lost 5% of her baseline weight over the past 6 months. Based on this assessment, E. N.'s signs and symptoms are most consistent with which one of the following?
   A. Malnutrition
   B. Anorexia
   C. Cachexia
   D. Depression

3. To minimize risk of the occurrence and severity of taste alterations during chemotherapy treatment, the oncology nurse should do which one of the following?
   A. Encourage the use of salt and pepper to enhance taste.
   B. Encourage the patient to drink one glass of alcoholic beverage prior to dinner.
   C. Instruct the patient to perform oral hygiene in the morning and at bedtime.
   D. Instruct the patient to suck on smooth, flat, tart candies or lozenges.

4. A risk factor for weight gain in patients with cancer is which one of the following?
   A. A multi-agent chemotherapy regimen
   B. Immunotherapy
   C. Adjuvant chemotherapy for lung cancer
   D. Bisphosphonate therapy

5. In patients with weight loss, an intervention to promote comfort while eating is which one of the following?
   A. Administer pain medications if needed, 3 hours before eating.
   B. Encourage patients to perform oral hygiene only after meals.
   C. Encourage patients to consume cold foods.
   D. Administer nystatin suspension 5 minutes prior to eating.

6. Dysgeusia is defined as which one of the following?
   A. The loss of taste
   B. An unpleasant taste sensation
   C. A decrease in acuity in taste sensation
   D. An increase in acuity in taste sensation

7. D.R. is a 51-year-old female patient with cancer who comes to the clinic with a 5-pound weight loss since her last treatment 4 weeks ago. D.R. states that she has lost her sense of taste. Which one of the following recommendations should the oncology nurse make that may help with this symptom?
   A. Have a glass of wine before dinner.
   B. Participate in cooking of meals.
   C. Encourage food intake without gravy or sauces.
   D. Avoid chewing gum.

8. The oncology nurse knows that anorexia can be caused by which one of the following electrolyte imbalances?
   A. Hypercalcemia
   B. Hyperkalemia
   C. Hypermagnesemia
   D. Hypernatremia

9. Enteral nutrition has been ordered for a patient with cancer. The oncology nurse anticipates that enteral nutrition therapy will be given by which one of these approaches?
   A. Nephrostomy tube
   B. Tracheostomy tube
   C. Urostomy tube
   D. Naso-gastric tube

10. A risk factor for weight loss in a patient with cancer would include which one of the following?
    A. Chemotherapy regimens containing steroids
    B. Use of biologic medications
    C. Diagnosis of non-Hodgkin lymphoma
    D. Presence of pleural effusions

93

11. A female patient being treated for ovarian cancer reports taste changes. The oncology nurse understands that taste alterations may occur due to which one of the following?
   A. Thin saliva following radiation therapy
   B. Excess zinc levels
   C. Tamoxifen therapy
   D. Candidiasis

12. Potential complications can arise from central line insertion for parenteral nutrition. Which one of the following is a nursing intervention for management of a pneumothorax?
   A. Ensure that chest radiography is done after insertion of subclavian catheter to verify proper placement.
   B. Regulate infusion on a volumetric pump for accuracy.
   C. Monitor the catheter for migration from the superior vena cava to another vein, while making a notation of patient complaint of pain in the neck and shoulder, as well as swelling in the surrounding area.
   D. Check each bottle or bag before and during infusion for color and clarity of solution.

13. The oncology nurse is caring for a patient who developed an air embolus as a complication from central line insertion for the use of parenteral therapy. Which one of the following is a nursing intervention for management of an air emboli?
   A. Observe for bright red blood pulsating from catheter.
   B. Clamp IV tubing immediately and place patient on left side in the Trendelenburg position.
   C. Infuse 10% dextrose in water solution peripherally or through other lumen of catheter at the same rate as with total parenteral nutrition (TPN) to prevent hypoglycemia.
   D. If sudden cessation of TPN occurs, infuse 10% dextrose in water solution peripherally at same rate as TPN.

14. Which one of the following nursing interventions would be most effective in the prevention of infection when administering parenteral nutrition?
   A. Check each bottle or bag before and during infusion for color and clarity of solution.
   B. Change all IV tubing per institutional or agency procedure, using aseptic technique, and avoid interrupting TPN for other infusions or blood collection.
   C. Change dressing, using clean technique, and following institutional procedure, while observing the site for redness, tenderness, swelling, and exudates.
   D. Check urine for sugar, ketones, and acetone every 6 hours.

15. The oncology nurse who is caring for a patient receiving enteral nutrition is aware that potential complications can arise from enteral tube placement and feedings. Which one of the following is a nursing intervention for prevention of abdominal distention, and for symptoms such as vomiting and diarrhea?
   A. Giving continuous rather than bolus feeding
   B. Flushing nasogastric tube with hot water or pulsating motions
   C. Giving formula at room temperature
   D. Verifying proper placement via chest radiography and check placement each time using tube

16. Which one of the following is an example of a physical assessment strategy a patient with cancer might undergo as part of an overall nutritional assessment?
   A. Measure of daily caloric intake
   B. Blood pressure and heart rate
   C. Measures of serum prealbumin, total protein, and serum transferrin to assess protein stores
   D. Current weight in comparison with ideal body weight

17. Which one of the following is an example of laboratory data that could be collected for a patient with cancer as part of an overall nutritional assessment?
   A. Measure of allergic reactions to proteins in certain foods
   B. Skin turgor
   C. Muscle mass
   D. Nitrogen balance

18. A patient visits the clinic and expresses concerns about metabolic changes caused by cancer. To best answer the question, the oncology nurse explains the impact of malignancy on the metabolism of which one of the following?
   A. Vitamins and minerals
   B. Pharmacologic agents including chemotherapy
   C. Protein and calories
   D. Mono- and polyunsaturated fats

45 Pain

1. A patient with metastatic cancer is currently receiving MS Contin twice a day and morphine immediate release every 4 hours as needed for bone pain, with good control of symptoms. The oncology nurse understands that the patient's pain is best categorized as which one of the following?
   A. Neuropathic pain with insidious breakthrough pain episodes
   B. Chronic cancer-related pain
   C. Acute cancer pain
   D. A combination of visceral, somatic, and neuropathic cancer-related pain

2. Which one of the following types of pain is poorly localized and results from nociceptor activation related to distention, compression, or infiltration of the thoracic or abdominal tissue?
   A. Somatic pain
   B. Sympathetically maintained pain
   C. Visceral pain
   D. Peripherally mediated neuropathic pain

3. Which part of the pain pathway involves the brain's attempt to modify the pain experience through the release of endogenous opioids, norepinephrine, and serotonin?
   A. Transduction
   B. Transmission
   C. Perception
   D. Modulation

4. An oncology nurse is seeing a patient who has been diagnosed with Stage III esophageal cancer. The patient has recently completed combined neoadjuvant therapy with chemotherapy and radiation. The oncology nurse would anticipate that the patient may experience the most pain symptoms from which one of the following?
   A. Postsurgical incision
   B. Lymphedema
   C. Mucositis
   D. Sinusitis

5. An oncology nurse is seeing a patient who has been diagnosed with Stage III colorectal cancer. The patient has recently completed combined neoadjuvant therapy with chemotherapy and radiation, complicated by a shingles outbreak. The oncology nurse would anticipate that the patient may experience the most pain symptoms from which one of the following?
   A. Post-herpetic neuralgia
   B. Chemotherapy-induced peripheral neuropathy (CIPN)
   C. Chemotherapy-induced lymphedema
   D. Complex regional pain syndrome (CRPS)

6. D.V. is a 62-year-old male patient with lung cancer and multiple liver metastasis. He reports intermittent pain rated 6 out of 10 in the area of the tumor. He has a history of renal failure and diabetes. Using the World Health Organization's analgesic ladder, the oncology nurse anticipates that which one of the following may be considered the best initial treatment for this patient's pain?
   A. Acetaminophen 1000 mg four times per day
   B. Morphine 15 mg every 3 hours as needed
   C. Fentanyl patch 25 mcg/hour
   D. Oxycodone 5 mg/acetaminophen 325 mg combination (1 to 2 tablets) every 4 hours as needed

7. L.M. is a 59-year-old male patient with end-stage pancreatic cancer. He is admitted to the hospital with intractable pain and is being treated with opioids. His wife has concerns of addiction and worries about withdrawal. The oncology nurse's best response to L.M.'s wife is which one of the following?
   A. "While addiction is a risk, the drugs are useful, and we consider them to be the primary method for pain control."
   B. "There is no need for you to worry about addiction because of your husband's advanced cancer."
   C. "The patient is experiencing tolerance, which means he has increased needs of medication due to his disease."
   D. "The patient will not go through withdrawal because he is not addicted to the medicine."

8. When the oncology nurse is conducting a comprehensive pain assessment, which one of the following best reflects an existential concern?
   A. Fear of addiction with the use of opioids due to recent media attention
   B. Depression related to the fatigue caused by the pain
   C. Lack of mobility caused by the pain
   D. Perception that pain is a punishment

9. When the oncology nurse is conducting a comprehensive pain assessment, which one of the following best reflects a psychological concern?
   A. Financial hardship as a result of paying for pain medication
   B. Influence of religion and prayer on coping with pain
   C. Use of traditional medicine in healing and pain relief
   D. The patient's history of illnesses such as anxiety and depression

10. When the oncology nurse is conducting a comprehensive pain assessment, which one of the following best reflects a social concern?
    A. The patient's experience with coping with pain in the past
    B. The patient's willingness to try nontraditional medicines
    C. How a family caregiver responds to a patient's pain
    D. The role of a spiritual community in a patient's ability to cope with pain

11. When the oncology nurse is conducting a comprehensive pain assessment, which one of the following best reflects a psychological concern?
    A. The role of pain in the everyday life of the patient
    B. The definition of how the patient differentiates pain and suffering
    C. The amount of support a patient receives, either at home or through their community
    D. The level of cognition of the patient, including any signs of confusion or delirium

12. In the pain assessment known as PQRST, which one of the following represents the "P" in the acronym?
    A. Pain
    B. Position
    C. Proximity
    D. Provocation/palliation

46 Respiratory Symptoms

1. An oncology nurse is administering a monoclonal antibody to a patient who develops a hypersensitivity reaction that includes bronchospasm. The nurse understands that the mechanism of action in bronchospasm is due to:
   A. abnormal fluid accumulation in the lung
   B. compression of tracheobronchial tree
   C. alveolar hemorrhage
   D. bronchitis

2. An oncology nurse is caring for a 59-year-old female patient with lung metastases who is complaining of shortness of breath. The nurse is preparing to educate the patient on measures that she can take to increase the effectiveness of her breathing. The nurse should include which one of the following in the patient's teaching?
   A. Keeping the house temperature warm
   B. Limiting activity to conserve energy
   C. Decreasing the amount of fluid intake
   D. Instructing the patient to use a walker

3. An oncology nurse is caring for a patient who develops immunotherapy-induced pulmonary toxicity. The oncology nurse is aware that this is caused by which one of the following?
   A. Release of hormones into the vascular system
   B. The signaling of an antigen response
   C. Equal amounts of dose and volume of drug administered
   D. An inflammatory process causing lung injury

4. A 52-year-old male patient with cancer is suspected of having pneumonitis. When assessing the patient, the oncology nurse caring for him is aware that the cardinal symptom of this condition includes which one of the following?
   A. An elevated heart rate
   B. Malaise
   C. Dyspnea
   D. Crepitus

5. T.S. is a 63-year-old female patient on an oncology unit who has developed chemotherapy-induced pulmonary toxicity. The nurse knows that the management of this condition includes which one of the following?
   A. The patient will be put on strict bedrest until resolution of symptoms.
   B. The patient might continue the chemotherapy at a reduced dose.
   C. Monitoring of electrocardiograms (ECGs) and echocardiogram (ECHO) will be required.
   D. Serial arterial blood gas (ABG) will be required.

6. A nurse in an outpatient clinic is assessing a 54-year-old male patient who is being seen for signs of dyspnea and poor oxygenation. Which of the following findings could indicate chronic hypoxemia?
   A. A carotid artery pulse on palpation
   B. Normal size lower extremities
   C. Clubbing of the fingers
   D. A ventilation rate 20/min

7. An oncology nurse on the thoracic oncology floor is caring for a patient with a benign pleural effusion. The patient questions the nurse as to why this may have occurred. The nurse responds that it is most likely due to the tumor causing which one of the following?
   A. Increased negative pressure in the pleural space
   B. Development of spontaneous hemopericardium
   C. Direct extension of primary tumor to the pleura
   D. Formation of pustules within the pleural space due to infection

8. On performing a physical examination on a patient with a pleural effusion, the oncology nurse is most likely to find which one of the following?
   A. Rhonchi and rales
   B. Tracheal shift to the left
   C. Egophony
   D. Resonance upon percussion

9. An oncology nurse is caring for a patient with a pleural effusion. The nurse is aware that the most efficacious, evidence-based treatment for this patient is which one of the following?
   A. Insertion of a peritoneal catheter to drain fluid
   B. Wedge resection to remove a portion of pleural effusion
   C. Immunotherapy to decrease the tumor
   D. Therapeutic aspiration with an intrapleural chemical agent

97

10. The oncology nurse knows that which one of the following chemotherapy or targeted therapy agents is associated with pulmonary and radiologic abnormalities and hemoptysis?
    A. Bortezomib
    B. Alpha-interferon
    C. Erlotinib
    D. Bevacizumab

11. Which one of the following chemotherapy or targeted therapy agents is associated with pulmonary and radiologic abnormalities most associated with acute pneumonitis?
    A. Sorafenib
    B. Busulfan
    C. Etoposide
    D. Doxorubicin

12. Which one of the following would a nurse anticipate for a patient with cancer who has just been given a diagnosis of empyema?
    A. Treatment will involve radiation therapy to the lung field(s).
    B. Systemic antibiotics will be used to treat the infection.
    C. Subcutaneous epinephrine 1:100 solution will be used.
    D. The patient will be placed in a semi-Fowler position and oxygen will be given at 30% face mask.

13. J.D. is a 52-year-old male patient with cancer, who has been receiving a combination of radiation therapy and bleomycin (Blenoxane) chemotherapy. The oncology nurse caring for him knows that he will be at risk for which one of the following types of pulmonary toxicity?
    A. Hemothorax
    B. Pulmonary empyema
    C. Pneumonitis
    D. Pleural effusion

47 Sleep Disturbances

1. The oncology nurse is doing a comprehensive patient assessment of symptoms, including sleep. Which one of the following best describes sleep-wake disturbances?
   A. An active biobehavioral process that causes night-time anxiety
   B. Actual or perceived interruption in sleep with resulting daytime impairment
   C. Transient inability to initiate or maintain sleep
   D. Circadian rhythm disorders

2. G.K. is a 58-year-old male patient who complains to his nurse that he is feeling very tired secondary to issues with falling asleep. However, once asleep, he sleeps soundly. Which one of the following classes of medications would be best to assist this patient in falling asleep?
   A. Antihistamines
   B. Antipsychotics
   C. Alpha-adrenergic receptor blockers
   D. Antidepressants

3. The oncology nurse is reviewing the patient's sleep habits and discussing ways to improve sleep. Which one of the following interventions will help to promote sleep hygiene?
   A. Make sure the patient has their last cup of coffee in the early evening.
   B. Have the patient go to bed even if they are not sleepy.
   C. Encourage the patient to watch TV prior to falling asleep to help calm down.
   D. Educate the patient to keep their room cool and dark.

4. F.J. is a 71-year-old male patient who tells the oncology nurse caring for him that he has not been sleeping well. He reports that he wakes up every day at 6 am and drinks a cup of coffee, he exercises each day, and then enjoys an afternoon nap. Which one of the following is the biggest risk factor for a sleep-wake disturbance in this patient?
   A. He wakes up at 6 am each morning.
   B. He drinks his coffee shortly after waking.
   C. He exercises each day.
   D. He enjoys an afternoon nap.

5. The oncology nurse is educating a patient about the physiology of sleep, including the sleep-wake cycle. Which one of the following best describes the sleep-wake cycle?
   A. Non-rapid eye movement phase of sleep until waking in the morning
   B. Rapid eye movement, non-rapid eye movement, and the awakening phase
   C. Rapid eye movement phase and non-rapid-eye movement phase, with repeat cycles approximately every 90 minutes
   D. Rapid eye movement phase and non-rapid eye movement phase, with repeat cycles lasting approximately every 180 minutes

6. The oncology nurse is orienting a new nurse and discussing the timing and process of assessment of sleep. Which one of the following represents the best time to assess a patient's sleep cycle?
   A. At the initial patient assessment
   B. After their first cycle of chemotherapy
   C. At the beginning and end of all treatment
   D. At regular intervals and with any changes in clinical status

7. A patient with cancer reveals that he is awake often at night and relates this condition to job concerns, feelings of anxiousness, and fear of what the future holds. He also reports having pain in his hip. Of his concerns, which one of the following describes a physical stressor?
   A. Job concerns
   B. Feelings of anxiousness
   C. Fear of the future
   D. Pain in his hip

8. A patient reports a sleep disturbance. The oncology nurse knows that which one of the following diagnostic tests is utilized to assess sleep?
   A. Electroencephalogram (EEG)
   B. Polysomnography
   C. NCCN Distress Thermometer
   D. Assessment of sleep patterns, including usual bedtime, bedtime routine, and usual time to sleep

48 Metabolic Emergencies

1. The oncology nurse is caring for M.L., a 74-year-old male patient with advanced prostate cancer, who has been admitted to the hospital for work-up of suspected disseminated intravascular coagulation (DIC). The oncology nurse explains to M.L. and his family that DIC is which one of the following?
   A. Systemic disorder of coagulation resulting in the consumption of platelets and coagulation factors
   B. Systemic disorder of hematopoiesis due to the lack of available hemoglobin
   C. Systemic disorder of coagulation related to the overproduction of platelets and coagulation factors
   D. Local disorder of coagulation leading to the consumption of platelets and coagulation factors within a single organ

2. The oncology nurse caring for M.L. should assess him for which set of signs and symptoms often associated with DIC?
   A. Bradycardia and dizziness
   B. Itching and flushing
   C. Diaphoresis and thirst
   D. Pallor and petechiae

3. Knowledge of the sequence of events that triggers the development of DIC helps the oncology nurse understand that successful treatment of M.L.'s DIC is aimed at which one of the following?
   A. Identifying and treating the underlying cause
   B. Administering platelet transfusions as the only source of treatment
   C. Identifying the precipitating genetic pathogenic variants
   D. Administering prophylactic anticoagulants to prevent clots

4. Thrombotic thrombocytopenic purpura (TTP) is a blood disorder characterized by widespread clotting in small blood vessels of the body, resulting in which one of these laboratory values?
   A. Low platelet count and microangiopathic hemolytic anemia
   B. High platelet count and microangiopathic hemolytic anemia
   C. Low platelet count and macroangiopathic hemolytic anemia
   D. High platelet count and macroangiopathic hemolytic anemia

5. In the medical management of a patient experiencing TTP, the oncology nurse would expect to receive an order for which of these interventions?
   A. Administer plasma exchange with fresh-frozen plasma.
   B. Withhold blood products.
   C. Initiate macrolide antibiotics for prophylaxis.
   D. Restrict fluids.

6. Syndrome of inappropriate antidiuretic hormone (SIADH) can be caused by a variety of malignant and nonmalignant conditions. The oncology nurse knows that the condition with the highest risk of SIADH is which one of the following?
   A. Small cell lung cancer
   B. Antitumor antibiotics
   C. Congestive heart failure
   D. Breast cancer

7. The oncology nurse caring for a patient with SIADH should monitor for all of these signs and symptoms of SIADH except:
   A. decreased serum sodium
   B. normal serum potassium
   C. increased urine output
   D. decreased mentation

8. The oncology nurse is monitoring the status of a patient being treated for breast cancer with a paclitaxel infusion. The oncology nurse knows that initial symptoms of a hypersensitivity reaction may include which one of the following?
   A. Peripheral edema
   B. Arrhythmia
   C. Stridor
   D. Flushing or rash

9. Which one of these complications occurs because the patient's immune system was previously sensitized to a particular allergen and produces severe symptoms when the patient is re-exposed to the same allergen?
   A. TTP
   B. Anaphylaxis
   C. DIC
   D. Sepsis

10. A patient is demonstrating signs of anaphylaxis minutes after the second cycle of paclitaxel is initiated. The chemotherapy nurse immediately stops the infusion and gets ready to administer which one of the following agents used for first line pharmacologic management of anaphylaxis?
    A. Epinephrine
    B. Inhaled alpha agonist
    C. IV antibiotics
    D. H2 receptor agonists

11. An oncology nurse in the oncology clinic examines M.A., a 77-year-old female patient who has chemotherapy-induced neutropenia. The oncology nurse is aware that M.A. is at increased risk for sepsis and notes that which one of the following findings may be an early sign of sepsis in this patient?
    A. Hypertension
    B. Thrombocytopenia
    C. Bradycardia
    D. Fever

12. The oncology nurse sends M.A. to have blood drawn and monitors the laboratory results. The nurse focuses on which one of the following laboratory values that may indicate that M.A. is experiencing sepsis?
    A. White blood cell (WBC) count with a left shift
    B. Increased platelets
    C. Normal prothrombin time (PT)/international normalized ratio (INR)
    D. Hypoglycemia

13. Patients at increased risk of tumor lysis syndrome (TLS) are those with malignancies associated with a high burden of rapidly proliferating cells, such as the leukemias. TLS is an oncologic emergency that occurs when cytotoxic treatment causes the rapid destruction of large numbers of tumor cells. The oncology nurse knows that diagnosis of TLS is typically based on the results of which one of the following tests?
    A. Complete blood count
    B. PT/INR
    C. Electrolytes
    D. Glucose

14. The oncology nurse knows that prevention of TLS in patients at high risk of the complication following initiation of antineoplastic therapies includes administration of which one of the following?
    A. IV hydration 24 to 48 hours prior to treatment initiation
    B. Potassium supplementation 24 hours prior to first infusion
    C. Antibiotics if WBC less than 4000
    D. Allopurinol beginning after initial chemotherapy cycle

15. The oncology nurse is reviewing information about oncologic emergencies. The nurse is aware that which one of the following is the most commonly seen oncologic emergency?
    A. DIC
    B. SIADH
    C. Hypercalcemia
    D. TLS

16. The oncology nurse learns that the tumors most often associated with hypercalcemia include which one of the following?
    A. Prostate, breast, and lung
    B. Multiple myeloma, colon, and brain
    C. Adrenal, kidney, and leukemia
    D. Stomach, thyroid, and pheochromocytoma

17. A patient with a history of cancer reports recent onset of symptoms to the oncology nurse. The nurse anticipates that the patient will be worked up for hypercalcemia because which one of the following set of symptoms indicates hypercalcemia?
    A. Increased appetite, fatigue, and frequent urination
    B. Nausea/vomiting, restlessness, and polydipsia
    C. Hyperactivity, nocturia, and anorexia
    D. Lethargy, frequent urination, and hypertension

101

18. The oncology nurse understands that which one of the following medications would be appropriate to use in the treatment of hypercalcemia of malignancy in a patient with renal insufficiency?
    A. Bevacizumab
    B. Infliximab
    C. Denosumab
    D. Pembrolizumab

19. The oncology nurse is caring for a 66-year-old female patient who has just presented with sepsis. The nurse anticipates receiving all of these orders to treat the patient, *except* which one of the following?
    A. Remove infected IV lines.
    B. Administer empiric antibiotic therapy within the first hour of presentation.
    C. Provide vasopressor therapy as ordered to maintain a mean arterial pressure (MAP) of 65 mm Hg.
    D. Withhold fluids until fever abates.

20. The oncology nurse is monitoring a patient receiving a monoclonal antibody infusion. The nurse should be alert to signs and symptoms of anaphylaxis that include which one of the following?
    A. Fatigue
    B. Urticaria
    C. Pain around an intravenous insertion site
    D. Itching around an intravenous insertion site

49 Structural Emergencies

1. An oncology nurse is caring for a patient with breast cancer and brain metastases who has recently been admitted to the ICU for management of increased intracranial pressure. The cause of the increased intracranial pressure in this patient is most likely due to which one of the following?
   A. Vitamin deficiency related to increased metabolic needs of tumor cells
   B. Increased brain tissue volume related to expanding tumor
   C. Head injury resulting in increased cerebral blood flow
   D. Increased hormone production by the brain cancer cells

2. A nurse is assessing H.C., a 68-year-old-female patient with lung cancer who has received cranial radiation therapy as prophylaxis for lung cancer metastases to the brain. The patient reports that she is having headaches, which are worse on awakening, and also nausea, vomiting, and weakness. The nurse caring for her suspects that the patient is exhibiting signs of which one of the following?
   A. Spinal cord compression
   B. Bowel obstruction
   C. Pleural effusion
   D. Increased intracranial pressure

3. H.C. is admitted to the oncology unit for work-up of possible increased intracranial pressure (ICP). The oncology nurse explains to the patient and caregivers that the most reliable method to diagnose ICP is which one of the following?
   A. Positron emission tomography (PET) with CT scan
   B. Bone marrow biopsy
   C. Labs to evaluate glucose and protein
   D. Epidural ICP monitoring

4. H.C. is diagnosed with elevated intracranial pressure and is transferred to the ICU for immediate treatment to rapidly decrease the ICP. The oncology nurse caring for the patient should anticipate an order for which one of the following?
   A. Radiation therapy to the head
   B. Administration of systemic biotherapy agents
   C. Intubation and hyperventilation
   D. Injection of steroids into the cervical spine

5. Which of these nursing measures should be included in the management of H.C.'s increased intracranial pressure?
   A. Monitoring for decreased cardiac output, including decreased urine output
   B. Assisting patient to lay on their stomach to relieve pressure on the head
   C. Keeping the patient's head of bed low to prevent headaches
   D. Frequent suctioning to prevent aspiration of saliva

6. An oncology nurse is assigned to care for F.P., a 75-year-old male patient who has just arrived on the unit for work-up of suspected spinal cord compression. The oncology nurse understands that which one of the following is the diagnostic procedure of choice for assessing the extent of F.P.'s spinal cord involvement?
   A. Computerized tomography of the spine
   B. Positron emission tomography of the whole body
   C. Diagnostic radiology films of the thoracic spine
   D. Magnetic resonance imaging of the entire spine

7. An oncology nurse is instructing the patient regarding management of his spinal cord compression. Education might include which one of the following?
   A. Add moderate exercise to improve motor function
   B. Report sensory and sexual changes
   C. Expect loss of appetite
   D. Take diuretic drugs as ordered

8. A nurse on the oncology unit is caring for a male patient diagnosed with lung cancer in the right lung. When assessing the patient, the nurse notes distended jugular veins and facial swelling. The nurse is aware that, based on his cancer history, this patient is at increased risk for which one of the following?
   A. Plaque deposition in the carotid vein
   B. Pulmonary embolism
   C. Superior vena cava obstruction
   D. Myocardial infarction

9. A patient with non–small lung cancer arrives at the oncology clinic for a follow-up visit. The patient reports that he has dyspnea, feelings of fullness in his head, dysphagia, and nasal stuffiness upon awakening, but improves throughout the day. The oncology nurse suspects the patient is experiencing signs of which one of the following?
A. Sinusitis
B. Pneumonia
C. Churg-Strauss syndrome
D. Superior vena cava syndrome

10. An oncology nurse makes a postdischarge phone call to a patient who recently had a colon resection. The patient reports nausea and vomiting of orange-brown material with a fecal odor. The nurse recognizes that the symptoms the patient is describing may be due to an obstruction of which one of the following?
A. Proximal small intestine
B. Distal small intestine
C. Small bowel
D. Gastric outlet

11. While caring for a patient with mesothelioma who has been admitted for cardiac tamponade, the nurse is aware that the fluid accumulation in the pericardial sac may be a result of which one of the following?
A. Comorbid coronary artery disease
B. Confirmed accurate insertion of a new triple lumen central line
C. Increased capillary permeability secondary to chemotherapy
D. Leakage of fluid into the chest from a pneumothorax

12. A patient with a history of colon cancer has been admitted to the oncology unit for treatment of a bowel obstruction. The oncology nurse anticipates an order to prepare the patient for which one of the following interventions?
A. Removal of the colon with anastomosis
B. Administration of hyperosmolar agents to stimulate the bowel
C. Insertion of a biliary stent to bypass the obstruction
D. Injection of methylnaltrexone to relieve constipation

13. The nurse in the oncology clinic is assessing a patient who has developed pneumonitis while undergoing therapy for advanced kidney cancer. The oncology nurse should recognize that the pneumonitis has most likely been caused by which of the following types of therapy?
A. Systemic hyperthermia
B. Platinum-based chemotherapy
C. Dendritic cell treatment
D. Checkpoint inhibitor immunotherapy

14. An oncology nurse is caring for a patient who recently had a colon resection. The patient is having new onset severe pain in the abdomen and states that the pain was initially manageable, but has gotten much worse. The oncology nurse reports to the physician that she believes the patient has developed which one of the following?
A. Constipation
B. Postsurgical ileus
C. Bowel perforation
D. Addiction to pain medication

15. A 66-year-old male with small cell lung cancer (SCLC) is emergently admitted to the ICU with significant upper torso and facial swelling and severe shortness of breath. The oncology nurse should recognize that the most effective initial treatment for this patient is which one of the following?
A. Radiation therapy
B. Chemotherapy
C. Percutaneous stent placement
D. Surgical resection

16. A 57-year-old female patient presents for her check-up 8 weeks after completing chest radiation and multimodality combination therapy for lymphoma. She reports that she is unable to take in a full breath, has chest pain, and a low-grade fever. Her oncology nurse recognizes these symptoms may be due to which one of the following?
A. Superior vena cava syndrome
B. Myocardial effusion
C. Cardiac tamponade
D. Pneumonitis

17. A 78-year-old patient with a history of mesothelioma is admitted to the hospital with complaints of dyspnea upon exertion, tachycardia, and chest pain that intensifies when lying down. The patient has comorbid heart disease and has been treated for mesothelioma with doxorubicin and more than 4000 cGy of radiation to the chest. Based on the data provided, the oncology nurse is aware that the patient is most likely experiencing which one of the following?
A. Superior vena cava syndrome
B. Cardiac tamponade
C. Costochondritis
D. Cardiomyopathy

18. A nurse on the oncology unit is caring for a male patient diagnosed with lung cancer in the right lung. When assessing the patient, the nurse notes distended jugular veins and facial swelling. The oncology nurse is aware that, based on his cancer history, this patient is at increased risk for which one of the following?
    A. Plaque deposition in the carotid vein
    B. Pulmonary embolism
    C. Superior vena cava obstruction
    D. Myocardial infarction

19. Early detection of spinal cord compression (SCC) is essential for prompt intervention and preventing loss of function. The most common presenting symptom of SCC in patients with cancer is which one of the following?
    A. Motor weakness and motor loss
    B. Sensory loss
    C. Back pain
    D. Bowel or bladder incontinence

20. Which one of the following are examples of early signs of SVCS?
    A. Muffled heart rate of 100 beats/min, abdominal distention, and fever
    B. Hypertension, bradycardia, widening of pulse pressure, and abnormal respirations
    C. Jugular vein distention and edema of the face, periorbital area, back, neck, upper thorax, breasts, and upper extremities
    D. Hypotension and Cheyne-Stoke respirations

50 | Body Image Considerations

1. An oncology nurse is explaining to a new nurse orientee about the ways a patient adjusts to a diagnosis of cancer and changes in body image. The nurse explains that altered body image is defined as which one of the following?
   A. As a change in a patient's perception of how friends react to the change
   B. As a change in a patient's perception of how they feel about themselves
   C. As a change in a patient's perception of how other individuals view them
   D. As a change in a patient's perception of how their children will respond or have responded to them

2. Which one of the following nursing interventions is the most supportive in facilitating a patient's acceptance of a change in body image?
   A. Providing a time frame for the patient to grieve and then quickly moving on
   B. Facilitating conversations between the patient and long-lost family members
   C. Encouraging the patient to take an antidepressant
   D. Educating the patient and family members preoperatively regarding body image changes

3. When describing chemotherapy-induced alopecia, which one of the following statements should the oncology nurse use as an explanation regarding the patient's condition?
   A. "Hair loss is total including eyebrows."
   B. "Hair loss typically starts 2 days after chemotherapy."
   C. "Hair regrowth is 2 to 4 weeks after treatment."
   D. "Hair regrowth may take more than 3 years."

4. When assessing for psychosocial adjustment the oncology nurse understands that cancer survivors who are at increased risk for altered body image are in which one of the following groups?
   A. Females
   B. Older
   C. Younger
   D. Recently diagnosed

5. The oncology nurse is caring for a newly diagnosed patient on a Phase III trial of a new chemotherapy agent. At the start of therapy the patient was not experiencing alopecia. One month after receiving the investigational agent the patient is experiencing moderate patchy hair loss. The oncology nurse documents that the WHO classification of this amount of hair loss is:
   A. Grade 1
   B. Grade 2
   C. Grade 3
   D. Grade 4

6. The nurse is caring for a 59-year-old female patient recently diagnosed with a brain tumor who is being treated with radiation therapy to the brain and high-dose corticosteroids. In addition to explaining the risk of alopecia in the radiation field, the nurse provides education and anticipatory guidance that the patient is at risk for which one of the following?
   A. Moon face
   B. Weight loss
   C. Neuropathic pain
   D. Cachexia

7. The oncology nurse is completing a comprehensive psychosocial assessment of a patient being treated for cancer that includes coping with body image changes. The nurse knows that which one of the following relates to altered body image?
   A. Is not impacted by the reactions of others
   B. Can result in role changes
   C. Is associated with increased self-confidence
   D. Is a short-term treatment-related concern

8. The oncology nurse is caring for a woman newly diagnosed with breast cancer. The patient understands that the planned chemotherapy will cause her hair to fall out and she is very distressed by this. She has read about scalp cooling. She asks the oncology nurse to tell her more about scalp cooling. The nurse should inform the patient that which one of the following is accurate?
   A. The scalp is cooled with a pneumatic machine.
   B. It is rarely effective in preventing alopecia.
   C. It is a very comfortable procedure.
   D. There is no evidence it increases risk of scalp metastases.

51 Caregiver Burden

1. The oncology nurse is presenting at a seminar on the basics of caregiving and caregiving burden. Which one of the following statements is true regarding caregiver burden?
   A. Caregiver burden is a continuum of health care activities for someone unable to independently care for themselves.
   B. Caregiver burden is provision of services and support and health management for the well-being of another person.
   C. Caregiver burden is a time-sensitive, life-changing commitment and experience.
   D. Caregiver burden is influenced by multiple patient and caregiver comorbidities and symptoms.

2. The oncology nurse is reviewing the legislative acts that address issues associated with caregiving. Which one of the following is true regarding the Caregiving, Advise, Record, and Enable (CARE) Act?
   A. CARE applies to the ambulatory setting.
   B. CARE supports family caregivers who work.
   C. CARE requires hospitals to record family caregiver name.
   D. CARE oversees a tax credit for qualified expenses to help a loved one.

3. The oncology nurse is caring for a 69-year-old man recently diagnosed with pancreatic cancer who requires assistance with medications, activities of daily living, and getting to appointments. The nurse inquires about who could serve as a caregiver. Which one of the following demographic features is associated with a higher level of caregiver burden distress?
   A. Male gender
   B. Holding a graduate degree
   C. Lives in a separate residence
   D. Younger in age

4. A 70-year-old male patient with leukemia arrives in the clinic with his wife, who is his primary caregiver. The caregiver states she is not feeling well. When assessing health risk factors of the caregiver, the oncology nurse understands that which one of the following would be a physiological factor?
   A. Cardiometabolic risk
   B. Weight gain
   C. Excessive sleep
   D. Social isolation

5. An oncology nurse asks a caregiver, "What medical problems does your care recipient have?" The nurse is assessing the caregiver's perception of the patient's:
   A. cognitive status
   B. health status
   C. caregiving needs
   D. caregiver values

6. The oncology nurse is providing a community education program on caregiving. The nurse begins by providing background on caregiving. The nurse explains that caregiving has become a major public health concern due to which one of the following?
   A. An aging and growing population
   B. Lack of formal caregiver training
   C. An economic burden
   D. Impact on long-standing relationships

7. The oncology nurse describes the role of the caregiver during a nursing continuing education program. The role of the caregiver is normally associated with which one of the following?
   A. Compensated work
   B. Time-limited care
   C. Assisting with daily care
   D. Financial responsibility to cover medical care

8. The oncology nurse knows there are many stressors associated with caregiving. Which one of the following creates an environmental stressor that can cause depression in both the caregiver and recipient?
   A. Involvement of secondary caregiver
   B. Caregiver resilience
   C. Plan of care not documented
   D. Dependency

9. The oncology nurse meets with a patient and her caregiver to assess the caregiving process, which includes therapeutic communication. Therapeutic communication between the caregivers and healthcare team should occur:
   A. at onset of caregiving experience
   B. continuously
   C. at advance care planning appointment
   D. through the patient

10. The oncology nurse is assessing caregiver burden in a caregiver who has been providing daily care for over 4 months to her husband with metastatic prostate cancer. Which one of the following caregiver clinical tools measures caregiver burden through such factors as employment, finances, physical, social, and time aspects, and includes 13 screening items?
    A. Caregiver Reaction Assessment
    B. Caregiver Strain Index
    C. Caregiver Burden Scale
    D. Zarit Burden Interview

11. The oncology nurse is assessing the caregiver profile. Which of the following information would be included?
    A. Length of time in the caregiver role
    B. Functional status of the care recipient
    C. Educational level of the caregiver
    D. Presence of additional paid caregivers

12. The oncology nurse is caring for a patient with metastatic lung cancer. He is 78 years old and has difficulty performing ADLs. His adult children are willing to serve as caregivers and will rotate the responsibilities but all of them have full time jobs which they are afraid of losing. The oncology nurse explains that which one of the following legislative acts provides job protections for caregivers?
    A. Recognize, Assist, Include, Support, and Engage Family Caregivers Act of 2017
    B. CARE Act
    C. The Credit for Caring Act
    D. The Family and Medical Leave Act

52 Social Determinants of Health and Financial Toxicity

1. The oncology nurse is completing an assessment of a newly diagnosed 67-year-old woman diagnosed with HER2-positive breast cancer. This assessment includes social determinants of health. The nurse knows that which of the following are considered domains of social determinants of health?
   A. Economic stability and education quality and access
   B. Federally qualified health centers
   C. Section 8 housing availability
   D. County public health vaccine program

2. The oncology nurse is attending a seminar on social determinants of health. The presenter discusses structural racism. The presenter describes and gives examples of structural racism as which one of the following?
   A. Assessment of race on admission
   B. Access to clinical trials regardless of race
   C. Restricted access to health care services
   D. Access to both pediatric and adult oncology care

3. The oncology nurse is presenting a program on social determinants of health. The nurse explains that socio-economic factors, environmental conditions, and health behaviors determine about what percentage of an individual's health?
   A. 20%
   B. 40%
   C. 60%
   D. 80%

4. The oncology nurse is orienting a new staff nurse on the oncology unit. The oncology nurse explains that financial toxicity is defined as the harmful personal financial burden faced by patients receiving cancer treatment. The nurse continues that it is a significant problem affecting what percentage of oncology patients?
   A. 23%
   B. 37%
   C. 48%
   D. 59%

5. During an assessment of a new patient, the oncology nurse inquires about where the patient lives. This is important information because the built neighborhood domain influences health through which one of the following?
   A. Transportation system
   B. School quality
   C. Health literacy
   D. Social isolation

6. The hospital administration is developing a patient-centered chemotherapy education program designed to be available to patients through telehealth. The oncology nurse questions the type of program access because the nurse knows that many individuals do not have access to broadband internet. The percentage of patients affected by lack of internet access is estimated to be which one of the following?
   A. 10%
   B. 20%
   C. 30%
   D. 40%

7. The oncology nursing education council is developing patient education fact sheets on chemotherapy and needs to consider health literacy. Which one of the following factors is correct regarding health literacy?
   A. Health literacy is dependent on high literacy levels.
   B. Health literacy is only a concern when developing written materials.
   C. Health literacy does not affect patient outcomes.
   D. Health literacy impacts patient decision-making.

8. As the oncology nurses prepare to develop the chemotherapy education sheets, they need to consider the wording. Ideally, patient education sheets should be written at which one of the following education levels?
   A. 2nd grade
   B. 4th grade
   C. 6th grade
   D. 8th grade

9. The oncology nurse is using a screening tool to make an assessment of a patient's social determinants of health. Which one of the following is a 15-item tool?
   A. PREPARE (Protocol for Responding to and Assessing Patient's Assets, Risks, and Experiences)
   B. YCLS (Your Current Life Situation)
   C. OCHIN
   D. WellRx Questionnaire

10. The oncology nurse understands that cultural humility is important in oncology care. Self-assessment of cultural humility is assessed using which one of the following instruments?
    A. AHC HRSN (Accountable Health Communities Health-Related Social Needs)
    B. Oncology Nurse Navigator (ONN) Patient Assessment
    C. EveryONE Project
    D. Harvard IAT

53 Cultural and Spiritual Care

1. An oncology nurse is attending a conference on cultural and spiritual care. The speaker states that culture is defined as which one of the following?
   A. Customary beliefs, social forms, material traits, and characteristic features of everyday existence shared by people of a racial, religious, or social group in a place or time
   B. A condition of being composed of differing elements, especially the inclusion of people of different races or cultures in a group
   C. A social construct based on expressed phenotype, in which people are categorized based on external, selective, and arbitrary physical features
   D. A heritage of historical, contextual, and geographic experiences of a specific community or population

2. An oncology nurse is attending an annual symposium on diversity and inclusion which includes a discussion of race and ethnicity, with a goal of increasing awareness to provide more sensitive and appropriate care. Race and ethnicity differ from each other in which one of the following ways?
   A. Race is identified in social definitions, whereas ethnicity is identified by biological foundations.
   B. Race is based in cultural heritage, whereas ethnicity is based in social construct.
   C. Race is based on external, selective, arbitrary physical features and genetic make-up, whereas ethnicity is based on historical, cultural, contextual, and geographic experience of community.
   D. Race is based in the identity of wide racial diversity within shared characteristics based on geographic, historic, contextual, and cultural group of origin, whereas ethnicity is based on the phenotype of a culture that expresses observable characteristics such as skin tone, hair texture, and eye color.

3. According to the U.S. Census Bureau, ethnicity and race are defined by the federal government via the Office of Management and Budget as two distinct concepts, shaping how American society and demographers conceptualize what are in practice social definitions without any biological foundations. Race may be defined by which one of the following?
   A. Shared physical traits
   B. Geographic experiences
   C. Cultural heritage
   D. Historical origins

4. As an oncology nurse, it is important to understand that cultural norms influence relationships between health care practitioners and patients and/or their caregivers. When communicating with patients, an oncology nurse may consider avoiding which one of the following?
   A. Folding hands in lap
   B. Planting feet solidly on the floor while seated
   C. Giving the "thumbs up" gesture
   D. Standing at least 2 feet away from the patient or caregiver

5. The oncology nurse is providing a community presentation on the early detection of cancer. A participant expresses concerns about the costs of screening. The oncology nurse understands that poverty may lead to late-stage diagnosis of cancer due to which one of the following?
   A. Lack of quality health care despite adequate access to facilities
   B. Necessity to prioritize basic needs over seeking cancer care
   C. Higher exposure to poor nutrition, workplace carcinogens, and modifiable risk factors
   D. Regular cancer screening

6. Responses to a diagnosis of cancer varies widely based on a person's cultural norms and behaviors. The oncology nurse is aware that which one of the following cultural factors may hinder a person's willingness to undergo cancer screening?
   A. Emphasis on traditional healers
   B. Fear of having to be in a clinical trial for treatment
   C. Ignorance of cancer treatment process
   D. Fatalistic view of a cancer diagnosis

7. F.L. is a 58-year-old female who was admitted for hematopoietic stem cell transplantation. She divulges to her oncology nurse the healing impact that caring for her rose garden has had on her life, and that she will miss her weekly ritual once discharged after her transplant. The oncology nurse realizes that her relationship with nature is rooted in which one of the following?
   A. Religion
   B. Spirituality
   C. Culture
   D. Ethnicity

111

8. Which one of the following terms is defined as protected knowledge, typically bestowed by a higher power, that exists outside the parameters of an established faith?
   A. Religion
   B. Sacred
   C. Spirituality
   D. Belief

9. An oncology nurse may assess the level of spiritual support that a patient or caregiver needs by doing which one of the following?
   A. Consulting pastoral services
   B. Praying with the patient
   C. Reading a passage from a holy scripture of the patient's religion
   D. Deep listening

10. The nurse is caring for a patient with cancer from a different culture than other patients on the unit and from her own. When the nurse enters the patient's room, the patient maintains a downward gaze and avoids eye contact. Which one of the following represents an indication of the most likely cause of the patient's actions?
    A. The patient is not comfortable with cultural diversity and health care providers.
    B. The patient's culture may view direct eye contact as a sign of disrespect.
    C. The patient is dealing with depression related to her cancer diagnosis.
    D. The patient wants the nurse to avoid close physical contact.

11. The oncology nurse is completing an admission assessment on a patient who is beginning chemotherapy. The nurse understands that which one of the following terms noted in the patient's hospital chart is associated with gender identity?
    A. Homosexual
    B. Lesbian
    C. Queer
    D. Nonbinary

54 Psychosocial Disturbances and Coping

1. One of the primary treatment approaches for patients experiencing cancer-related distress is the use of which one of the following?
   A. Psychotherapy interventions
   B. Anti-anxiolytic agent every 4 hours and imagery
   C. Psychotherapy and a benzodiazepine agent
   D. Psychotropic medications and hydrotherapy

2. An oncology nurse is caring for a 60-year-old female patient with metastatic disease. She is on third-line therapy and has difficulty concentrating, frequently cancels appointments, and has had emotional outbursts with family and the medical team. There is no history of past mental illness or unusual behavior. The oncology nurse recognizes that the correct course of action is which one of the following?
   A. Discuss hospice with the health care team as the patient does not want to continue treatments.
   B. Ask to be removed from the patient's care because the patient refuses to cooperate with the medical team.
   C. Consider asking the health care team if the patient should be seen for a psychology/psychiatry evaluation.
   D. Her behavior is a normal symptom in patients receiving third-line treatment and the patient should be treated with an anti-anxiolytic.

3. The oncology nurse is completing an admission assessment for a patient with a cancer diagnosis. The nurse considers that possible nonpsychiatric causes of depression may include which one of the following?
   A. Well-controlled HTN
   B. Hypocalcemia
   C. Vitamin B12 deficiency
   D. Hyperglycemia

4. An oncology nurse is teaching a patient with cancer about how to take their new antidepressant medication (SSRI). The oncology nurse knows that teaching has been successful when the patient verbalizes which one of the following?
   A. "If I do not feel differently after 2 weeks, I should stop my medication immediately and see my doctor at the first available visit."
   B. "It may take several weeks to months for this medication to work, and I need to keep taking it as prescribed, and see my therapist regularly."
   C. "This medication will work right away, and I will be able to get better sleep and wake up feeling refreshed."
   D. "This medication can have interactions with other drugs, and I should talk to my doctor before starting any new medications, but herbal supplements are okay to take."

5. When caring for a pediatric patient, which one of the following interventions will assist in preventing their loss of personal control while being treated for cancer? Pediatric patients should:
   A. be provided opportunities to indicate choices through art therapy
   B. be distracted with books, toys, and TV
   C. defer to their parents as the decision-makers
   D. be kept out of the room when treatment options are discussed

6. Practical and effective nursing strategies to address multiple aspects of psychological distress and impaired coping include which one of the following?
   A. Provide educational materials about the patient's diagnosis, treatment, and care plan.
   B. Automatically have all patients screened by a social worker before beginning treatment.
   C. Screen patients as needed only if they are displaying symptoms of psychological distress.
   D. Avoid asking questions about potentially sensitive subjects, because this will impair coping.

7. The oncology nurse realizes that many persons with a diagnosis of malignancy experience distress. The best nursing intervention to identify cancer-related distress in the cancer patient is to do which one of the following?
   A. Screen for distress within the first several visits and regularly.
   B. Ask the family about the patient's distress during each clinic visit.
   C. Screen for distress when symptoms are identified.
   D. Observe the patient's behavior and screen as necessary.

8. The oncology nurse is presenting a program on grief and bereavement. The nurse discusses that a risk factor for complicated grief includes which one of the following?
   A. An expected death for a terminal condition
   B. A deep emotional relationship to the deceased
   C. A large multi-generational family
   D. An ambivalent relationship to the deceased

113

9. The oncology nurse is orienting a new nurse to the unit and is discussing cancer-related distress. They discuss risk factors for distress. Which one of the following types of patients are at the highest risk for emotional distress?
   A. Diagnosis of breast cancer, newly promoted to manager at work, history of anxiety
   B. Diagnosis of lung cancer, employed for 35 years in same company, history of arthritis
   C. Diagnosis of stage 1 breast cancer, recently retired, and history of depression
   D. Diagnosis of lung cancer, newly promoted to vice president of company, and poor pain control

10. An oncology nurse is completing an assessment for a 69-year-old male recently diagnosed with lung cancer. The nurse reviews his medication history and notes that the patient is at increased risk for experiencing anxiety because he is receiving which one of the following medications?
    A. Beta-adrenergic stimulants
    B. Angiotension receptor blockers
    C. Angiotensin-converting enzyme inhibitors
    D. Beta blockers

11. The oncology nurse understands that there are several types of depression. Which one of the following statements is true regarding reactive depression?
    A. Reactive depression is more common in elderly persons.
    B. Reactive depression is a normal response to a precipitating event or situation.
    C. Reactive depression commonly occurs in people taking corticosteroids for cancer treatment.
    D. Reactive depression is more common in persons who have experienced domestic abuse.

12. A 35-year-old single mother with two young children is receiving chemotherapy after recently learning the malignancy has metastasized to her liver. The oncology nurse knows she is experiencing multiple stressors including a loss of control. The nurse suspects this because a person experiencing loss of control might manifest in which one of the following?
    A. Excessive house cleaning
    B. Frequent questions about therapy
    C. Frequent compliments to staff on care delivery
    D. Reluctance to express emotions

13. A 32-year-old father of two is dying from colon cancer. He is concerned about how his 6-year-old daughter is coping with this information. Developmentally, a 6 year old might view the death of a parent as which one of the following?
    A. As a punishment for bad behavior
    B. As a temporary situation
    C. As a separation
    D. As a threat to independence

14. The oncology nurse is orienting a new nurse to the unit. They are discussing psychosocial concerns and that there are many symptoms of grief. Symptoms of grief include which one of the following sets of terms?
    A. Hyperactivity, distractibility, and avoidance
    B. Intrusive thoughts, sleep disturbances, and occupational lapses
    C. Preoccupation with loss, hyperactivity, and increased energy
    D. Changing beliefs or views, increased energy, and rumination

15. J.W. is a 55-year-old male patient who is undergoing chemotherapy. He is experiencing problems with coping. To help, he decides to engage in a weekly support group and see a counselor. This is an example of which one of the following?
    A. Problem-focused coping
    B. Emotion-focused coping
    C. Primary-appraisal coping
    D. Meaning-focused coping

16. The oncology nurse is providing a community seminar on coping with cancer. The nurse discussed that anxiety is a common reaction in individuals diagnosed with malignancy. Symptoms of anxiety include which one of the following sets of symptoms?
    A. Feelings of suffocation, dizziness, fatigue, or exhaustion
    B. Palpitations, eating disturbances, feeling of worthlessness or guilt
    C. Difficulty swallowing, crying easily, insomnia
    D. Sense of impending doom, easily overwhelmed, psychomotor agitation

17. A patient has been admitted to the oncology unit in preparation for an autologous bone marrow transplant. As part of the admission process, the oncology nurse performs a psychosocial assessment for anxiety, distress, and depression. Symptoms of depression include which one of the following pairs of symptoms?
    A. Easily overwhelmed, change of appetite
    B. Unable to relax, insomnia
    C. Sense of impending doom, hypersomnia
    D. Decreased energy, recurrent thoughts of death or suicide

18. H.K. is a 49-year-old female who has been recently diagnosed with cancer. She has reported having trouble coping with her diagnosis and has said she feels "sad." Her oncology nurse is evaluating H.K.'s condition to determine if she is at risk for a diagnosis of a major depressive disorder. Which one of the following symptoms should the nurse recognize as a potential sign that H.K. should be referred for further evaluation?
    A. Complaining of a sense of impending doom
    B. Feeling highly agitated and easily overwhelmed
    C. Having trouble swallowing and often feels suffocated
    D. Reporting that she'll sleep well into the afternoon on a regular basis

114

19. H.K.–the 49-year-old female patient with cancer from the previous question–is being evaluated to determine if she is at risk for diagnosis of a major depressive disorder. As part of her evaluation, her nurse knows that H.K. will be evaluated for both subjective and objective symptoms. Which one of the following is an example of an objective symptom?
    A. Report of depressed mood
    B. Report of insomnia
    C. Measurement of weight loss or gain
    D. Report of feeling worthless or guilty

20. The oncology nurse is using a formal tool to assess the level of distress in a patient newly diagnosed with cancer. Which one of the following is a characteristic of the Hospital Anxiety and Depression Scale (HADS) assessment tool for distress?
    A. 0 (no distress) to 10 (severe distress) measurement, with accompanying simple questions identifying source of distress
    B. 14-item scale (7 questions: anxiety; 7 questions: depression)
    C. Recommendation that score of 4 or more triggers further physician or nurse evaluation, referral to psychosocial services, or both
    D. Score from 0 to 25 (0–5 per question) to evaluate anxiety or depression levels

21. The nurse is orienting a new nurse to the ambulatory infusion center The oncology nurse explains that distress is a multidimensional construct that:
    A. is impacted by developmental stage, phase of disease, past coping skills, and available resources
    B. does not require routine screening, because patients will self-identify if they need help
    C. has a simple straightforward process for management
    D. is a normal response to a diagnosis of cancer and seldom needs additional intervention

22. The family of a patient who died 2 months ago is planning a visit to the cancer center to meet with staff. Which one of the following grief responses by the family would cause the nurse who had cared for the deceased patient the greatest concern?
    A. Crying, angry outbursts, and accusations
    B. Preoccupation with the deceased family member
    C. Somatic symptoms similar to the deceased
    D. Withdrawal or social isolation

55 Sexuality and Sexual Dysfunction

1. An oncology nurse is teaching a class about how to open communication about sexual changes with patients with cancer. The nurse explains that the PLISSIT model of sexual health communication stands for which one of the following?
   A. Patient to discuss the topic, provide limited information, provide specific suggestions, request intensive therapy
   B. Permission to discuss the topic, provide limited information, provide specific suggestions, refer for intensive therapy
   C. Push to discuss the topic, provide written and detailed information, provide general suggestions, refer for intensive therapy
   D. Permission to discuss the topic, provide detailed information, provide general suggestions, refer for intensive therapy if patient requests

2. The oncology nurse teaches that which one of the following is an example of a nonpharmacologic intervention for sexual concerns in cancer?
   A. Using Eros therapy device for clitoral stimulation
   B. Applying lubricant oil to the vaginal opening
   C. Ingesting natural herbs to increase libido
   D. Referring to couple's counseling targeting communication and relationship dynamics

3. Oncology nurses and physicians may hesitate to ask about sexuality because of which one of the following?
   A. They may hold biased beliefs about the patient's age, prognosis, or partner availability.
   B. They assume that sexuality questions were already asked at the initial patient assessment.
   C. They think that patients do not want to be asked questions about this topic.
   D. They think patients have access to internet information and do not need further information.

4. The oncology nurse explains that a sexual practice that can be safely practiced by patients who are immunocompromised or thrombocytopenic is which one of the following?
   A. Stoma coitus
   B. Vaginal stimulation without lubrication
   C. Massage, caressing, kissing
   D. Nipple or penile rings

5. The oncology nurse meets with a young woman diagnosed with cancer who is scheduled to begin a chemotherapy regimen and explains that the patient's fertility may be affected. The nurse is aware that which one of the following is true regarding fertility preservation?
   A. Does not affect quality of life
   B. Does not affect sexual function
   C. Does constitute a key survivorship issue
   D. Does not affect treatment decision-making

6. J.M. is a 41-year-old female patient with breast cancer who is getting ready to begin chemotherapy. Her oncology nurse knows that the patient should be aware of which one of the following?
   A. She may be affected by menopausal changes.
   B. Her libido may be increased.
   C. She cannot engage in sexual intercourse.
   D. She will have increased vaginal secretions

7. The oncology nurse understands that which one of the following statements is true about serum anti-Müllerian hormone (AMH)?
   A. AMH is the most reliable strategy to assess ovarian reserve, but only in women under the age of 25 years.
   B. AMH is the most reliable strategy to assess ovarian reserve and predict onset of menopause, but only in women under the age of 25 years.
   C. AMH is the most reliable strategy to assess ovarian size, but only in women over the age of 25 years.
   D. AMH is the most reliable strategy to assess ovarian reserve and predict onset of menopause, but only in women over the age of 25 years.

8. A 28-year-old female patient has just completed therapy for Hodgkin lymphoma. She tells the oncology nurse that she and her husband are planning to try to get pregnant. The oncology nurse replies that general recommendations suggest waiting at least which one of the following periods of time before attempting to conceive after cancer treatment is complete?
   A. 3 to 6 months
   B. 6 to 12 months
   C. 12 months
   D. 24 to 36 months

9. The oncology nurse is aware that in the "5 A's" discussion model to enhance sexual health communication, which one of the following examples is the definition of the "advise" step?
   A. Bring the topic up.
   B. Ask about sexual functioning.
   C. Provide information and resources.
   D. Normalize symptoms and acknowledge the problems.

10. The oncology nurse understands that which one of the following is a potential change that would affect sexuality or sexual functioning in either male or female patients with cancer who are being treated with steroids?
    A. Alopecia to include the loss of pubic hair
    B. Peripheral neuropathy
    C. Development of infertility
    D. Reduced sexual function and desire

11. The oncology nurse should explain to a male patient being treated with pelvic radiotherapy for prostate cancer that which one of the following is a potential side effect of the treatment that could affect his sexual functioning?
    A. Vascular or nerve damage causing erectile dysfunction
    B. Decreased or loss of libido
    C. Flu-like symptoms that could affect libido
    D. Mouth sores that could affect sexual behavior

12. The oncology nurse understands that which one of the following is a potential change that would affect sexual functioning in a female patient with cancer being treated with chemotherapy?
    A. Vaginal stenosis
    B. Chronic constipation
    C. Vaginal stomatitis
    D. Chest pain

13. C.K. is a 27-year-old female who has just been diagnosed with cancer. She asks the oncology nurse if the diagnosis means that she will not be able to have children. She adds, "Will I even live long enough to see my first baby?" The response of the nurse caring for her would be guided by which one of the following?
    A. Awareness of the need to address preservation of fertility prior to treatment initiation
    B. Stressing to her patient at diagnosis the improvements that have been made in survival with cancer treatment and the need to focus on care
    C. Understanding that, at the patient's current age, there will be a variety of fertility options available to her in the future
    D. Providing the reassurance to her patient that when she survives the treatment, adoption will always be an option

117

56 Standards of Practice and Professional Performance

1. To best understand the standards for professional practice in various oncology settings, the oncology nurse should refer to which one of the following?
   A. *Standards of Oncology Nursing Education: Generalist and Advanced Practice Levels*
   B. *Oncology Nursing Society: Scope and Standards of Practice*
   C. American Society of Clinical Oncology (ASCO)/ Oncology Nursing Society (ONS) Chemotherapy Administration Safety Standards
   D. A nurse recruiter at a Commission on Cancer Accredited Cancer Center

2. An oncology nurse unit educator is updating a policy. In this role the nurse is responsible for which one of the following?
   A. Their own self-assessment to guide professional growth
   B. Integrating evidence-based science into practice
   C. Determining if staff affected by the policies are in agreement with changes
   D. Supporting continuing education programs

3. The ASCO/ONS Chemotherapy Administration Safety Standards are recognized by oncology nurses as which one of the following?
   A. A two-tiered system for nurses and physicians to report unsafe practices
   B. An evidence-based resource for locating current clinical trials
   C. Interprofessional standards outlining best practices for reducing errors in administration
   D. A document for patients to better understand efficacy and side effects of antineoplastic therapy

4. An effective way for institutions to evaluate the required documentation of oncology care is to perform which one of the following?
   A. Survey the staff about ease in locating the policies related to documentation of care.
   B. Hire a compliance consultant to review documentation policies.
   C. Send all documents to the compliance department for review.
   D. Do a side-by-side comparison of standards to current processes.

5. Standards of Oncology Practice include which one of the following set of components?
   A. Planning, coordination of care, ethics, and outcomes identification
   B. Assessment, diagnosis, coordination of care, health teaching, and health promotion
   C. Communication, collaboration, leadership, quality of practice
   D. Coordination of care, health teaching and health promotion, resource utilization, ethics

6. Which one of the following is a definition for standards for professional nursing practice?
   A. Statements that include recommendations for optimal patient care
   B. Authoritative statements of the duties that subspecialties of nurses are expected to perform with competence
   C. Authoritative statements of the duties that all registered nurses are expected to perform with competence
   D. Recommendations of the duties that all registered nurses are expected to perform with competence

7. Which one of the following statements is a definition of the education component in the Standards of Professional Performance?
   A. The oncology nurse partners with the patient and family, the interprofessional team, and community resources to optimize cancer care.
   B. The oncology nurse seeks and expands personal knowledge and competence that reflect the current evidence-based state of cancer care and oncology nursing.
   C. The oncology nurse identifies clinical dilemmas and problems appropriate for study while supporting research efforts.
   D. The oncology nurse considers factors related to safety, efficiency, effectiveness, and cost in planning and delivering care to patients.

118

8. An oncology nurse navigator is orienting a new navigator to the role. They discuss the Oncology Navigation Standards of Practice. All of these statements about nurse navigation standards are correct *except* which one of the following standards?
   A. Educate physicians about the essential role of nurse navigators.
   B. Enhance the quality of navigation services provided to people impacted by cancer.
   C. Mandate affiliation with oncology nurse practitioners in providing patient care.
   D. Promote participation in quality improvement projects.

57 Evidence-Based Practice

1. Which one of the following statements accurately describe evidence-based practice (EBP)?
   A. EBP has been implemented throughout the United States consistently.
   B. EBP contradicts pay-for-performance programs.
   C. Evolution of evidence is limited.
   D. Nonpayment for complications model exists when EBP is not followed.

2. Which one of the following statements accurately describes an element of the PICOT format?
   A. P = Patient
   B. I = Improvement
   C. O = Opportunity
   D. T = Theory

3. Which one of the following levels represents the highest level of strength of the evidence?
   A. Level 1
   B. Level 2
   C. Level 5
   D. Level 7

4. To ensure feasibility and sustainability, practice changes in a clinical setting should first be which one of the following?
   A. Incorporated into policy
   B. Published
   C. Piloted
   D. Reviewed by the Institutional Review Board (IRB)

5. EBP is most valuable when which one of the following occurs?
   A. Outcomes are disseminated
   B. Clinical practice is changed
   C. Incorporated into EBP grand rounds
   D. Presented at a national conference

6. A characteristic of qualitative research is which one of the following?
   A. Focus on outcome
   B. Focus on objective
   C. Focus on generalizable results
   D. Focus on process

7. Which one of the following represents the highest level of evidence in a quantitative study?
   A. Single-site randomized control studies (RCT) studies
   B. Case or cohort studies
   C. Single descriptive study
   D. Systemic review of RCTs

8. An oncology nurse is interested in creating a culture of EBP at her workplace and begins a journal club with her colleagues. Which one of the following is a journal club in the multistep process of using evidence to support clinical practice?
   A. Identifying a problem or trigger
   B. Creating a sense of inquiry and creating an EBP culture
   C. Searching and critiquing the literature for relevant studies
   D. Identifying information and stakeholders needed to solve the problem

58 Principles of Education and Learning

1. The oncology nurse understands that before the development of a targeted education program or material, a focus group is appropriate when assessing which one of the following populations?
   A. Individuals
   B. Caregivers
   C. Survivors
   D. Community

2. The oncology nurse is preparing a staff education program and is writing learning objectives using the SMART method. The SMART methodology for writing objectives includes which one of the following components?
   A. S = Survey
   B. M = Measurable
   C. A = Action
   D. R = Results

3. The oncology nurse understands that performance analysis is helpful with which one of the following phases of staff education?
   A. Development of the teaching plan
   B. Determination of teaching objectives
   C. Evaluation
   D. Content identification

4. The oncology nurse is providing discharge education on nutrition to a patient who had a colon resection and will soon be starting chemotherapy. The nurse is aware that which one of the following nutritional goals are focused on an objective outcome?
   A. Understand nutritional impact on the body.
   B. Prepare low-fat foods.
   C. Maintain adequate sodium intake.
   D. List four vegetables with high-fiber content to avoid.

5. The oncology nurse understands that diagnostic methods are frequently used as an assessment for which one of the following groups?
   A. Staff
   B. Patient
   C. Caregiver
   D. Community

6. The oncology nurse understands that the learning that takes place by watching and imitating others is based on which one of the following learning theories?
   A. Social
   B. Cognitive
   C. Behavioral
   D. Humanistic

7. H.R. is a 50-year-old male who has recently been diagnosed with prostate cancer. To learn more about his disease, he conducts an internet search prior to his next appointment. A patient performing an independent internet search for their specific cancer diagnosis is an example of which one of the following learning theories?
   A. Operant conditioning
   B. Motivational
   C. Adult learning
   D. Pedagogic learning

8. Learning that is activated through internal and external cues is based on which one of the following learning theories?
   A. Social
   B. Cognitive
   C. Motivational
   D. Humanistic

59 Legal Issues

1. The enforcement of Nurse Practice Acts that guide nursing practice is regulated by which one of the following?
   A. National Council of State Boards of Nursing (NCSBN)
   B. Nurse Practice Acts
   C. State Boards of Nursing (BoN)
   D. National Council Licensure for Registered Nurses (NCLEX)

2. The Affordable Care Act advocates for patient's rights in the health care environment to include which one of the following?
   A. Requiring insurers to provide coverage to dependent children if enrolled in college
   B. Providing coverage to patients with a history of cancer
   C. Placing annual limits on coverage provided
   D. Placing limits on lifetime coverage

3. Which one of the following is a national oncology-specific accreditation program?
   A. The Joint Commission (TJC)
   B. National Institutes of Health (NIH)
   C. Centers for Medicare and Medicaid (CMS)
   D. Quality Oncology Practice Initiative (QOPI)

4. Legal issues for individuals with cancer include which one of the following?
   A. Ensuring insurance coverage for a bone marrow transplant
   B. Obtaining reimbursement for prescribed oral chemotherapy
   C. Filing for bankruptcy
   D. Accepting a promotion at work because they are a cancer survivor

5. In being oriented to a new position, the oncology nurse learns that breach of duty is best defined as which one of the following?
   A. Deviation from a professional standard of care
   B. Failure to meet an acceptable standard of care
   C. Deviation from the acceptable standard of care that a reasonable person would use in a specific situation
   D. A cause that directly produces an event and without which the event would not have occurred

6. During the job orientation, the oncology nurse is told that reasons for litigation against nurses include which one of the following?
   A. Following established standards of care and hospital policies and procedures
   B. Performing a patient assessment and reporting the findings to a physician
   C. Advocating for a patient's right to refuse treatment
   D. Witnessing an informed consent when the nurse didn't hear what was explained to the patient

7. Oncology nurses can utilize strategies for minimizing risk of malpractice or disciplinary action. Which one of the following strategies involves the development of skills in interpersonal communication?
   A. Attending relevant continuing education programs
   B. Obtaining specialty certifications
   C. Becoming involved in patient advocacy programs and listening to patient concerns
   D. Communicating clearly when educating patients and families

8. Which one of the following legal terms is defined as the "deviation from the acceptable standard of care that a reasonable person would use in a specific situation?"
   A. Malpractice
   B. Negligence
   C. Defamation
   D. Breach of duty

9. Which one of the following legal terms is defined as the "deviation from a professional standard of care?"
   A. Negligence
   B. Slander
   C. Malpractice
   D. Duty

10. The Oncology Nursing Society's Practice Standard named "Statement on the Scope and Standards of Oncology Nursing Practice Generalist and Advanced Practice" is described by which one of the following statements?
    A. Describes the scope of oncology nursing practice, standards of care for RNs and advanced practice RNs, and professional performance issues
    B. Describes formal and informal education standards that oncology nurses can use for planning and evaluating education for patients and significant others
    C. Describes survivorship care plan requirements, including documentation, implementation, and key elements of the care plan
    D. Describes pathways for chemotherapy/biotherapy course and/or certificate completion based on administration volume or number of chemotherapy and/or biotherapy agents

60 Ethical Issues

1. A patient who has recently undergone a bone marrow transplant is in the intensive care unit (ICU) receiving aggressive treatment. A source of moral distress in the oncology nurse caring for the patient may include which one of the following?
   A. Availability of technology that may result in overtreatment
   B. Collaboration between physician and nurse about treatment
   C. A request by the patient to continue treatment
   D. Actively helping the patient to complete an advance directive

2. An oncology nurse is about to administer a clinical trial drug and asks the patient if he has signed an informed consent and if he understands the treatment. By doing so, the nurse is requesting of the patient which one of the following?
   A. That he must complete the entire treatment plan and follow-up
   B. That he acknowledges that no harm will become him during treatment
   C. That he understands the risks, benefits, and consequences of treatment
   D. That he understands that the treatment will ultimately cure him of his disease

3. According to the American Nurses Association Code of Ethics, which of the following is a provision that represents nursing's core values, duties, and accountabilities? An oncology nurse who:
   A. calls a physician for additional medications for a patient in pain
   B. joins a research group to study the effects of pain medication
   C. decides to go back to school to study palliative care
   D. arrives on time for work and completes tasks in a timely manner

4. An oncology nurse working on a bone marrow transplant unit is caring for M.R, a 75-year-old patient who had an allogenic transplant. The nurse questions why they are treating a patient of his age group. This statement by the nurse is an example of the ethical theory of which one of the following?
   A. Utilitarianism
   B. Ethical egoism
   C. Deontology
   D. Divisibility

5. G.R. is a 39-year-old male who has been newly diagnosed with leukemia. During his office visit, he discusses treatment options for therapy with the physician. The oncology nurse understands that this type of decision making is an example of which one of the following?
   A. Informed consent
   B. Shared decision-making
   C. Power of attorney
   D. Combined decision-making

6. The oncology nurse is answering a patient's questions about a clinical trial protocol. The nurse understands that which one of the following ethical principles is defined by the duty to not harm others?
   A. Beneficence
   B. Autonomy
   C. Justice
   D. Nonmaleficence

7. The oncology nurse understands that which one of the following is an example or a definition of the ethical principle of justice?
   A. Ensuring the benefits of a patient's treatment outweighs the harm
   B. Showing compassion toward a patient in a nurse's care
   C. Respect for a person's right to choose their own destiny, or, in medical terms, their own plan of care
   D. Allocating the same resources to each patient, no matter their socioeconomic status, race, religion, or moral standing

8. Which one of the following is the third step in identifying ethical concerns?
   A. Explore practical alternatives.
   B. Analyze the problem using ethical theories.
   C. Gather the information from key participants and obtain the facts.
   D. Evaluate the process and outcome.

9. The staff nurses on an oncology inpatient unit are initiating an improvement project. They ask the advanced practice oncology nurse (APN) to provide teaching. The APN explains the concept of *everyday ethical comportment*. Which one of the following is included in this concept?

A. Respect for the autonomy of patients and their caregivers

B. Identify the type of ethical problem that exists and define what makes this an ethical problem.

C. Acquire practice-based knowledge, skills, and reasoning through lived clinical experiences of caring for patients

D. Consider social determinants of health to develop group interventions for vulnerable populations

10. The APN on the oncology unit describes the concept of self-care to the staff nurses. Which one of the following best describes self-care in nursing?

A. Self-care is a priority to promote mental health, build resilience, and decrease burnout.

B. In self-care, nurses should take responsibility and ownership for their words, and practice.

C. Self-care involves acting on concerns about patients' decision-making abilities.

D. In self-care, nurses can use social media platforms to learn and conduct research.

61 Professional Issues

1. Collaborative partnerships are critical in optimizing the care of oncology patients. Which one of the following is an example of an obstacle to building a collaborative relationship?
   A. Interdisciplinary team meetings involving doctors, nurses, social workers, and leadership
   B. Lack of recognition of the knowledge and expertise of the oncology nurse
   C. Relationship building with team members other than the physician
   D. Initiation of change of shift reporting guidelines

2. Certification in oncology nursing is critical for which one of the following examples?
   A. Obtaining higher pay
   B. Mandated for relicensure
   C. Representation of the knowledge and qualifications unique to oncology
   D. Required by the Board of Registered Nursing (BRN) by 2020

3. The oncology nurse is planning a quality improvement project. Which model would be helpful and typically seeks to answer three fundamental questions about the project?
   A. PICOT
   B. SMART
   C. PDSA
   D. PLISSIT

4. Medical errors have significant financial and nonfinancial costs to the health care system. Which one of the following represents an opportunity for the oncology nurse to minimize this risk?
   A. Obtain certification.
   B. Recognize and remove faulty equipment.
   C. Participate on an evidence-based care committee.
   D. Read journals in their specialty area regularly.

5. The oncology nurse is caring for an older frail patient who falls when trying to get up from bed without assistance. The oncology nurse knows this is which one of the following types of error?
   A. Diagnostic
   B. Treatment
   C. Preventive
   D. Other communication

6. An oncology nurse learns that there is a mandate to improve the culture of safety in the institution. Which of the following might be a strategy that is implemented?
   A. Punitive investigatory processes involving peers
   B. Confidential investigatory processes involving administrators
   C. Review of selected errors and near misses on a quarterly basis
   D. Policies and procedures that support safe care

7. The oncology nurse is attending a seminar on quality improvement which includes a discussion of Patient Family Advisors (PFAs). The oncology nurse knows that PFAs are recognized by which one of the following agencies?
   A. Institute of Medicine
   B. Joint Commission
   C. Centers for Medicare and Medicaid Services
   D. College of Surgeons Commission on Cancer

8. The oncology nurse is attending a seminar on budgets and related legislation. The nurse knows that the American Rescue Plan Act of 2021 includes which one of the following?
   A. Mandates all Americans have some form of health insurance
   B. Sets uniform standards for Medicaid payment
   C. Lowers health care premiums
   D. Increases traditional Medicare payments through alternative payment model

62 Compassion Fatigue

1. An oncology nurse's coworker has been exhibiting increased behaviors of emotional distress after several patient deaths. The oncology nurse is concerned that these symptoms may be signs of which one of the following?
   A. Chronic job stress
   B. Compassion fatigue
   C. Moral distress
   D. Hyperactivity

2. An oncology nurse working on a bone marrow transplant unit may be at risk for developing compassion fatigue. A factor that may increase the nurse's risk includes which one of the following?
   A. Being married with children
   B. Overconfidence in caring for patients
   C. Caring for high-acuity patients over a long period of time
   D. Having more than 10 years oncology nursing experience

3. Suggested activities for a female oncology nurse displaying symptoms of compassion fatigue might include which one of the following?
   A. Going out for drinks and staying out late with friends
   B. Scheduling a day at a spa for a massage and facial
   C. Avoid talking with anyone about issues with work
   D. Frequent resting in bed when not at work

4. An oncology nurse is concerned about a long-time coworker who has become distant and distracted. When questioned, the coworker states that they are just overwhelmed and exhausted. The coworker may be experiencing which one of the following?
   A. Chronic fatigue syndrome
   B. Compassion fatigue
   C. Burnout
   D. A cognitive disorder

5. An oncology nurse working on a unit where there is a heavy caseload and high levels of stress may best be assessed for secondary distress disorders through use of which one of the following?
   A. Montreal Cognitive Assessment Scale
   B. Mini-Mental State Exam
   C. Professional Quality of Life Scale (ProQOL)
   D. Maslach Burnout Inventory—Human Services Survey MBI-HSS

6. Which one of the following is an example of a self-reflection exercise that a nurse could try as part of self-care management?
   A. Indulging in a massage
   B. Exercise (recommend three to four times weekly for 20 to 30 minutes)
   C. Enjoying a hobby, listening to music, humor, and enjoying nature
   D. Making time for prayer and meditation

7. Which one of the following is an example of managing self-care through mindfulness-based interventions?
   A. Establishing good nutrition and eating well
   B. Sending cards to the family, reminiscing about time spent with patients, sometimes attending funerals of patients with whom there has been a close bond
   C. Engaging in activities that focus attention on the present experience, and becoming more aware of one's physical, mental, and emotional condition in a way that is nonjudgmental
   D. Scheduling preventive and medical care appointments

CHAPTER 1

1. *Answer:* C

   Rationale: Cancer epidemiology is defined as the study of the distribution and determinants of cancer in population groups and assists in the development of population-based profiles. The rates of cancer occurrence in a population indicate the incidence of cancer, usually reported for a given period of time. Number of deaths is the mortality rate for cancers over a given period of time.

2. *Answer:* A

   Rationale: Female breast cancer incidence has increased 0.5% per year for the last 20 years due to declining fertility rates and increasing obesity rates. Colorectal cancer incidence increased by 1.5% in people younger than 50 years of age. Prostate cancer incidence dropped rapidly from 2004 to 2017 due to early detection and screening. Lung cancer incidence dropped 3% in males and 1% in females from 2009 to 2018, reflecting trends in smoking prevalence. Colorectal cancer incidence declined by 2% in people aged 50 years and older.

3. *Answer:* A

   Rationale: According to the American Cancer Society, as of January 1, 2019, 64% of cancer survivors are 65 years of age or older. Only 1 in 10 cancer survivors are younger than age 50. Since the 1960s, the 5-year relative survival rate for all cancers has increased from 39% to 68% in white people and from 27% to 63% in Black people. The chronic myeloid leukemia relative survival rate has increased from 22% in the mid-1970s to 71% in 2017. For all stages combined, 5-year survival is highest for prostate (98%), melanoma of the skin (93%), and female breast cancer (90%). Survival is lowest for lung (22%), liver (20%), and pancreas (11%).

4. *Answer:* B

   Rationale: For prostate cancer, African American men have the highest incidence and mortality rates as compared with other ethnic groups in the United States and are more than twice as likely as white men to die from prostate cancer. Asians/Pacific Islanders have the highest incidence and death rates of all groups for cancers of the liver and stomach, not kidney cancer. For both lung and colorectal cancers, Blacks/African Americans have the highest incidence and mortality compared with other ethnic groups in the United States. Hispanic/Latina women have the highest incidence rate for cervical cancer, but the highest mortality rate is seen among African American women.

5. *Answer:* C

   Rationale: Tobacco use is the single largest preventable cause of disease and premature death in the United States and is associated with at least 30% of cancer-related deaths each year. Smokeless tobacco is not a safe alternative to cigarettes. It is associated with increased risk of oral, pancreatic, and esophageal cancers. Adults without a high school degree are two to four times more likely to be current smokers than those with a college degree. Those who are uninsured are twice as likely to be tobacco users as insured persons.

6. *Answer:* B

   Rationale: Cancers of the gastrointestinal system (i.e., those of the esophagus, liver, stomach, pancreas, gallbladder, and colorectum) are among cancers linked to overweight and obesity. Lung cancer risk is not elevated in obesity. Overweight and/or obesity contribute to an estimated 16% of all deaths due to cancer. Approximately 5% of cancers in males and 11% of cancers in females are attributed to obesity.

7. *Answer:* D

   Rationale: Recommended HPV vaccination age is 9 to 12 years for girls and boys (and as early as 9 years and as late as 26 years) because a higher immune response is seen at this age than later adolescence. A two-dose series is recommended for children before age 15. After age 15, a three-dose series is recommended.

8. *Answer:* A

   Rationale: Tamoxifen and raloxifene are FDA approved for use as chemoprevention agents to reduce risk of breast cancer. These agents have been shown to reduce breast cancer incidence by up to 50% among high-risk women. The other drugs are not indicated for chemoprevention of breast cancer. In the past, diethylstilbestrol use during pregnancy has been associated with cancer of the vagina in female offspring. Anabolic steroids may be associated with liver cancer. Menotropins are fertility drugs that may increase the risk of ovarian cancer.

9. *Answer:* D

   Rationale: When accessing Ms. P for motivation for preventative behavior as per the health belief model, she should be asked the question, "How difficult do you think it will be to decrease your risk for cancer by quitting your smoking habit?" Since Ms. P is a smoker, her health care provider would have recognized that smoking is an unhealthy behavior that could lead to a diagnosis of cancer. Under the health belief model, her health care provider would want to know what barriers exist in her overcoming harmful habits. Asking about current medical conditions and medications, her own and her family's history cancer diagnoses, and previous treatments, such as chemotherapy, radiation therapy, and immunotherapy, would all be done during earlier medical history and physical examinations.

10. *Answer:* C

Rationale: According to the American Cancer Society, a fact that is true regarding cancer mortality in populations with low socioeconomic status (SES) is that there is a higher rate of advanced disease found at diagnosis among poorer populations and those who live in rural regions than in the rest of the U.S. population. Instead of high socioeconomic status being associated with increased risk of lung cancer, cervical cancer, stomach cancer, and cancer of the head and neck, it is low socioeconomic status that is a contributor. The use of alcohol is not a leading cause of cancer mortality in poorer populations, but tobacco use is and is increasing in persons from lower socioeconomic status. High socioeconomic status is associated with increased risk of breast, prostate, and colon cancers.

11. *Answer:* A

Rationale: As of 2020, more than 3 million middle and high school age students were identified as e-cigarette users, with a variety of appealing flavors cited as the primary reason for use. This increase in use by teens and young adolescents has given rise to parental warnings of school-age students over the use of e-cigarettes and a restriction on the types of flavors that can be manufactured and sold to minors. As of 2020, the U.S. Food and Drug Administration (FDA) has not approved e-cigarettes as a cessation aid. Nicotine is found in e-cigarettes, in which the inhaled vapor is produced from cartridges that contain flavoring and other chemicals. Use of e-cigarettes has been linked to leading nonsmokers and children to begin smoking.

12. *Answer:* B

Rationale: For smokers unwilling to quit, the U.S. Public Health Service (USPHS) recommends brief motivational interventions that can help increase attempts. (1) Ask patient about smoking status. (2) Advise to quit. (3) Assess for willingness or readiness to quit. (4) Assist in quitting. (5) Arrange a follow-up visit.

13. *Answer:* C

Rationale: *Helicobacter pylori* is associated with 31% of stomach cancers. About one third of the U.S. population is infected, often without symptoms. It is transmitted through fecal-oral and oral-oral routes. Hepatitis B virus and hepatitis C virus are associated with cirrhosis, liver cancer, and non-Hodgkin lymphoma. Growing evidence suggests that Type 2 diabetes is associated with increased risk for liver, endometrium, pancreas, colorectal, kidney, bladder, breast, and ovary cancers.

14. *Answer:* B

Rationale: Rubber workers have increased rates of prostate cancer. Steel workers have increased rates of lung cancer. Chemical workers have increased rates of bladder cancer. Miners have increased exposure to uranium and radon with a subsequent increase in gastric cancer and birth defects

15. *Answer:* B

Rationale: Current American Cancer Society recommendations for physical activity are that adults should have 150 to 300 minutes of moderate-intensity activity per week or 75 to 150 minutes of vigorous-intensity activity per week. Children should have at least 60 minutes of moderate- or vigorous-intensity activity each day, with vigorous activity on at least 3 days each week.

CHAPTER 2

1. *Answer:* C

Rationale: Sensitivity of a test measures the test's ability to correctly identify individuals with the disease. Reliability of a test is the level of agreement between measurements taken at different times. Negative predictive value is the percentage of persons who screen negative and who do not have the disease (true negatives). Specificity of a test measures the test's ability to correctly identify individuals who do not have the disease. Both sensitivity and specificity can show how accurate the results are, but they do not measure reliability.

2. *Answer:* A

Rationale: Between ages 21 to 29, cytology (Pap test, also known as a Pap smear) is recommended every 3 years. It is the primary screening tool for cervical cancer. Cervical cancer screening, endorsed by ACOG, ASCCP, and SGO, recommends cytology alone every 3 years for average risk individuals aged 21 to 29 years of age. Women age 30 to 65 can have screening with cytology alone every 3 years, FDA-approved hrHPV every 5 years, or co-testing (cytology + hrHPV) every 5 years. No screening is recommended over age 65 or in individuals with hysterectomy with cervix removed and no history of high-grade cervical precancerous lesions or cervical cancer.

3. *Answer:* D

Rationale: Average risk for breast cancer is defined as those with no personal history of breast cancer, no strong family history, or no known genetic pathogenic variant known to increase the risk. In average-risk women aged 45 to 54 years of age, an annual clinical breast exam with an annual mammography is recommended per NCCN guidelines. Women age 40 to 44 have the option to begin annual mammography. Women age 45 to 54 are recommended to have annual mammography. For those who are 55 years of age and older with an average risk, they have the option to switch to mammography every other year or choose to continue yearly mammogram. High-risk women are considered to be those with a greater than 20% lifetime risk, a pathogenic variant in a gene associated with an increased risk for developing breast cancers, or a first-degree relative. An annual mammography should start at age 30, along with an MRI screening, clinical breast exams every 6 to 12 months, and consideration of risk reduction strategies such as bilateral salpingo-oophorectomy, or chemoprevention per NCCN guidelines.

4. Answer: B

Rationale: The AUA Panel does not recommend routine PSA screening in men age 70+ years or any man with less than a 10- to 15-year life expectancy. Some men age 70+ years who are in excellent health may benefit from prostate cancer screening. The AUA panel recommends against PSA screening in men under age 40 years. The AUA panel does not recommend routine screening in men between ages 40 to 54 years at average risk. For men younger than age 55 years at higher risk, decisions regarding prostate cancer screening should be individualized. Those at higher risk may include men of African American race and those with a family history of metastatic or lethal adenocarcinomas (e.g., prostate, male and female breast cancer, ovarian, pancreatic) spanning multiple generations, affecting multiple first-degree relatives, and that developed at younger ages. For men ages 55 to 69 years the Panel recognizes that the decision to undergo PSA screening involves weighing the benefits of reducing the rate of metastatic prostate cancer and prevention of prostate cancer death against the known potential harms associated with screening and treatment. Digital rectal examination (DRE) should not be used as a stand-alone screening test. DRE is a complementary test to be used with PSA in asymptomatic individuals.

5. Answer: B

Rationale: The USPSTF recommends annual screening for lung cancer with low-dose computed tomography (LDCT) in adults aged 50 to 80 years who have a 20 pack-year smoking history and currently smoke or have quit within the past 15 years. Screening should be discontinued once a person has not smoked for 15 years or develops a health problem that substantially limits life expectancy or the ability or willingness to have curative lung surgery. Screening with chest x-ray or sputum cytology is not recommended.

6. Answer: C

Rationale: Screening tests are used to detect early stages of cancer in people who are otherwise healthy without any symptoms. Screening should be directed toward an important health problem and there should be effective treatment available to reduce cause-specific mortality. Treatment is more effective if initiated during the pre-symptomatic stage. Diagnostic tests are usually done to find out what is causing certain symptoms that have already become noticeable. However, not all screening tests are safe as there are some which may expose the body to radiation and others can potentially be invasive. Therefore, it is always important to outweigh the risks and benefits of a screening test.

7. Answer: A

Rationale: The goal of primary prevention is to reduce the risk factors of cancer or increase an individual's resistance to them. This is considered to be the most effective management for cancer. Secondary prevention prevents disease progression by the early detection and treatment of cancer. Tertiary prevention is the application of effective therapy to improve the outcomes and disease morbidity and mortality in affected individuals.

Quaternary prevention refers to avoiding consequences of unnecessary or excessive interventions.

8. Answer: A

Rationale: A positive predictive value (PPV) identifies the percentage of persons who screen positive who actually have the disease. Negative predictive value (NPV) is the percentage of persons who screen negative who do not have the disease. The higher the prevalence of a disease, the higher the PPV and lower the NPV. Sensitivity measures a test's ability to recognize persons who have the disease, also referred to as true positives. In other words, it does not miss any people who are ill. Specificity measures a test's ability to recognize persons who do not have the disease, also referred to as true negatives.

9. Answer: D

Rationale: Prevalence is the percentage or number of all individuals affected with the disease at a given point in time. Incidence is the number of new cases identified in a specified population occurring in a particular time period (such as 1 year). Mortality is the number of deaths identified in a specified population occurring in a particular time period (such as 1 year). Epidemiology is the study of the distribution and determinants of health-related states.

10. Answer: A

Rationale: Fatigue, malaise, recent weight gain, or weight loss are considered to be constitutional symptoms which can affect many different systems of the body. Dyspnea, orthopnea, and chest pain are considered cardiac symptoms. Increased urination, thirst, and perspiration are considered endocrine symptoms. Joint stiffness, vertigo, and limited movement are neurologic and musculoskeletal symptoms.

11. Answer: B

Rationale: The correct answer is B, a screening mammogram. This woman is asymptomatic. If a problem is detected on physical examination or on the screening mammogram, a diagnostic mammogram will be ordered. Women who have a known symptom of breast cancer (lump, nipple discharge, nipple deviation, skin changes, bulge, or puckering), women with a personal history of breast cancer, or women with breast implants will need a diagnostic mammogram. Screening mammography is recommended for women age 45 and over but may be started at age 40. A breast ultrasound and breast MRI are part of a diagnostic evaluation. Breast MRI can be used for screening in women at a 20% or higher risk of developing breast cancer, such as women with a strong family history of malignancy or a known pathogenic variant in a gene associated with an increased risk for developing cancer.

12. Answer: B

Rationale: A benefit of colonoscopy is the ability to visualize and remove precancerous polyps at the time of screening, thus preventing that polyp from turning into cancer. Risk of harm with colonoscopy or flexible sigmoidoscopy includes bleeding, infection, and perforation, which occurs in less than 1% of persons screening with direct visualization. For adults at average risk (e.g., those without a personal or family history of colorectal cancer, polyps, etc.), the age to begin colorectal

130

screening has been lowered to age 45, rather than age 50. Although colonoscopy is the preferred screening method, there is no direct evidence that suggests that colonoscopy improves mortality associated with colon cancer.

CHAPTER 3

1. *Answer:* A

Rationale: A cancer diagnosis impacts not only the affected individual, but also family and friends who may experience challenges in dealing with the illness and its sequalae. The National Comprehensive Cancer Network (NCCN) states that patients diagnosed with cancer are considered survivors from the time of diagnosis through the rest of their lives. Survivorship does extend to family, significant others, and children of patients with cancer. Survivorship is not limited to an early-stage cancer diagnosis. In addition, a time frame is not placed upon survivorship. A person does not have to wait a certain number of years before being considered a survivor. Survivorship is not limited to younger individuals.

2. *Answer:* C

Rationale: Late effects are absent or subclinical during treatment and occur months or years later, requiring focused follow-up care and monitoring. Long-term effects do not begin at least 1 year after treatment completion. In fact, long-term effects begin during treatment, persist throughout treatment, and may continue long after treatment has been completed. The first year after treatment has no impact on treatment for sequelae development and is not the most critical period of time. A patient who is of a younger age at the time of diagnosis—such as an adolescent or a young adult—does place the patient at higher risk for significant late effects, such as cardiomyopathy, where the cumulative incidence increases over time. Other late effects seen in adolescent and young adult survivors are fatigue, altered cognition, sexual dysfunction, and impaired fertility.

3. *Answer:* B

Rationale: Female survivors who have received chest radiation prior to age 30 should have annual breast imaging including mammography, breast MRI, or both starting at age 25 or at least 8 years after radiation, whichever occurs last. Lifestyle and age do contribute to risk for second malignancy and should be considered in planning second malignancy screening and health promotion counseling. PET scans are not routinely ordered in female breast survivors who have received chest radiation prior to age 30.

4. *Answer:* C

Rationale: Essential components of survivorship care include surveillance for recurrence, monitoring for late treatment effects, health promotion, and communication with other health care providers. Other health care providers such as urologists, primary care physicians, and nurse practitioners can assume the care of cancer survivors with transition care and communication of care plan. To promote care coordination, survivorship care plans should be provided to the patient and nononcology providers after treatment completion. This provision should be automatic and not require a patient request.

5. *Answer:* C

Rationale: Cancer survivors may experience a range of psychosocial challenges, making assessment an important component of follow-up care. Past coping skills, social support, and social history also help to guide the assessment. Fatigue, insomnia, and pain may be contributing factors to risk for depression, anxiety, and fear of recurrence. Reliable and valid screening tools such as the NCCN distress thermometer, Patient Health Questionnaire, or Hospital Anxiety and Depression Scale should be considered for anxiety and depression assessment, and, instead of being avoided, should be utilized regularly. Frequent changes in occupation and living arrangements should not be considered as a positive sign and could be seen as a sign that a person is having a difficult time adapting to life as a cancer survivor. While personal questions can be difficult for both the patient and the health care provider, they should not be avoided, as learning details about a patient's personal life can assist a health care provider in accessing how a person is coping with their life as a survivor.

6. *Answer:* B

Rationale: Since Mr. S. had led a previously active lifestyle, the recommendation should be for 150 minutes of moderate-intensity or 75 minutes of vigorous-intensity exercise per week as tolerated. Patients should be encouraged to remain or become physically active as soon as possible and to avoid sedentary behaviors so rest would be discouraged. Stretching is recommended for muscle health. Two to three weekly sessions of strength training that involves major muscle groups and tendons is recommended.

7. *Answer:* D

Rationale: Achieving and maintaining a healthy weight requires healthy eating habits, including portion control and a plant-based diet. Routine weight checks are helpful in assessing progress and should not be discouraged. Fast food, fried foods, and red meat consumption should be limited or avoided altogether, even once a healthy goal weight has been achieved.

8. *Answer:* C

Rationale: Adolescent and young adult survivors are at higher risk for physical and psychosocial sequelae, including limited access to follow-up care and insurance, as well as increased reports of medication nonadherence due to cost and limited financial resources. Special attention should be paid to survivors that are of school age so that cognitive issues such as altered attention, concentration, and processing speed are addressed.

9. *Answer:* B

Rationale: General health recommendations, such as those adapted from the American Cancer Society, are important for all survivors and should be reviewed or provided in writing to survivors to promote optimal health, even if unrelated to cancer history and treatment exposures. These include sun protection, safe sex, tobacco prevention, and abstinence, as well as information on the risks of vaping, bone health, and immunizations.

10. *Answer:* B

Rationale: The number of cancer survivors in the United States is predicted to increase to more than 22.1 million persons by 2030. Sixty-four percent of cancer survivors are 65 years of age or older. Sixty-five percent of cancer survivors have survived 5 years or more.

11. *Answer:* D

Rationale: Long-term cardiovascular effects include cardiomyopathy, congestive heart failure, carotid artery disease, valvular heart disease, arrhythmias, and pericardial disease. Pulmonary long-term effects include pulmonary fibrosis, restrictive lung disease, dyspnea, and pneumonitis. Being at a younger age at the time of treatment increases the risk for late physical sequalae. Prompt evaluation and a plan for long-term management are indicated.

12. *Answer:* B

Rationale: Fear of recurrence and anxiety are common around testing/surveillance appointments. It is important to encourage patients to keep their regularly scheduled follow-up appointments and let them know feelings of anxiety and fear are not unusual. Regular surveillance appointments afford the opportunity to detect and treat late effects and monitor/treat long-term effects to improve quality of life. This also includes assessment of psychosocial functioning. Symptoms should be reported if they are occurring with greater frequency or intensity as they may negatively impact quality of life and adherence to follow-up recommendations.

CHAPTER 4

1. *Answer:* A

Rationale: Palliative care is the concept that includes delivering ancillary therapy to treat side effects of treatment and the disease so that quality of life (QOL) is improved. It is defined as patient- and family-centered care that optimizes QOL by anticipating, preventing, and treating suffering as well as addressing physical, intellectual, emotional, social, and spiritual needs. The goal of palliative care is to facilitate patient autonomy, access to information, and choice with respect to treatment and symptom management throughout the continuum of illness. Palliative care is a structured approach that improves the QOL of patients and their families facing the problem associated with life-threatening illness, through the prevention and relief of suffering by means of early identification and focused assessment and treatment of pain and other physical, psychosocial, and spiritual problems. Key components of palliative care include patient- and family-centered care across the serious illness trajectory. Articulating goals of care and shared decision-making are essential elements of the palliative care approach.

B is incorrect because palliative care is not focused on the actual treatment of the cancer, but on the other issues surrounding it. C is not correct because palliative care is most commonly delivered by an interdisciplinary team of providers and ancillary staff. D is incorrect because

palliative care can be instituted at the time of diagnosis; it is not only reserved for use during end-of-life care.

2. *Answer:* C

Rationale: Although other insurance plans may have different parameters, Medicare maintains a parameter of 6 months life expectancy as a requirement for patients to access Medicare hospice benefits. Eligibility criteria should not be confused with length of service; patients can receive hospice care for as long as they meet eligibility criteria.

3. *Answer:* C

Rationale: Tertiary palliative care is provided by physicians and other team members who have specialty palliative care training. Tertiary palliative care is offered by a interprofessional team composed of physician (board-certified or fellowship-trained specialist), advanced practice registered nurse (APRN), nurse, social worker, and spiritual care provider. Tertiary palliative care addresses the most complex cases. There is typically formal involvement of the interprofessional team in teaching, ongoing quality improvement and safety initiatives, and research to further the palliative care field, as well as use of evidence-based national guidelines or expert consensus to support patient care processes. Secondary palliative care is offered in the form of a consultation by specialist physicians and their medical team and is typically provided within a hospital or treatment center/cancer center. Primary palliative care is provided by general practitioners and includes communication regarding advance care planning and prognosis and basic symptom management. Primary palliative care is typically provided in community settings such as a home or clinic.

4. *Answer:* C

Rationale: Two physicians must certify that the patient is terminally ill. This typically includes the referring provider and the hospice medical director. This is made after independent assessment of the patient and based on the best judgment of the two physicians.

5. *Answer:* C

Rationale: Patients must agree to cessation of aggressive therapy in order to enroll in hospice care. Getting a second opinion, being intubated for respiratory distress, and receiving chemotherapy are not included in a hospice care plan.

6. *Answer:* C

Rationale: Providers tend to be optimistic and usually estimate the patient's survival as four times longer than the patient actually survives.

7. *Answer:* C

Rationale: Patients live on average 18 days after admission to hospice. Hospice referrals may be delayed in pursuit of potentially curative therapies. Rapid clinical decline at end of life may also make transition to hospice logistically difficult. Physicians often are reluctant to discuss hospice, as it may be perceived by patients as "giving up."

8. *Answer:* A

Rationale: The first modern hospice, St. Christopher, was founded in 1967 in England, and based on the work of Dame Cicely Saunders, whose work with terminally ill, starting in 1948, is credited as starting the modern hospice movement. The first hospice program in the United States was opened in 1974 in Branford, CT and was founded by Dr. Florence Wald, Yale School of Nursing dean, and an early pioneer in the hospice movement in the United States. The Medicare hospice benefit was approved by Congress in 1982 after demonstration projects demonstrated that interdisciplinary team care focusing on quality of life and addressing symptom burden of terminal illness improved outcomes and cost less than usual care. The Medicare benefit became permanent in 1986, which provided a stable source of payment for hospice care and resulted in a steady growth of hospice programs throughout the United States.

9. *Answer:* D

Rationale: Grief benefits are offered to the family of hospice patients after the death of the patient so that they do not have to rely on only other family members, clergy, or therapists. Grief counseling is a large part of hospice care, is the responsibility of the entire interdisciplinary team, and support groups should be offered to all family members whenever possible.

10. *Answer:* B

Rationale: SWAT, or the Social Work Assessment Tool, is the tool most commonly used by social workers to evaluate the patient/family environment and assess their sociocultural needs. Patients, family members, and/or caregivers are rated on their coping in the following domains: End-of-life care decisions consistent with patients' religious and cultural norms; patients' thoughts of suicide or wanting hastened death; death anxiety; environmental preferences, social support, financial resources, safety, comfort, complicated anticipatory grief, denial, and spirituality. NCCN stands for the National Comprehensive Cancer Network, ECOG is the abbreviation for the Eastern Cooperative Oncology Group, and EQOL is the abbreviation for an evaluation of the quality of life of the patient.

11. *Answer:* B

Rationale: Positioning the patient on their side can often decrease the noise and distress caused by secretions pooling in the back of the oropharynx. These can also be alleviated by anticholinergic drugs and suctioning, but these interventions are more invasive. Cool wash cloths do not help terminal secretions.

12. *Answer:* C

Rationale: If the score of the Distress Screening tool is lower than a 4, then the tool suggests that the primary oncologist and their staff can manage the distress. If the score is 4 or higher, the patient should be referred to specialty services such as psychiatrist, support group, clergy, social worker, counselor, or palliative care team.

13. *Answer:* C

Rationale: Describing the quality of Cheyne-Stoke breathing to the patient's family can help them recognize this as one of the signs of impending death. Other clinical signs of impending death which families should be aware of include pulselessness of the radial artery, respiration

with mandibular movement, decreased urine output, terminal secretions, nonreactive pupils, and a decreased response to visual stimuli. Rapid breathing, restless movements, and bounding pulse are less likely to be signs of eminent death, though restless movement may precede the more terminal phases.

14. *Answer:* A

Rationale: In end-of-life situations, MANH is unlikely to prolong life and can lead to complications that increase physical suffering and is not known to reduce the sensation of thirst or dry mouth. According to the Hospice and Palliative Nurses Association, many patients experience the sensation of dry mouth but this symptom is associated with other factors besides lack of fluids, and, as a result, the introduction of parenteral fluids is unlikely to alleviate thirst. The use of MANH may increase the likelihood of aspiration and MANH given through a feeding tube is associated with an increased chance of infection and fluid overload.

15. *Answer:* D

Rationale: According to the NCCN's standards of palliative care in oncology, symptom burden from disease or treatment is anticipated, prevented, and skillfully managed. This standard is best exemplified in how the palliative care team treated G.T.'s symptom of pain and is reflected in D. A is incorrect because developing a treatment plan for cancer is not a standard of palliative care, even though respecting the autonomy of the patient is a standard. B is also incorrect. A standard of palliative care in oncology is treating psychosocial and spiritual distress with the same importance as a physical condition, but, in this example, the palliative care team was dealing with the symptom of pain, making B an incorrect response. C is also incorrect. End-of-life care is not a standard of palliative care identified by the NCCN.

16. *Answer:* C

Rationale: Advance directives include Living Will documents and Durable Power of Attorney for Health Care documents. Living Will documents specify patient preferences around life-sustaining treatments and resuscitation and typically take effect in the event of irreversible or terminal illness. Durable Power of Attorney for Health Care documents specify the choice and authorization of a surrogate medical decision maker if needed.

17. *Answer:* C

Rationale: Specialty palliative care is offered in five major service delivery models which include (1) acute inpatient consultative teams; (2) acute inpatient palliative care units (APCUs); (3) outpatient palliative care or supportive care clinics integrated within ambulatory care, oncology specialty clinics, radiation oncology, or infusion centers; (4) community-based palliative care programs; and (5) hospice care.

18. *Answer:* C

Rationale: The top five principal diagnosis categories of patients enrolled in the hospice benefit in fiscal year 2019 were (1) Alzheimer's/Dementia/Parkinson's disease (20.9%); (2) respiratory (7.1%); (3) circulatory/heart (6.4%); (4) stroke/CVA (5.4%); and (5) cancer (4.9%).

19. *Answer:* D

Rationale: Inpatient respite care is provided in an approved inpatient facility on a short-term basis for up to 5 consecutive days to give the caregiver a rest. While scheduled rest breaks, increasing nurse visits, and help from a neighbor may help, they will not be adequate to relieve exhaustion.

20. *Answer:* B

Rationale: Complicated or prolonged grief is an intense, intrusive, maladaptive response that persists greater than 1 year beyond the loss. Anticipatory grief is the psychological, social, and somatic responses to an anticipated loss and is an unconscious process. Disenfranchised grief occurs when the loss cannot be openly acknowledged, socially validated, or publicly mourned. Examples include death of a person in an unsanctioned relationship such as an extramarital affair or outside of a legally recognized union, loss from miscarriage or abortion, or loss of the essence of the individual before actual death (e.g., severe dementia). Grief is a normal response to loss.

21. *Answer:* D

Rationale: Medical aid in dying may also be known as physician-assisted dying, physician-assisted suicide, or request for hastened death. Euthanasia occurs when another individual administers lethal medication to a person with intent to end life, at that person's voluntary and competent request. Palliative care is an interdisciplinary care delivery system designed to anticipate, prevent, and manage physical, psychological, social, and spiritual suffering to optimize quality of life for patients, their families, and caregivers. Hospice is a philosophy of care, a care delivery system, and a regulated insurance benefit for individuals with a prognosis of less than 6 months.

22. *Answer:* C

Rationale: The Edmonton Symptom Assessment System–Revised (ESAS-r) measures nine common symptoms in palliative care including pain, tiredness, drowsiness, nausea, lack of appetite, depression, anxiety, shortness of breath, and well-being.

23. *Answer:* C

Rationale: Nonpharmacological management of delirium includes ensuring the patient has their glasses and hearing aids to decrease disorientation. Decreasing disturbances in sleep/wake cycle can be helpful, including avoiding awakening the patient unless necessary. Pharmacological interventions include utilizing haloperidol or other antipsychotics. Since P.T. has delirium, antidepressants and opioids are not likely to be helpful and may further aggravate the delirium.

24. *Answer:* D

Rationale: In some cases, symptoms may be so severe that they cannot be adequately managed despite comprehensive conventional treatments. Palliative sedation, the intentional lowering of wakefulness towards, and possibly including, unconsciousness, may be considered to treat refractory, uncontrolled severe symptoms. Palliative sedation utilizes nonopioid medications such as benzodiazepines, barbiturates, or propofol.

25. *Answer:* B

Rationale: The Palliative Performance Scale (PPS) is a validated tool which measures both performance status and predicts survival of palliative care patients with cancer. PPS measures five essential functional domains: ambulation, activity level and burden of disease, self-care, oral intake, and level of consciousness. Each domain is divided into 11 levels from 0% to 100% and scored in 10%-point increments. A score of 0% indicates death and 100% indicates fully independent and healthy. The PPS does not measure pain, orientation, or hydration.

CHAPTER 5

1. *Answer:* A

Rationale: Created by Dr. Harold Freeman in New York City in 1990, the first patient navigation program targeted women with breast cancer. Fifty percent of these women were uninsured. Many of these women were black. Today navigators work with oncology patients with a variety of diagnoses.

2. *Answer:* A

Rationale: The goals are to: serve as a patient's advocate, identify and resolve barriers to care, provide education about a treatment plan that empowers patients to actively engage in decision-making and self-care, provide education on symptom and side effect management to reduce early and late treatment associated complications, reduce distress, and provide psychosocial support. This care can occur throughout the cancer trajectory and can be in person or by other communication methods. Only A represents a goal of care.

3. *Answer:* A

Rationale: The lay navigator is a trained nonprofessional or volunteer who provides individualized assistance to patients, families, and caregivers to help overcome health care system barriers and facilitate timely access to quality health and psychosocial care from prediagnosis through all phases of the cancer experience. A novice nurse navigator is a nurse who has worked 2 years or less in the ONN role and is building upon his or her academic preparation, nursing knowledge, and oncology navigation experience to develop in the ONN role. An expert ONN who has worked at least 3 years, is proficient in the role, and has the education and experience to use critical thinking and decision-making skills pertaining to the evolution of navigation processes and the individual ONN. There is no community clinic navigator.

4. *Answer:* C

Rationale: There was a significant increase in 5-year survival rates by 39% to 70%. The goal of the program was to reduce cancer mortality by improving access quality care.

5. *Answer:* C

Rationale: The AONN+ was incorporated in 2009.

6. *Answer:* A

Rationale: A PNRP study showed that delays in diagnosing cancer can be overcome with patient navigation, addressing unemployment, housing type, and marital status.

7. **Answer:** C

Rationale: Provider, patient, and family satisfaction scores directly assess ONN value. Other measures of value include timeliness of care/access to care, management and monitoring of the plan of care, clinical trial accrual, and reduced hospital readmissions. The other answers are the responsibility of inpatient nurses.

8. **Answer:** A

Rationale: The nurse navigator should assess the patient's psychosocial distress during each clinic visit. A psychologist does not need to be present to assess for psychosocial distress. While patients might experience psychosocial distress at the end stage of disease, patients can experience psychosocial distress at any time during the cancer continuum.

9. **Answer:** C

Rationale: In order to evaluate navigation services, it is necessary to examine processes that link navigation to improved patient outcomes by using standardized instruments. The limitations to determine effectiveness are associated with studies with relatively small sample sizes, poor response rates to questionnaires, not using valid instruments to gather data, and lack of data about patients who have used navigation services.

10. **Answer:** A

Rationale: This is a transportation barrier because the patient does not have the capability or resources to reach the facility for appointments and treatment. These are many different types of barriers to care. There is no indication that there is a cultural or language barrier, or a lack of family support.

11. **Answer:** B

Rationale: Navigators can communicate with a financial assistance team or designated financial assistance experts to help decrease the financial burden to patients. There are options to offer patients: medication assistance programs, charity care, copay assistance programs, as well as assistance with transportation and lodging expenses. This is not a transportation barrier. It is not realistic for the treating facility's staff to pay for medications and patients cannot donate medications to other patients.

12. **Answer:** D

Rationale: AONN+ offers the ONN-Certified Generalist and Certified Generalist Thoracic certifications, as well as the Oncology Patient Navigator-Certified Generalist. ONS offers certifications but they are not designated as certifications in nurse navigation. ONC stands for Oncology Certified Nurse and is not specific to patient navigation. ACOS stands for American College of Surgeons; although they require navigation for credentialing and certification of an institution, they do not offer individual certification for nurse navigators.

13. **Answer:** D

Rationale: Coordination of the care of patients with a past, current, or potential diagnosis of cancer includes timely scheduling of appointments, diagnostic testing, and procedures to expedite the plan of care and to promote continuity of care. The communication competency includes assisting patients with cancer, families, and caregivers to overcome health care system barriers, (e.g., transportation, child care, elder care, housing, language, culture, literacy, role disparity, psychosocial, employment, financial, insurance) and facilitates referrals as appropriate to mitigate barriers. Education and resources competencies facilitate informed decision-making and timely access to quality health and psychosocial care throughout the cancer care continuum. The fourth competency is to establish and maintain the professional role of the ONN such as through quality improvement of an organization's navigation program.

CHAPTER 6

1. **Answer:** C

Rationale: Shared decision-making is a model of care delivery that requires collaboration between the patient and the clinician. Key elements include that there are at least two participants, which include the clinician and patient. It can also include other treatment team members and patient's family. Both parties share information. Provider(s) define/explain the health care problem and present options. Both parties take steps to build consensus about preferred treatment, weighing risks, and benefits. Parties discuss benefits/risks/costs, clarify patient values/preferences, and discuss patient ability/self-efficacy. Provider(s) present what is known and make recommendations. Provider(s) clarify the patient's understanding. Decision is made via mutual agreement between patient and clinician on treatment approach (verbal and/or written). SDM can be implemented in a variety of health care settings; location does not matter. It has been validated with research. The focus is to improve communication, not necessarily to lower health care costs.

2. **Answer:** C

Rationale: Step 1 of AHRQ's shared decision-making process requires the clinician to inform the patient of choices as well as explicitly invite and involve the patient in the decision-making process. Step 2: Assist the patient in comparing and evaluating treatment options by discussing the risks and benefits of each option. Step 3: Assess the patient's goals, values, and priorities and incorporate what matters most to the patient. Step 4: Make a decision with the patient. Step 5: Evaluate the treatment decision: plan to follow-up and revisit the decision, monitor progress, and revise as needed.

3. **Answer:** C

Rationale: Options A, B, and D are all long-term benefits of shared decision-making. C is a short-term benefit. Short-term benefits include increased confidence in treatment decisions, higher satisfaction with treatment decisions, enhanced trust with providers, improved self-efficacy, and less stress and anxiety related to treatment decision-making. Long-term benefits relate to adherence to treatment, improved quality of life, and remission.

4. *Answer:* C

Rationale: Oncology nurses reported the following barriers to shared decision-making implementation: scope of practice, limited time, limited resources devoted to shared decision-making education and training, lack of institutional policy that protects time and allows the nurse to engage in SDM, noisy environments that are not conducive to discussion and lack of leadership support for shared decision-making. A lack of systemic alerts/triggers in the electronic medical record (to incorporate decision aids) is another structural/system barrier.

5. *Answer:* C

Rationale: Older adults with cancer reported that convenience of treatment, trust in their physician and their recommendations, and seeing the necessity of treatment were influential in their treatment decisions. Access to patient decision aids and educational videos, as well as the number of infusion nurses has not been reported as an influential factor for treatment decisions in older adults with cancer.

6. *Answer:* B

Rationale: Two published systematic reviews on preferred and actual preferences for patient participation in decision-making found that the Degner and Beaton's Pattern of Treatment Decision-making questionnaire (Control Preferences Scale) was the most frequently used instrument to measure the patient's preferences for participation in decision-making.

7. *Answer:* D

Rationale: D is the correct answer because it addresses uncertainty and the complexity of a diagnosis. A reflects the advocacy role, B reflects the patient education role, and C reflects the information sharing to multidisciplinary team role of the oncology nurse during the treatment decision-making process.

8. *Answer:* A

Rationale: An oncology nurse's role in shared decision-making can be complex and take on many different aspects. The oncology nurse meeting with S.T. provided both patient education material and psychosocial support for the patient. In the future, the oncology nurse might provide advocacy for the patient, but at this time in their nurse and patient relationship, the nurse is offering patient education and psychosocial support. The oncology nurse did not complete a patient needs assessment, nor perform an outcome evaluation, so answers B through D are incorrect.

CHAPTER 7

1. *Answer:* D

Rationale: Proto-oncogenes that are pathogenically altered, such as *Ras*, can enable a cancer cell to become self-sufficient in growth, and are common in pancreatic and colorectal cancers. In chromosome translocations, one chromosome moves to another as the cell divides, thereby activating an oncogene, such as occurs in CML where the BCR gene on chromosome 9 is fused to the *Abl* gene on chromosome 22, making a protein called tyrosine kinase, which proliferates myeloid cells. Missense

pathogenic variants change a DNA base pair that results in the substitution of one amino acid for another in the protein made by a gene and is typically the cause of sickle cell disease. An insertion pathogenic variant is the addition of one or more nucleotide base pairs into a DNA sequence, such as occurs in Huntington's disease or fragile X syndrome.

2. *Answer*: B

Rationale: Tumor suppressor genes control cell proliferation by preventing uncontrolled growth. When pathogenically altered, these genes no longer suppress proliferation; it is as though the brakes of a car have been released and the car cannot stop. Caretaker genes function to repair mistakes in DNA and maintain chromosome stability during replication of normal cells. Sex-linked genes are genes that are located on the x and y sex chromosomes inherited from the mother and father. Senescence is the irreversible arrest of cell division in normally proliferating cells that allows for the inactivation of diseased or damaged cells.

3. *Answer:* A

Rationale: A germline pathogenic variant is an altered inherited gene that is passed from a parent to their offspring through the x or y chromosome and becomes incorporated into every cell in the offspring. A somatic pathogenic variant develops due to exposure to carcinogens that alter the DNA in body cell; it is not inherited. Microsatellite refers to a series of randomly repeated nucleotides. The variation in the number of these tandem repeated nucleotides can be identified in pathology report. Normal cells have a consistent length of nucleotides. A carcinogen is any substance that can cause cancer, such as repeated exposures to toxic environmental or occupational substances.

4. *Answer:* B

Rationale: During carcinogenesis, normal cells are transformed into cancer cells through a complex and dynamic process that starts with pathogenic alterations in regulatory cells and is promoted by genomic instability, inflammation, and interactions within the tumor microenvironment. Angiogenesis is the creation of new blood vessels from existing ones to provide nutrients and remove waste products. Normal cells have a developmental regulatory program called epithelial mesenchymal transition (EMT). This process causes epithelial cells to lose cell polarity and cell–cell adhesion and have invasive properties so that they can become mesenchymal cells. This process is involved in mesoderm formation and neural tube formation during embryogenesis. It has also been found to play a role in wound healing and organ fibrosis. Epigenetics describes a mechanism that may change the activity of a gene without changing the sequence of DNA.

5. **Answer**: A

Rationale: Epigenetic changes in cellular DNA are a type of genetic reprogramming whereby the activity of a gene becomes changed without changing the sequence of DNA in the gene. Lifestyle factors may induce epigenetic changes, including diet, obesity, tobacco use, and alcohol consumption, as well as toxic environmental exposures.

The cells containing the modified DNA are passed from parent to offspring. Polymorphic microbiomes refer to the variability in the microbiomes of individuals that can impact their cancer phenotype, including cancer development, malignant progression, and response to therapy. Stimulation of angiogenesis refers to the ability of cancer cells to secrete substances that lead to the creation of new blood vessels that support continued tumor growth by providing nutrients and removing waste products from tumors. Tumor necrosis factor is a cytokine released by white blood cells in response to inflammation. This cytokine may have an antitumor effect (in immune surveillance); however, it plays a role in carcinogenesis as well.

6. *Answer:* C

Rationale: The acquisition of cancer hallmarks is classified as the second phase of the process of tumor formation. A tumor is formed from a single precursor cell containing genetic alterations that undergoes clonal expansion. Clonal evolution is the process by which cells within a tumor accumulate genetic changes over time that differ from one cell to the next. An initiating pathogenic alteration is considered the first step in the process, acquisition of cancer hallmarks is next, and, finally, the cell undergoes further genetic evolution.

7. *Answer:* D

Rationale: Cancer cells can acquire characteristics that give them a growth advantage over normal cells. The ability to resist programmed cell death, a feature that regulates the life span of normal cells, allows cancer cells to continue proliferating and become immortal. Cancer cells do not inhibit angiogenesis; they are able to secrete substances that stimulate angiogenesis. A hallmark of cancer cells is their ability to continue dividing unchecked by constraints such as contact inhibition. In normal cells, contact with one another inhibits further cell growth.

8. *Answer:* B

Rationale: Epidermal growth factor receptors participate in colon cancer development and play a role in some colon cancer metastases. Vascular endothelial growth factors may cause tumor cells to spread to regional lymph nodes. Nerve growth factors are primarily involved in the regulation of growth, maintenance, proliferation, and survival of certain target neurons, especially those that transmit pain, temperature, and touch sensations. There is no medial growth factor.

9. *Answer:* A

Rationale: Clonal evolution describes the process of cells within a tumor accumulating genetic changes over time that differ from one cell to the next and are heterogeneous for different traits. Even though a tumor may consist of cells that arose from the same mother cell, clones of cells may have arisen within the tumor that are genotypically different from one another and possess more aggressive growth abilities. This characteristic forms the basis for using combination therapies to destroy tumor cells. Convergent evolution and changes and coevolution are two of the six important patterns of macroevolution, which are not involved in the

development of carcinogenesis. Perseverance is a term to indicate steadfastness and does not relate to the process of carcinogenesis.

10. *Answer:* D

Rationale: Angiogenesis is the creation of new blood vessels from existing ones. A tumor cannot grow larger than a few millimeters in size without the presence of new blood vessels that can deliver an adequate supply of oxygen and nutrients to the tumor cells and remove their waste products. Carcinogenesis is the formation of a cancer where normal cells are transformed into cancer cells. Glycolysis is the breakdown of glucose by enzymes, releasing energy and pyruvic acid, and is not involved in metastases. Pathogenesis of a disease is the biological mechanism that leads to the disease state and can describe the origin and development of the disease.

11. *Answer:* B

Rationale: Among the survival methods that cancer cells circulating in the bloodstream may use to avoid detection and destruction by immune cells is to combine with platelets to form platelet–tumor aggregates or tumor cell emboli. Cancer cells can secrete proteases or other substances to break down solid nearby tissues, but this does not help to avoid detection. Cancer cells that enter nearby lymph nodes are typically destroyed by the immune cells that are present there. Senescent cells are old cells that no longer participate in cell division. Normal cells become senescent; cancer cells are able to overcome the tumor suppressor action of senescence and continue proliferating. Senescence does not apply to cancer cells avoiding detection while in the bloodstream.

12. *Answer:* C

Rationale: "Skip metastasis" is an example of tumor cell dissemination throughout the lymphatic system. "Skip metastasis" occurs when cells bypass the first lymph node and reach more distant sites. Tumors bypassing one organ and metastasizing in another is not an example of a pathway in which tumor cells disseminate. Tumor cells spreading through pulmonary capillary beds or pulmonary arteriovenous (AV) shunts is an example of arterial spread. Arteries have thick walls and are not able to be penetrated as veins are.

13. *Answer:* A

Rationale: Non–small cell lung cancer (NSCLC) accounts for 85% of lung cancer diagnoses. It is also the most common type of primary tumor metastasizing to brain, with about 9% of patients with NSCLC developing brain metastases. Prostate cancer commonly metastasizes to the adrenal gland, bone, liver, and lung. Liver cancer is often the site of metastatic cancer. Colorectal cancer typically metastasizes to the liver, lung, and peritoneum.

14. *Answer:* D

Rationale: A history of sunburns and tanning parlor use is a key association and cause of cancer. Too much fiber in a person's daily diet is not identified as a key association and cause of cancer; rather, lack of fiber is identified as a cause for cancer. Other key associations and causes of cancer include lack of exercise and daily intake of processed red meat. Five to nine servings of fruits and vegetables are recommended daily. Lack or limited intake of fruits and vegetables is a key association and cause of cancer.

15. *Answer:* C

Rationale: Metastatic disease spread to distant organs or tissues is the major cause of death from cancer. The presence of primary disease located within the breast or in nearby lymph nodes is not a major cause of cancer death. The presence of existing comorbid disease conditions would not be a cause of death from cancer.

CHAPTER 8

1. *Answer:* C

Rationale: The appearance of new lesions in this patient represents the escape phase of the extrinsic tumor suppressor mechanism. The escape phase occurs when persistent tumor clones that have evaded the innate and adaptive immune systems result in clinically measurable disease, as seen in this patient. The elimination phase represents ongoing immune surveillance, where the host is cancer free. In the situation above, the patient has relapsed. The equilibrium phase is a phase by which a rare tumor clone undergoes cellular alterations to avoid elimination by the innate immune system. There is no evidence of clinically measurable disease in this phase. This does not apply to the patient's situation, as he/she has new lesions. Progression is not a phase of the proposed tumor suppression mechanism.

2. *Answer:* A

Rationale: Immune surveillance is carried out by both the innate and adaptive immune response systems which act to destroy clinically unmeasurable tumors. Innate and adaptive immunity is the elimination phase of extrinsic tumor suppression mechanism, where the host's immune system responds to microscopic invasion by destroying circulating tumor cells. This is a homeostatic process ongoing in hosts with an intact immune system. B is an example of the equilibrium phase of tumor suppression where the first line of defense with natural barriers and inflammatory response have been overcome. Humoral and cell-mediated immunity mechanisms are now holding tumor growth in check. C is incorrect as the equilibrium phase occurs once resistant tumor clones escape immune surveillance and innate immunity has been overcome. D is incorrect as the mechanism of action with chemotherapeutic agents is cell death through cytotoxic cellular processes that inhibit mitosis. Immunotherapy agents function to increase immune surveillance through modification of the adaptive immune system.

3. *Answer:* A

Rationale: Only the adaptive immune system possesses memory. The adaptive immune system provides a long-lived immune response by creating antibodies and T lymphocytes that can recognize and respond rapidly to repeat exposures to specific antigens. The innate immune system is a rapid cellular response to invasion of pathogens and/or tissue damage and does not rely on previous exposure to initiate an immune response.

Humoral immunity uses antibodies produced by B lymphocytes, which respond to a specific antigen. Cell-mediated immunity uses T lymphocytes to active immune responses. Inflammatory response is controlled by the innate immune system, not adaptive immune system. Nonspecific processes for immune defense is related to innate immunity.

4. *Answer:* B

Rationale: Tumor cells can acquire the ability to evade the adaptive immune system by promoting T-cell exhaustion and dysfunction. Clones of tumor cells can emerge within a tumor that are able to promote T cells to increase PD1/PDL1 on their surfaces, which allows them to "hide" from T-cell immune surveillance. Thus tumor growth and cancer progression continues. Recently developed immunotherapeutic medications, called checkpoint inhibitors, use this known concept of tumor biology to block tumor cells from promoting hosts' T-cell exhaustion, which stimulates the adaptive immune system. Chemotherapy resistance occurs as a result of changes in tumor biology, such as drug inactivation, drug target alteration, drug efflux, DNA damage repair, and cell death inhibition. These are changes that occur with the tumor's interaction with the chemotherapeutic agent and not with the host's immune system. The innate immune system is the body's first line of defense against host invaders and works with the adaptive immune system in tumor surveillance. When the innate immune system can no longer keep the tumor in check (equilibrium phase), the adaptive immune system can function independently to perform ongoing immune surveillance. Another method of immune system evasion is decreasing or losing antigens, not increasing, on the tumor's surface. When this occurs, the adaptive immune system can no longer recognize the tumor cell. This leads to ongoing progression/reproduction of cancer.

5. *Answer:* D

Rationale: An example of humoral immunity is the production of plasma cells. Humoral immunity involves antibodies produced by B lymphocytes. Each B cell reproduces and differentiates to become either a memory B cell or plasma cell. Plasma cells then circulate and bind to specific antigens, which starts a cascade of cytokine reactions to attract macrophages and NK cells. Antigen presentation refers to the process of activating T cells, which is called cell-mediated immunity. T lymphocytes activation by APCs leads to T-cell multiplication immune surveillance/ response. T lymphocytes are involved in cell-mediated immunity as part of the adaptive immune system. Neutrophils are a part of the innate immune system, not adaptive immune system.

6. *Answer:* A

Rationale: Cytokines assist with cell signaling during immune responses. Cytokines are proteins secreted by immune cells to facilitate communication between cells of the immune system to aid in rapid response. Macrophages are immune cells of the innate immune system that recognize, ingest, and kill microbes. They release cytokines to produce a nonspecific inflammatory response and present antigens to T cells. Plasma cells are differentiated B cells, which produce one specific antibody against a specific antigen as part of the humoral immune response. Erythrocytes or red blood cells develop in the bone marrow and transport oxygen to the body's tissues.

7. *Answer:* C

Rationale: The bone marrow functions as both a primary and secondary lymphoid tissue. The thymus is a primary lymphoid organ and allows for the maturation of the lymphocytes. The spleen, lymph nodes, and tonsils/adenoids are examples of secondary lymphoid tissue. The spleen responds to bloodborne antigens, while the lymph nodes initiate immune responses to antigens circulating in the lymph, skin, or mucosal surfaces.

8. *Answer:* C

Rationale: The T cells migrate to the thymus gland for maturation and are integral to immune surveillance and response. T cells are named for the thymus gland in which they mature. NK cells are large granular cells that release cytokines, migrate rapidly to the site of the inflammation, and directly kill tumor or viral-infected cells without previous antigen exposure. B cells develop in the bone marrow (for which they are named) and include memory B cells and plasma cells. Dendritic cells capture foreign cells and process antigens.

9. *Answer:* A

Rationale: Granulocytes have granules in cytoplasm with enzymes that aid in digestion of foreign particles (phagocytosis) and cause inflammation. Neutrophils are the most abundant granulocytes, but they only live about 6 hours. Neutrophils cause inflammatory response due to engulfing and destroying foreign particles and debris. Basophils have IgE receptors that are involved in allergic responses and cause release of histamine and prostaglandins. Eosinophils attack parasites and secrete cytokines that cause inflammation during allergic responses. Macrophages rapidly recognize, ingest, and kill microbes; macrophages are not granulocytes.

CHAPTER 9

1. *Answer:* B

Rationale: Precision medicine is the use of specific information about a person's genes, proteins, and environment to prevent, diagnose, and treat disease. Tumor size, treatment history, and laboratory values may affect response but are not the primary consideration when applying precision medicine. Expression of programmed death-ligand 1 (PD-L1) is an example of using genomic information from the tumor and impacts treatment decisions in head and neck squamous cell, Hodgkin lymphoma, Merkel cell carcinoma, and urothelial carcinomas. Targeted therapies that might be utilized in those with high PD-L1 expression include atezolizumab, avelumab, durvalumab, nivolumab, and pembrolizumab. The patient has cancer of the bile duct (cholangiocarcinoma), and the presence of a large mass in the right lobe of the liver is important to consider when planning therapy but is not a part of precision medicine.

2. *Answer:* A

Rationale: Biomarkers do not provide information on the origin of a tumor or low long it has been present. Biomarkers can determine disease severity and outcomes and aids in treatment planning. A biomarker is a molecule found in blood, tissues, or other body fluids that signals the presence of a condition or disease; can be used to evaluate response to treatment. Predictive biomarkers provide information on the effect of a therapeutic intervention. A prognostic biomarker provides information about the patient's overall cancer outcome, regardless of therapy. Germline pathogenic variants are biomarkers that provide information about cancer risk for the individual and family and can guide treatment if risk-reducing surgery is appropriate.

3. *Answer:* C

Rationale: ER/PR/Her-2 Neu are examples of biomarkers used to guide treatment decisions. Germline genetic testing might confirm the presence of a hereditary cancer predisposition syndrome. ER/PR/Her2 Neu status does not alter the dose of the drug but it might alter the choice of agent. Adjuvant chemotherapy decisions might also be based on tools that assess a combination of genes on a tumor to determine the potential efficacy of chemotherapy (e.g. Mammaprint, Endopredict, or Oncotype). Er/PR/Her2Neu status might be one criteria utilized to determine if a patient is eligible for a clinical trial but it will not be the sole criteria.

4. *Answer:* D

Rationale: Pharmacogenomics is the integration of pharmacology and genomics in developing safe and effective medications. Pharmacogenomics can determine safe doses based on genomic data. It can help reduce the use of drugs with serious or toxic side effects, thereby increasing rates of adherence to therapy. It does not necessarily decrease the cost of medications or increase enrollment in clinical trials.

5. *Answer:* C

Rationale: Clinically relevant biomarkers are associated with specific cancers; ideal targets are present in cancer cells but are absent from normal cells. Targeted therapies can provoke severe adverse reactions, albeit different from traditional chemotherapy. Targeted therapies can be classified as hazardous drugs and can be delivered orally (small molecule drugs) or parenterally (monoclonal abs).

6. *Answer:* A

Rationale: Genetic testing results may take up to 8 weeks and cause waiting-related patient anxiety when treatment is dependent on results. Germline genetic testing has implications for both the patient and family members. It can be expensive and insurance preauthorization is often required. Informed consent issues include how privacy will be maintained and use of the specimen after testing is completed.

7. *Answer:* B

Rationale: Gene deletion is defined as the loss of all or part of a gene found in cancer cells, and other genetic diseases. Deletion is a type of variant involving the loss of genetic material. It can be small, involving a single missing DNA base pair, or large, involving a piece of a chromosome. Answer A is epigenetic. A heritable change that does not alter the DNA sequence but changes gene expression is defined as an epigenetic alteration. Gene overexpression is the increase in the copies of a protein made from a gene that may play a role in cancer development. Gene amplification refers to the increase in the number of copies of a gene that may cause cancer cell growth or resistance to anticancer drugs.

8. *Answer:* D
Rationale: Patients provide biospecimens for biorepository and research purposes in addition to use in clinical decision-making, and an ethical consideration for a patient undergoing treatment with precision medicine is whether or not their personal information is safe and secure from cybercrime as well as intrusions from the government. Adverse events and side effects are clinical concerns and not necessarily ethical considerations, and, while financial toxicity is a major concern for patients and families undergoing expensive treatments, the cost of treatment may not be an ethical concern, especially if costs were explained before treatment begins. It also may not be an ethical concern if the patient received education prior to treatment of potentially serious side effects that could compromise quality of life and that unexpected life-threatening events can occur.

CHAPTER 10

1. *Answer:* B
Rationale: The "central dogma" of molecular biology, that is, "DNA makes RNA, and RNA makes protein," guides the production of protein for all bodily functions. This knowledge aids in the education of patients and families about their genetic testing results and the pathophysiology of carcinogenesis. A is incorrect because, while this is an accurate statement, it is not necessary information for oncology nursing practice. C is false as RNA contains uracil instead of the thymine contained in DNA. All humans are actually 99.9% identical in their genetic make-up and 0.1% different.

2. *Answer:* D
Rationale: Chromosomes are threadlike structures of DNA containing the genetic information of the cell. There are 46 chromosomes per cell. Humans have 23 pairs of chromosomes—22 pairs of numbered chromosomes, called autosomes, and one pair of sex chromosomes, X and Y. Each parent contributes one chromosome to each pair so that offspring get half of their chromosomes from their mother and half from their father.

3. *Answer:* B
Rationale: HBOC is associated with ovarian cancer especially when it occurs before age 50. HBOC is also associated with early onset breast cancer (before age 50) especially when there are multiple family members diagnosed with breast cancer, triple negative breast cancer diagnosed before age 60, or a family history of pancreatic

cancer or metastatic prostate cancer. A is incorrect because these individuals are each from both maternal and paternal lineages. C is also incorrect, because even though her brother is young, testicular cancer is not associated with HBOC and testicular cancer is usually diagnosed in younger men. D is incorrect because childhood leukemia is not typically associated with HBOC.

4. *Answer:* C
Rationale: Germline pathogenic variants occur in the reproductive cells of a person with an inherited predisposition to cancer. A is incorrect because single nucleotide polymorphism (SNVs) occurs in both germline and somatic cells. They can be pathogenic or benign. B is incorrect as both males and females develop pathogenic variants in their somatic cells over a lifetime. Only females have a monthly reproductive cycle. D is incorrect as somatic pathogenic variants occur in body cells (except the gametes) after conception and are acquired over a lifetime.

5. *Answer:* A
Rationale: A malignant tumor is derived from genetic instability and genetic alterations in genes that control cell growth and proliferation. B is incorrect as proto-oncogenes are normal genes essential for normal cell growth and proliferation. Pathogenic changes occurring in proto-oncogenes convert to oncogene activation to cause uncontrolled cell division. C is incorrect because driver pathogenic variants offer a selective growth advantage to cancerous cells, while passenger variants do not. D is incorrect as pathogenic variants in DNA repair genes may be inherited from a parent or acquired over time due to aging or impact of carcinogens from the environment.

6. *Answer:* C
Rationale: Most hereditary cancer syndromes are inherited in an autosomal dominant fashion. This typically includes multiple close relatives (first, second, and third degrees) with the same or related types of cancer. A is incorrect because in most cases the altered gene is passed from one side of the family. B is incorrect as a deleterious germline pathogenic variants in a cancer susceptibility genes is suggestive of risk for hereditary cancer. D is incorrect as cancer types are similar in multiple generations, usually from one side of the family, with a risk for hereditary cancer.

7. *Answer:* D
Rationale: Any individual with a diagnosis of cancer should provide information about treatments, age at onset, and other pertinent medical history that might explain the diagnosis of cancer, such as risk factor exposures. This might include tobacco usage history, an early hysterectomy, or use of a chemoprevention agent such as tamoxifen. A is an incorrect answer as only three generations of cancer information for both lineages is required. B is incorrect as females are designated as circles while males are designated as squares. C is incorrect as race, ethnicity, and age of individuals should be included for all of the individuals in a 3 generation pedigree.

8. *Answer:* C
Rationale: When an individual is tested for a known family germline pathogenic variant and tests negative,

the individual did not inherit the increased risk associated with the pathogenic variant from the side of the family with the known pathogenic variant. The history from the other side can also influence risk. A negative test result in a family with a known pathogenic variant implies at least population risk for developing malignancy, and if there is risk from the other side of the family risk could be increased. A is incorrect because even with a negative test for a known pathogenic variant the individual still has at least population risk for developing malignancy. B is incorrect because inherited risk comes from germline not somatic pathogenic variants. D is incorrect because if the family history is consistent with the risks associated with the known pathogenic variant, the pathogenic variant likely explains the family history of malignancy.

9. **Answer:** B

Rationale: A VUS is a change in the genetic material for which there is not enough data to determine if it is a harmful or harmless change in the genetic material. A is incorrect as a VUS is identified when a cancer risk has NOT been established. C is also incorrect as a VUS label can change to pathogenic or benign based on information identified in new types of genetic testing. D is incorrect as a VUS can be a fairly common finding occurring as often as 20% to 40% on larger germline panels.

10. **Answer:** A

Rationale: "23 and Me" is a direct-to-consumer test that includes only the three *BRCA1/2* (selected variants) pathogenic variants most common in persons of Ashkenazi descent. These are the most common out of thousands of pathogenic variants which are *not* included in the direct-to-consumer test. B is incorrect as it is FDA approved. C is incorrect as it is not FDA approved for diagnosis or clinical decision-making in breast cancer. D is incorrect as only 23 and ME is FDA approved but there are other types of direct to consumer genetic testing.

11. **Answer:** A

Rationale: Cytogenetic reports include the number of chromosomes, the sex chromosome designation, and abnormality abbreviations (first chromosome separated with a semicolon from the second chromosome, then the arm and band number). Sanger sequencing is a form of gene sequencing that determines the sequence of a gene being tested and detects sequence changes in regions being analyzed. A limitation of this testing is that it may miss pathogenic variants outside the coding region or pathogenic variants that are large genomic rearrangements or large deletions The genome-wide association studies (GWAS) sequencing reviews for changes with specific disease (cancer type) versus people without the cancer. D is incorrect as transcriptome analysis analyzes the entire collection of RNA sequences in a cell.

12. **Answer:** C

Rationale: A de novo pathogenic variant is a change in a gene and is present for the first time in one family member due to harmful change in a germ cell (egg or sperm) of one of the parents or in the fertilized egg. A is incorrect as a germline pathogenic variant is passed from generation to generation. The genetic change will henceforth be inherited in an autosomal-dominant fashion in the family. B is incorrect as germline pathogenic variants are present in the reproductive cells (the eggs and sperm). D is incorrect as it only occurs in the gametes: eggs and sperm at conception. Acquired somatic changes occur after conception

13. **Answer:** C

Rationale: Heightened anxiety may result when patients learn that they are at a substantially increased risk for developing cancer. A is incorrect as, although there can be depression, a sense of relief has not been reported; in fact they experience more anxiety. B is incorrect as this relates to family members versus the patient as it occurs when family members pass on the pathogenic variant to one of their offspring. D is incorrect as you see this type of guilt in persons who have not inherited the pathogenic present in other close family members.

14. **Answer:** D

Rationale: The Genetic Information Nondiscrimination Act (GINA), federal legislation enacted in 2008, applies to health insurance and employment discrimination based on genetic information. GINA does not apply to active duty military personnel, Veterans Administration, or Native American Health Service because the laws amended for GINA do not apply to these groups. Health insurance protections with GINA include protections against accessing an individual's genomic information, requirements for an individual to undergo a genetic or genomic test, and using genomic information against a person during medical underwriting. Employment protections include prohibiting employers from accessing an individual's genetic information, use of genomic information to deny employment, or collecting genomic information without consent. GINA does not supersede state legislation that provides for more extensive protections.

15. **Answer:** D

Rationale: Genetic testing cannot determine longevity of life so it is not part of the informed consent process. Answers A, B, and C are parts of the informed consent. Elements of informed consent include discussion of the purpose of the test, motivation for testing, risks and benefits of testing, potential limitations of testing, risk of misidentified paternity, inheritance pattern of the gene and likelihood of a pathogenic variant being detected, accuracy of the test, potential outcomes of testing, how confidentiality will be maintained, the possibility of discrimination, alternatives to testing, how testing will influence health care decision-making, costs of testing, and considerations for testing in children.

16. **Answer:** A

Rationale: All the listed are genetic diseases, but the only one that is not associated with risk of developing brain cancer is Peutz-Jeghers syndrome, which is associated with hamartomatous polyps, and colorectal, pancreatic, and breast cancers. Neurofibromatosis type 1 is associated with malignant peripheral nerve sheath tumors, optic gliomas, meningiomas, hamartomatous intestinal polyps other gliomas, and leukemias. Li-Fraumeni syndrome is associated with soft tissue sarcoma, osteosarcoma, premenopausal breast cancer, brain tumors, adrenocortical carcinoma (ACC), and leukemias. Von Hippel-Lindau disease is associated with renal cancers, pancreatic neuroendocrine tumors, hemangioblastomas, and pheochromocytomas.

17. *Answer:* B

Rationale: The small arm is known as the petite arm and is labeled as "p." The long arm is labeled as "q" because "q" comes after "p" in the alphabet. There is no "o" or "s" arm.

18. *Answer:* A

Rationale: Exons are protein-coding segments of a gene. Introns are non–protein-coding segments, the sequence-interrupting piece of a gene. A codon is a sequence of three mRNA nucleotides (e.g., ACG) yielding one (threonine) of the 20 amino acids. An autosome is any chromosome that is not a sex chromosome.

19. *Answer:* B

Rationale: MUTYH-associated polyposis (MAP) is an autosomal recessive hereditary cancer syndrome and is associated with colon cancer and duodenal cancer, as well as colon, duodenal, and gastric fundic gland polyps, osteomas, sebaceous gland adenomas, and pilomatricomas. Polyp counts range from a few to >1000 with biallelic MUTYH pathogenic variants. Hereditary retinoblastoma, hereditary diffuse gastric cancer, and multiple endocrine neoplasia are all inherited in an autosomal dominant fashion. Hereditary diffuse gastric cancer found on the CDH1 gene is associated with diffuse gastric cancer, lobular breast cancer, adenocarcinoma and epithelial ovarian cancer, and prostate and signet ring colon cancer. Hereditary retinoblastoma is found on the RBI gene and is associated with malignant tumors of the retina, usually occurring before age 5. A family history of retinoblastoma, bilateral retinal tumors, and multifocal tumors have the highest chance to have hereditary retinoblastoma. Individuals with hereditary retinoblastoma also have an increased risk for pinealoblastoma, osteosarcomas, sarcoma, and melanoma. Multiple endocrine neoplasia type 1 (MEN1) is found on the MEN1 gene. It is associated with endocrine and nonendocrine tumors, including tumors of the parathyroid glands, pituitary gland, and the pancreas.

20. *Answer:* B

Rationale: Lynch syndrome is associated with pathogenic variants in the following genes: MLH1, MSH2 (including methylation due to EPCAM deletion), MSH6, and PMS2. Lynch syndrome is characterized by microsatellite instability (MSI) due to defective mismatch repair. Cancers associated with Lynch syndrome include cancers of the ovary, colon, rectum, stomach, small intestine, esophagus, biliary tract, brain, and endometrium. Other cancers at elevated risk are transitional cell carcinoma of the ureters and renal pelvis and pancreatic cancer. Lynch syndrome is not typically associated with cancers of the lung or thyroid or sarcomas.

CHAPTER 11

1. *Answer:* D

Rationale: In an observational study, the goal is to understand a situation in order to develop a hypothesis that can be evaluated using a clinical trial. Participants in an observational study are not assigned to a specific intervention, and their health care outcomes are assessed. In an experimental study, participants receive specific interventions, and each type is designed to answer different research questions. Participants in clinical trials involving human beings are called *subjects*. An interventional study is another name for an experimental study, as described above. Expanded access occurs when a clinical research study provides a means for patients to receive an investigational drug outside of a designated clinical trial. In expanded access, the investigational agent is restricted to patients with a serious condition or disease who no longer have satisfactory medical options available and who may benefit from the investigational therapy. This also may be referred to as "compassionate use."

2. *Answer:* A

Rationale: A screening trial evaluates the effectiveness of new techniques for early detection of cancer in the general population. A diagnostic trial evaluates tests or procedures that may better identify cancer in symptomatic individuals. A quality of life trial explores pharmacologic or nonpharmacologic therapies to minimize cancer-related toxicities. A prevention trial evaluates the safety and efficacy of various risk reduction strategies such as chemoprevention or actions such as increasing fruit and vegetable intake, adding exercise, avoiding tobacco, or limiting alcohol use.

3. *Answer:* A

Rationale: Expanded access provides a means for patients and their physicians to use an investigational drug outside of a designated clinical trial. Off-label use of a drug is not a characteristic of expanded access. Expanded access is restricted to patients with a serious condition or disease who no longer have satisfactory medical options available. Treatment or therapeutic trials are studies that are designed to evaluate the safety and efficacy of an intervention.

4. *Answer:* B

Rationale: The principal investigator ensures the ethical conduct of the research study. The study coordinator, statisticians, and data managers are all important members of the research team, but not responsible for the research study as a whole. The responsibilities of these other research members may vary from study to study.

5. *Answer:* D

Rationale: The Belmont Report focused on three major principles: beneficence, respect for persons, and justice. The Nuremberg Code focused on voluntary consent. The Declaration of Helsinki focused on informed consent, therapeutic versus nontherapeutic research, and surrogate decision-making. The Common Rule, also known as the Protection of Human Research Subjects, focused on informed consent and the responsibilities of institutional review boards in protecting human subjects.

6. *Answer:* B

Rationale: The performance status of participants considered for entry into an oncology clinical trial is often part of the eligibility criteria that must first be met. Eligibility criteria are characteristics that potential participants must meet to be enrolled into the trial and includes demographic, disease-specific, and treatment-related variables. These include inclusion and exclusion criteria. Common inclusion criteria that must be satisfied before an oncology patient can enter a trial includes performance status using indicators such as their scores on the Eastern Cooperative Oncology Group (ECOG) or Karnofsky Performance Status Scales. Other common inclusion criteria include stage and/or status of tumor, presence of measurable disease, and presence or absence of biomarkers. Geography or place of residence is not usually an eligibility criteria, although proximity to the trial may make participation easier. Some studies may not allow previous research participation; this can vary from study to study. The number of children a potential study participant has is seldom an eligibility criteria.

7. *Answer:* B

Rationale: On average, 20 to 100 subjects will be enrolled in a Phase I study. Phase I studies often include subjects with many cancer types (e.g., solid tumors), subjects with tumors refractory to standard therapy, and subjects with adequate organ function, specifically bone marrow, liver, and kidney function. Ten to 12 subjects are needed to conduct a Phase 0 study, while 80 to 300 subjects are needed for a Phase II study on average. In contrast, hundreds to thousands of subjects are needed for Phase III and IV studies, on average.

8. *Answer:* C

Rationale: The definition of overall survival is the time from randomization until the time of death. Disease-free survival is the time from randomization until recurrence of tumor or death from any cause. The objective response rate refers to the proportion of patients with a reduction of tumor size of a predetermined amount and for a minimum time period. The definition of the time to progression is the time from randomization until objective tumor progression, excluding death.

9. *Answer:* D

Rationale: The example of "A, B, A and B, placebo" represents a factorial design. Factorial design allows for multiple factors, such as multiple treatments, to be studied simultaneously so that two or more research questions can be answered with one clinical trial. The example of "A or B" represents a parallel design. In parallel design, a participant is randomized to one of several treatment groups. The example of "A→outcome→B" represents a crossover design. A crossover design allows participants to receive more than one treatment. A, B, A and B requires placebo (neither A nor B) to be added to represent a factorial design.

10. *Answer:* C

Rationale: A cohort study is a type of observational study in which subjects who do not have the outcome or condition to be studied (such as lung cancer) are followed over a period of time and compared related to who develops cancer and who does not based on their exposures. In an experimental or interventional study, participants receive specific interventions. Each type of clinical trial in an experimental or interventional study is designed to answer a different research question. Studies defined as outcomes research explore the results of health care practices and interventions, and feature patient-based outcomes, as well as the study of populations and different health care delivery methods.

11. *Answer:* B

Rationale: Outcomes research explores the results of health care practices and interventions, and feature patient-based outcomes, as well as the study of populations and different health care delivery methods. The clinical trials in experimental studies are designed to answer a different research question. Cohort studies are defined as clinical trial studies where subjects who have no reported outcomes or conditions are followed and compared, based on exposure. In a cross-sectional study, described is the association between a condition and other characteristics that may exist in a specific group.

12. *Answer:* C

Rationale: J.L. is participating in a quality of life study. This type of clinical trial explores pharmacologic or nonpharmacologic interventions to minimize toxicities related to cancer and cancer treatments. In contrast, screening trials are meant to evaluate the effectiveness of new techniques for early detection of cancer in the general populous. Diagnostic trials evaluate types of procedures or tests that may better help identify cancer in individuals who present with symptoms of the disease. Treatment or therapeutic trials evaluate the safety of new drugs, vaccines, biological agents, approaches to surgery or radiation therapy, treatment combinations, or other interventions. Even though J.L. is enrolled in a study exploring drug treatments, his trial explores treatments to minimize cancer-related toxicities, rather than exploring the safety and efficacy of new drugs or treatments.

CHAPTER 12

1. *Answer:* A

Rationale: Common primary tumors associated with metastases to bone include cancers of the prostate, lung, breast, kidney, and thyroid. Prostate cancer commonly spreads to the bone in advanced stages. Primary cancers that do not spread to the bone include brain cancer, leukemia, and ovarian cancer.

2. *Answer:* C

Rationale: A possible bone or soft tissue mass may or may not be visible or palpable. The mass may be firm, nontender, and warm. Its size should be compared bilaterally to the tibia of the other leg. This type of mass is not described as pus filled or pockmarked. Anemia is a condition related to the patient's blood, not the bone or soft tissue mass. A needle aspiration is part of a biopsy workup.

3. *Answer:* D

Rationale: Nursing management following reconstruction of bone after tumor removal includes assessment for infection, postsurgery union of nonmalignant tissue, healing, and functional concerns (especially with limb salvage). Thrombocytopenia is a condition of decreased platelets (clotting blood cells). Pruritis is an allergic reaction to topical or systemic treatment. For some targeted systematic treatments, cytokine response is when cytokines and other inflammatory mediators are released.

4. *Answer:* D

Rationale: Soft tissue tumors can be radiosensitive and radioresponsive. So, adjuvant radiotherapy can be a component of treatment before or after surgery, when the tumor is localized or after the tumor has been surgically debulked or removed. Radiotherapy is not a treatment for distant metastatic spread of disease. For soft tissue tumors, radiotherapy is not used as the primary treatment nor considered a standard of care. Radiotherapy may be considered as an adjuvant treatment.

5. *Answer:* C

Rationale: Phantom limb pain or sensation can occur 1 to 4 weeks postoperatively. This type of pain can resolve in a few months or can become chronic. The patient may describe phantom limb pain as itching, pressure, tingling, severe cramping, throbbing, and/or a burning pain. Phantom limb pain occurs over a period of time and not just when the patient intermittently stands.

6. *Answer:* B

Rationale: Most cases of Kaposi Sarcoma occur in people who have HIV and AIDS. Kaposi Sarcoma is caused by an infectious virus known as *human herpesvirus 8*. It is in the same family as the Epstein-Barr virus. Prevention includes protected sex, daily antiviral drugs for those at high risk for HIV, using clean needles to inject recreational drugs, and treating HIV-positive pregnant mothers and baby with anti-HIV drugs and avoiding breastfeeding. The occurrence of Kaposi Sarcoma is not especially associated with men younger than age 45, postmenopausal women, and those in high socioeconomic groups.

7. *Answer:* B

Rationale: The treatment of choice for chondrosarcoma is surgery, which includes amputation or limb salvage. Radiation therapy is an adjuvant therapy or used for palliative care or pain relief. Chemotherapy or immunotherapy can be used as adjuvant or neoadjuvant therapy with surgery.

8. *Answer:* A

Rationale: According to the American Cancer Society and the National Cancer Institute, treatment with radiation therapy is an identified risk factor for developing a soft tissue sarcoma. An individual's age and lifestyle habits, including smoking, poor diet, and lack of physical exercise are not listed as risk factors for soft tissue sarcoma.

CHAPTER 13

1. *Answer:* B

Rationale: Family history of a first-degree relative having breast cancer is a consideration for genetic evaluation. This is especially important in women with a first degree or second-degree relative with breast cancer diagnosed before the age of 50, multiple family members with breast cancer, or a family history of ovarian cancer. Breast biopsy, reproductive factors such as nulliparity or age at menarche, first pregnancy, or menopause are personal, not hereditary, risk factors for developing breast cancer.

2. *Answer:* A

Rationale: Male breast cancer is an indication for referral for genetic evaluation. Women diagnosed with breast cancer at age 50 or under should be given consideration for genetic evaluation, as well as women aged 60 and under with triple negative breast cancer. Answers B, C, and D reflect on women with average or older age of onset. These women would not be considered for referral for genetic evaluation unless there was a family history of breast, ovarian, melanoma, pancreatic, prostate, or colon cancer, or possibly a diagnosis of two primary breast cancers.

3. *Answer:* C

Rationale: Raloxifene is a selective estrogen receptor modulator (SERM) that may be used to reduce risk of developing breast cancer in high risk postmenopausal women. Premenopausal and postmenopausal women can also consider utilizing tamoxifen to reduce the risk of developing breast cancer. Metformin, retinoids, and cox-2 inhibitors are under investigation to determine if they are effective for the primary prevention of breast cancer.

4. *Answer:* C

Rationale: Basal cancers, known as triple negative breast cancer (ER-negative, PR-negative, HER-2/Neu-negative), tend to have a worse prognosis. Luminal A tumors have a high ER/PR expression and tend to respond well to endocrine therapy and are often associated with a better prognosis. The prognosis of lobular carcinoma is similar to that of ductal carcinoma. A poorer prognosis is associated with lymph node involvement.

5. *Answer:* A

Rationale: The nurse teaches the patient how to measure the circumference of the affected arm (where lymph nodes were removed) and to notify the health care provider if it increases, which may indicate the presence of lymphedema. Prevention of lymphedema is far easier than treatment. Prevention measures include avoiding constriction to the arm from tourniquets and blood pressure cuffs as well as trauma or injuries that could lead to infection. Exercise should be supervised and gradually be added into the patient's daily routine. A temperature of greater than 100.5°F could be suggestive of a postoperative infection. Sodium intake has not been shown to impact lymphedema risk. However, a person who has lymphedema should reduce their sodium intake.

6. *Answer:* C

Rationale: The Oncotype DX test is a 21-gene assay used to predict the benefit of adding chemotherapy to breast cancer therapy and estimate the 10-year risk of distant recurrence in women with early-stage ER/PR-positive, HER2-negative breast cancer. The recurrence score is calculated from gene expression in the cancer cells. For postmenopausal patients, such as our 67-year old patient, a recurrence score of < 26 indicates no benefit from the addition of chemotherapy. When the recurrence score is ≥26, then chemotherapy would be recommended. The

144

MammaPrint test is a 70-gene microarray-based assay that reports low or high risk of metastasis.

7. *Answer:* D

Rationale: T.K., a 27-year-old white woman, has a 1 in 8 chance that she will develop breast cancer in her lifetime. J.L., who is Hispanic, has a lower rate than the other races. Breast cancer is 100 more times likely in woman than in men, so D.C. has the smallest chances of the four choices. Finally, B.R., a 37-year-old African American woman, has a 1 in 10 chance of developing cancer. However, more African American women are diagnosed with breast cancer before the age of 45 compared to white women.

8. *Answer:* D

Rationale: The terminal duct lobular units (TDLUs) produce breast milk. Adipose tissue becomes more prominent after menopause. Sebaceous tissues are microscopic glands in the skin that secrete an oily substance known as sebum. There are no primary duct units.

9. *Answer:* A

Rationale: Luminal A tumors have the highest levels of ER expression: ER-positive and/or PR-positive, these tumors tend to be low grade, are most likely to respond to endocrine therapy, are responsive to chemotherapy, and have a favorable prognosis. Luminal B tumors are typically ER-positive, PR-negative, HER2-positive, and may have an unfavorable subset with aggressive behavior that can be tamoxifen resistant. Basal tumors are negative for ER, PR, and HER2 (triple-negative). They tend to be high grade and often have a poor prognosis; therefore these tumors will likely benefit from chemotherapy

10. *Answer:* B

Rationale: In the Bloom-Richardson or Nottingham histological grading systems for breast cancer, Grade 1 reflects a low-grade or well-differentiated breast cancer. Grade 2 represents an intermediate grade and moderately differentiated breast cancer. Grade 3 represents a high grade and poorly differentiated breast cancer.

CHAPTER 14

1. *Answer:* B

Rationale: Endoscopy of the upper gastrointestinal tract, termed esophagogastroduodenoscopy, is an endoscopic examination to visualize the lining of the esophagus, stomach, and first part of the small intestine. Biopsies may be taken to evaluate for the presence of malignancy. Colonoscopy is a screening test for colorectal cancer. An MRI of the brain and abdominal ultrasound are not part of a routine work-up for esophageal cancer. Other diagnostic modalities for esophageal cancer include a CT or a PET scan of the chest and abdomen, endoscopic ultrasound, thoracoscopy, and bronchoscopy.

2. *Answer:* A

Rationale: Modifiable risk factors are those within the control of the individual. An individual's risk for stomach cancer can be modified by avoiding the following lifestyle factors: alcohol use greater than 4 drinks per day, a diet high in salted and smoked foods and low in fruits and vegetables, smoking, being obese, and developing gastric ulcers. Individuals cannot control their family history nor can they control a history of genetic risk, such as Lynch syndrome. Other nonmodifiable risk factors include increasing age especially after age 60 to 80 years of age, being male, family history, Epstein-Barr virus, previous gastric surgery, gastric polyps, and inherited cancer syndromes (hereditary diffuse gastric cancer, familial adenomatous polyposis, Peutz–Jeghers syndrome, juvenile polyposis syndrome, and Lynch syndrome).

3. *Answer:* D

Rationale: Screening tests for colon cancer include guaiac-based stool testing, fecal immunochemical test, fecal occult blood test (FOBT), barium enema, flexible sigmoidoscopy, colonoscopy, or CT colonography. A CT of the abdomen, abdominal ultrasound, and a CT of the pelvis are all staging and diagnostic procedures used in the evaluation of colon cancer, often following a positive biopsy.

4. *Answer:* B

Rationale: Molecular classification in colon cancer includes KRAS/NRAS (in patients with metastatic disease), BRAF (in patients with metastatic disease), and MMR or MSI. PDL-1 and EGFR are used in the molecular classification of lung cancer. ER/PR (estrogen/progesterone) are used in the molecular classification of breast cancer.

5. *Answer:* C

Rationale: Risk factors for anal cancer include human papillomavirus infection (HPV) infections, human immunodeficiency virus (HIV) infection, anal sex, and lowered immunity. Human herpes virus (HHV-8) is associated with Kaposi sarcoma. Human T-lymphotrophic virus (HTLV-1) is a retrovirus that can infect T cells, B lymphocytes, monocytes, and fibroblasts.

6. *Answer:* A

Rationale: Risk factors for hepatocellular cancer include infections with hepatitis C virus (HCV) or hepatitis B virus (HBV), cirrhosis, diabetes, and obesity. Influenza is not a known risk factor for malignancy. Human papillomavirus infection (HPV) and human immunodeficiency virus (HIV) are risk factors for anal cancer. *H. pylori* infection is a risk factor for gastric cancer.

7. *Answer:* D

Rationale: Transplantation is a potentially curative option for early-stage HCC as it removes both detectable and undetectable tumor lesions and treats underlying cirrhosis. Treatment before transplantation may include bridge therapy or downstaging therapy with transarterial chemoembolization (TACE) or thermal/radiofrequency ablation (RFA). Partial hepatectomy is also potentially curative in patients with early-stage HCC, only in setting of preserved liver function and a Child–Pugh score A (assess prognosis of chronic liver disease). Local-regional therapies include ablation and arterially directed therapies. Ablation therapies include RFA, microwave ablation (MWA), and cryoablation. Arterially directed therapies include transarterial bland embolization (TABE), TACE, yttrium-90 transarterial radioembolization (TARE), and TACE with drug-eluting beads (DEB). Sorafenib is a systemic first-line therapy.

8. *Answer:* D

Rationale: Pancreatic adenocarcinoma is the most common form of pancreatic cancer. It accounts for almost 95% of cases and arises from the exocrine pancreas, where digestive enzymes are produced. It is the fourth most common cause of cancer death in the United States. Pancreatic adenocarcinoma is commonly found in the head of the pancreas but may also be found in the body and the tail. It is often found at advanced stages. When it is found in the tail it does not typically produce symptoms until it has spread. It typically first metastasizes to regional lymph nodes, then to the liver and, less commonly, to the lungs. It may also directly invade surrounding visceral organs such as the duodenum, stomach, and colon. It may also spread via the peritoneal cavity causing peritoneal carcinomatosis. Pancreatic neuroendocrine is less common.

9. *Answer:* C

Rationale: Regorafenib is a targeted therapy for metastatic colon cancer. FOLFOX, FOLFIRI ± bevacizumab, or cetuximab/panitumumab, depending on KRA/NRAS status are also used for metastatic colon cancer. Gemcitabine/cisplatin is used to treat pancreatic cancers that are due to *BRCA1* and *BRCA2* or *PALB2* pathogenic variants. Carboplatin and paclitaxel are commonly utilized to treat esophageal and gastric cancers. Trastuzumab added to chemotherapy for HER2+ metastatic esophageal adenocarcinoma.

10. *Answer:* D

Rationale: Primary prevention includes actions to prevent cancer from developing. The American Cancer Society recommends that all adults engage in at least 150 minutes of exercise weekly to reduce the risk of developing malignancy. The nurse should recommend to T.J. that he should limit alcohol intake to fewer than two drinks per/day as a course of action to prevent colorectal cancer. The recommendation is no more than two drinks per/day for a male and one drink/per day for a female. Treating *H. pylori* and gastric ulcers is a recommendation for the prevention of stomach cancer. Treating GERD and/or Barrett's esophagitis is a prevention recommendation for esophageal cancer. Other recommendations for the prevention of colorectal cancer include maintaining a healthy weight, limiting red and processed meat consumption while introducing more fruits and vegetables into a daily diet, and avoiding tobacco.

11. *Answer:* C

Rationale: Colorectal cancer is highest in Black communities; it is higher than any other racial/ethnic groups in the United States. African Americans are 20% more likely to be diagnosed with colorectal cancer and have about a 40% risk of mortality.

12. *Answer:* A

Rationale: L.M.'s pancreatic cancer is classified as resectable by surgery because it was diagnosed at an early stage (Stage 1). Due to late presentation, 15% to 20% of patients are unable to have surgery. Pancreatoduodenectomy (known as the Whipple procedure) is the most common surgery procedure done. It removes the head of the pancreas, duodenum, a portion of the common bile duct, gallbladder, and sometimes part of the stomach. Palliative radiation is not a consideration for patients with early-stage disease. Gemcitabine/cisplatin (for persons with *BRCA1*, *BRCA2*, or *PALB2* pathogenic variants) is utilized in persons with metastatic or unresectable pancreatic cancer. Immunotherapy utilizing pembrolizumab is a second line therapy for persons with metastatic or unresectable pancreatic cancer.

CHAPTER 15

1. *Answer:* D

Rationale: Clear cell carcinoma is a common type of kidney cancer that comprises 75% to 85% of all kidney cancer cases. Clear cell carcinoma is thought to arise in the proximal renal tubule and is not a tumor of the renal pelvis, which is considered to be very rare. Clear cell carcinoma does not have the worst prognosis among types of kidney cancers; rather, collecting duct carcinomas are aggressive tumors that are associated with rapid metastasis.

2. *Answer:* A

Rationale: Having a history of non-Hodgkin lymphoma and being overweight is the correct answer. The other choices are not correct because they are not known risk factors for kidney cancer, which include lifestyle risk factors such as tobacco use, obesity, and occupational exposure to petroleum products or heavy metals. Dietary risk factors include diets high in fats and protein. Finally, a history of non-Hodgkin lymphoma or sickle cell disease is also considered a risk factor.

3. *Answer:* C

Rationale: Intravenous pyelogram is the correct answer. This diagnostic test is commonly used to evaluate patients presenting with hematuria. Colonoscopy visualizes the colon and is not used to determine the cause of hematuria. The kidney is not biopsied to determine the cause of hematuria, and blood chemistry results would not be diagnostic for hematuria.

4. *Answer:* A

Rationale: Partial nephrectomy is the preferred treatment whenever feasible, especially in patients with limited renal function, bilateral tumors, or a solitary kidney. Cytoreductive nephrectomy is a procedure that may be performed in patients with surgically resectable primary tumor and multiple metastatic sites prior to systemic therapy. Renal cell cancers are unresponsive to radiation therapy. Chemotherapy has not been shown to improve survival in kidney cancer.

5. *Answer:* D

Rationale: The correct answer is immunotherapy agents. These agents, such as interleukin-2 and interferon-alpha, have produced response rates of 10% to 15% when used as single agents for treating cancer of the kidney. Systemic radiation therapy, in which radioactive drugs are delivered either orally or intravenously, is not used to treat renal cell cancers which are not radiation sensitive. Antibody-drug conjugates, in which an antibody is linked to a cytotoxic agent, are not used to treat kidney cancer because the malignant cells do not express specific antigens that would be the target of antibodies. Cytotoxic chemotherapy has not been shown to improve survival.

6. *Answer:* B

Rationale: Urothelial carcinoma of the bladder is the most common type of bladder cancer and comprises about 95% of bladder tumors. In 70% to 80% of cases, this type of tumor is generally diagnosed before it has become invasive and invaded the muscle wall of the bladder. Urothelial tumors are not associated with changes to *chromosome 9*, which are associated with papillary bladder cancers.

7. *Answer:* B

Rationale: Tobacco use is the most significant risk factor, accounting for 50% to 66% of all bladder tumors in men and 25% in women. Weight loss is not a risk factor; rather, a high BMI may increase risk and contribute to risk of disease recurrence. Excessive fluid intake does not increase bladder cancer risk, but not drinking enough fluids is reported to be a risk factor. Consuming a diet low in processed meats may be somewhat protective for bladder cancer.

8. *Answer:* C

Rationale: The correct answer is that AUA (American Urological Association) guidelines indicate that PSA screening between ages 55 and 69 years provides the greatest benefit. Therefore, it is not correct that results of PSA screenings are not useful for men at any age. Routine screening in men 40 to 54 years at average risk is not recommended. Men who decide to initiate PSA screening should have repeat screenings at intervals of 2 or more years.

9. *Answer:* B

Rationale: The Gleason score is based on microscopic examination of the prostate tumor tissue specimen. The pathologist determines the most common cell grade seen in the largest portion of the specimen (the primary cell grade) and in the second largest portion (the secondary cell grade). The two grades are then added together to determine the Gleason score. This score provides information about the aggressiveness of the disease in the prostate and serves as a guide for treatment strategies. Imaging tests using MRI or CT provide information about the extent of the disease but are not part of the process for determining the Gleason score, which is based on characteristics of the malignant tumor cells. PSA levels are not used for computing the Gleason score but may be useful as a marker for disease progression. Bone marrow aspiration is not used as a screening or diagnostic measure for prostate cancer.

10. *Answer:* B

Rationale: Hormonal manipulation is the accepted standard for treating patients with metastatic prostate cancer. The other options listed—radical prostatectomy, brachytherapy with radioactive seed placement into the prostate, and cryosurgery—are used to treat patients with early-stage prostate cancer.

11. *Answer:* C

Rationale: Impotence is the correct answer. Some form of impotence has been seen in 6% to 61% of men following brachytherapy to treat prostate cancer. Diarrhea, rather than constipation, is associated with both radiation therapy and brachytherapy. Anemia is not a side effect of brachytherapy because little bone marrow is exposed to radiation with this treatment. Decreased, not increased libido is associated with hormonal manipulation for metastatic prostate cancer.

12. *Answer:* B

Rationale: A recommendation to maximize patient safety postoperatively is monitoring vital signs, hemoglobin, hematocrit, kidney function tests, and urine output. These are critical measures when determining a patient's condition after surgery. Teaching a patient to manage and identify symptoms, including providing recommendations on when to report symptoms, occurs during patient education regarding follow-up care and surveillance, and not as a safety measure after surgery. Teaching patients how to perform coping skills to control anxiety and fear is also not a safety measure; however, nurses do teach patients about pulmonary hygiene, including how to perform coughing and deep breathing exercises. Finally, monitoring patients for signs of distress is not a safety measure, though nurses must monitor a patient's pain level after surgery in order to provide adequate pharmacologic and nonpharmacologic pain relief measures.

13. *Answer:* B

Rationale: For a radiographic examination of the kidneys, ureter, and bladder (KUB), the nurse should instruct the patient to lie flat on the examination table. Accessing the patient for a history of allergies to iodine dyes or contact media before testing is a nursing intervention instruction for an excretory urography test. For a retrograde urography diagnostic test, nurses are instructed to observe the patient for a reaction to anesthetic or analgesic, and monitor for bleeding, symptoms of a urinary tract infection, dysuria, or difficulty voiding after the test has been completed.

14. *Answer:* D

Rationale: External beam radiation therapy is a bladder preservation therapy. The bladder cancer is treated with radiation therapy rather than a surgical procedure. Radical cystectomy is major surgery that involves removal of the bladder and prostate gland and surrounding lymph nodes. An ileal conduit is a urinary diversion performed with cystectomy. Orthotopic neobladder is a technique that provides for the creation of a new bladder that is made from the intestine; better quality of life is reported compared with ileal conduit.

15. *Answer:* A

Rationale: Screening guidelines exist for prostate cancer although controversy continues at the national level with regard to routine screening for prostate cancer with PSA testing. The American Urologic Association published new guidelines for prostate cancer screening in 2019. Recommendations include no PSA screening for men younger than 40 or for men between the ages of 40 and 54 at average risk. Shared decision-making about PSA screening for men ages 55 to 69 years is recommended; the greatest screening benefit is seen in this age group No screening tests are available for kidney cancer. Screening for bladder cancer is not currently recommended by any major preventive group in the United States. The testes are part of the male reproductive system and are also an endocrine organ, secreting testosterone. No routine screening test exists for early detection of testicular cancer.

CHAPTER 16

1. *Answer:* B
Rationale: The patient has been diagnosed with thyroid cancer, which is considered a cancer of the head and neck. The category of head and neck cancers include cancers of the oral cavity, oropharynx, nasal cavity, paranasal sinuses, nasopharynx, larynx, hypopharynx, and salivary glands; as well as cancers of the thyroid and parathyroid. The category of head and neck cancers does not include cancers of the esophagus, brain, or bone.

2. *Answer:* A
Rationale: Known risk factors for head and neck cancer include infection with the human papillomavirus (HPV), tobacco use, excessive alcohol intake, indigestion, gastroesophageal reflux, history of neck radiation, and environmental exposure (wood, dust, asbestos). Sixty percent to 70% of cancers of the oropharynx may be linked to human papillomavirus (HPV). The rate of HPV oral cancer is increasing. Diabetes, menopause, and dental implants are not known risk factors.

3. *Answer:* D
Rationale: Tumor biopsy results are needed to develop a treatment plan for a patient with head and neck cancer. A definitive diagnosis of a cancer is arrived at through pathological evaluation of the tumor tissue, which provides information about the histology, molecular profile, and other pathological features of the cancer. Hereditary testing is not the first step needed to establish a treatment plan for head and neck cancer. Family history is important to assess, but it is not directly related to the treatment plan. After the patient has a treatment plan of care that includes chemotherapy, a neutrophil count may be calculated.

4. *Answer:* B
Rationale: Radiologic studies for head and neck cancer include computed tomography (CT) and magnetic resonance imaging (MRI). CT is used to assist in determining the extent of the primary tumor and to identify metastasis to the cervical lymph nodes. MRI is superior to CT in staging nasopharyngeal primaries. Positron emission tomography (PET) with CT (PET-CT) is useful in determining specific areas for biopsy, lymph node involvement, and the extent of disease to aid in treatment planning. PET is ordered to document metastatic spread of tumor cells. When providers order diagnostic radiologic studies, they do not order only chest X-ray or ultrasound. Intravenous pyelogram is used to evaluate kidneys, ureters, and bladder. A gallium scan is useful in evaluating patients with potential lymphoma, infection, osteomyelitis, or pulmonary problems. Barium enema is used to provide information about the lower GI tract.

5. *Answer:* A
Rationale: Focused nursing care of head and neck cancer patients includes monitoring of swallowing ability, respiration, speech, presence of trismus (restriction in the opening of the mouth), and hormone regulation. Depending on the patient's overall health maintenance, nursing care can also include attention to neutropenia, skin care, and lymphedema. However those conditions are not the specific focus of nursing care for a patient with head and neck cancer.

6. *Answer:* D
Rationale: Before laryngectomy surgery, the patient should have been taught a variety of communication strategies to utilize postsurgery, such as paper and pencil, magic slate, picture board, nonverbal cues, electronic communication board, or a speech device. Preoperative teaching for patients with a head and neck cancer covers discussion of the disease, treatment, side effects, and anticipated postoperative changes. It also includes instruction about equipment (tracheostomy tube, drains, nasogastric tube, tonsil-tip suction catheter). Specific for laryngectomy, the focus of preoperative teaching does not include ambulation, endurance, or opioid addiction.

7. *Answer:* A
Rationale: Following head and neck surgery, perfusion of blood supply to the surgical graft site is an essential nursing assessment. After a patient undergoes head and neck surgery that includes skin or muscle grafts to cover the removed tumor site, postoperative wound care assessment is done every 3 to 4 hours, noting color (pink versus cyanotic), temperature, and capillary refill after blanching of the skin and muscle. Flap perfusion and viability is maintained by avoiding excess pressure to the flap; the wound is assessed for infection and fistula formation. Nursing assessment of surgical grafts does not include range of motion, necrotic tissue removal, or regular lavage.

8. *Answer:* B
Rationale: During neck dissection, the patient's spinal accessory nerve and the sternocleidomastoid muscles may be resected. For the patient to regain range of motion and strength, the patient is referred to physical therapy. The patient is not likely to have significant pain issues by time of discharge nor do they require a gastroenterology consult as a routine referral. Occupational therapy is not a typical referral for neck dissection patients. Speech therapists play an integral role both preoperative and postoperatively to assist with issues in speech and swallowing.

9. *Answer:* C
Rationale: During a supraglottic laryngectomy the structures above the false vocal cords are resected. Thus, A.P. becomes at risk for aspiration until he learns swallowing techniques to protect the airway. Postoperative care of any patient includes risk of falling, maintaining hydration, and assessing somnolence, but these are not the primary concern of nurses caring for patients who are postoperative following supraglottic laryngectomy.

10. *Answer:* D

Rationale: Signs and symptoms of head and neck cancer include a persistent lump or sore that does not heal in the mouth, lip, throat, or jaw; a sore throat that does not go away; a change or hoarseness in the voice that does not resolve; difficulty chewing, swallowing, or moving the jaw or tongue; and a pain in one ear without hearing loss. A temperature of >100°F does not suggest a sign of head and neck cancer.

11. *Answer:* C

Rationale: The oropharynx extends from the circumvallate papillae below and hard palate above to the level of the hyoid bone. Structures of the oropharynx include the base of the tongue (posterior one-third), soft palate, the tonsils, and posterior pharyngeal wall. The oral cavity extends from the lips to the hard palate above and the circumvallate papillae below, with structures including the lips, buccal mucosa, floor of the mouth, and upper and lower alveoli. The nasopharynx is located below the base of the skull and behind the nasal cavity and continuous with the posterior pharyngeal wall. Finally, the larynx extends from the epiglottis to the cricoid cartilage and is protected by the thyroid cartilage.

12. *Answer:* B

Rationale: A hemilaryngectomy involves a vertical excision of one true and one false cord and the underlying cartilage. This procedure can give the patient a hoarse voice but leads to minimal to no swallowing problems. Laser therapy treatment is associated with little to no physical alterations and minimal bleeding. A maxillectomy involves partial or total en-bloc resection of the cavity. This procedure may include the ethmoid sinus, lateral nasal wall, palate, and floor of the orbit. Preoperatively, a maxillofacial prosthodontist makes a dental obturator to fill the large surgical defect and to facilitate swallowing. Postoperative nursing care requires daily care to the cavity and placement of the obturator. A craniofacial or skull base resection is a surgical treatment to inaccessible midfacial and extensive paranasal sinus and nasopharyngeal lesions. This procedure may create facial defects and cranial nerve (III, IV, V) deficits.

13. *Answer:* C

Rationale: The hypopharynx extends from the hyoid bone to the lower border of the cricoid cartilage, and structures include the pyriform sinuses, the postcricoid region, and the lower posterior pharyngeal wall. The oropharynx extends from the circumvallate papillae below and hard palate above to the level of the hyoid bone; and structures include the base of the tongue (posterior one-third), soft palate, and the posterior pharyngeal wall. The supraglottis is located below the base of the tongue, extending to but not including the true vocal cord, and includes the epiglottis, the aryepiglottic folds, the arytenoid cartilages, and the false vocal cords. Finally, the nasal cavity and paranasal sinuses include the nasal vestibule; paired maxillary, ethmoid, and frontal sinuses; and a single sphenoid sinus.

14. *Answer:* B

Rationale: Men have twice the incidence of cancers of the head and neck compared to women. Human papilloma virus infection accounts for 60% to 70% of cancers of the oropharynx and there is a higher incidence of HPV infection in men than women. Incidence rates for cancers of the head and neck also increase after age 40. Use of hair dye is not reported to be associated with head and neck cancer risk.

15. *Answer:* D

Rationale: Screening for cancers of the oral cavity is often part of the physical examination by a dentist or primary care physician. Standard screening guidelines for cancers of the head and neck do not exist. Radiographs of the mouth and evaluation of sputum are not recommended as screening strategies for cancers of the oral cavity.

16. *Answer:* C

Rationale: Thyroid cancer has the highest 5-year relative survival rate at 98%. The 5-year relative survival rate for all stages of oral cavity and pharynx cancers combined is 68% but is much lower in Black patients (36%) than in white patients (56%). Studies indicate that survival is better for patients with cancer who test positive for HPV. The rate of new cases of laryngeal cancer is decreasing by about 2% to 3% a year, most likely because fewer people are smoking.

17. *Answer:* C

Rationale: In the anatomy of the head and neck, the nasopharynx and the paranasal sinuses are located close to the brain. The nasopharynx is located below the base of the skull and behind the nasal cavity, continuous with the posterior pharyngeal wall. The vocal cords are located in the larynx, and the floor of the mouth lies in the oral cavity. The soft palate is located in the oropharynx. Structures in the oropharynx include the base of the tongue (posterior one-third), the soft palate, tonsils, and posterior pharyngeal wall.

18. *Answer:* A

Rationale: Important risk factors for developing cancer of the head and neck include excessive alcohol intake that increases the risk of developing oral or pharyngeal cancer. Use of tobacco and alcohol together poses a greater risk of developing these cancers than use of either tobacco or alcohol alone. Infection with human papilloma virus is associated with 60% to 70% of cancers of the oropharynx. Epstein-Barr virus infection is a risk factor for nasopharyngeal cancer and cancer of the salivary glands.

CHAPTER 17

1. *Answer:* A

Rationale: The average time from human immunodeficiency virus (HIV) infection to symptomatic disease depends on inoculation method, exposure, preexisting health, and prompt initiation of treatment for antiretroviral disease, so A would be the best representative answer. The average time of infection is not dependent on the patient's age at time of exposure nor is it dependent on the number of sexual partners. The average time from infection to active AIDS is approximately 10 years. It can be shorter in older adults and children.

2. *Answer:* C

Rationale: Acute infection occurs, then proceeds to a chronic/progressive infection before manifesting into AIDS. During the chronic/progressive infection stage, qualitative and quantitative T4-lymphocyte dysfunction occurs, with resultant defects in both cellular and humoral immunity as immunoregulatory function of T4 cells is gradually impaired. The order in answer A of chronic/progressive disease, AIDS, and acute infection is incorrect since acute infection would come before either of the two steps. B is also incorrect. While acute infection occurs first in the progression of the disease, contracting AIDS is the final step and does not come prior to chronic/progress infection. Finally, D is also incorrect, and also incomplete, as the answer omits the final stage of AIDS.

3. *Answer:* B

Rationale: Lifestyle factors including inadequate nutrition, general poor health, and tobacco use may influence the course of infection. There is an increased risk of infection in uncircumcised males related to dendritic cells on the foreskin. Other factors that might influence the progression of the disease might include the presence of cytomegalovirus (CMV), Epstein-Barr virus (EBV), hepatitis C virus, human papillomavirus (HPV), herpes simplex 6 (HSV-6), herpes simplex 8 (HSV-8), and other viruses.

Approximately 67% of cases in gay, bisexual, and other men who have sex with men comprise half of newly infected HIV infection and half of people living with the disease, and not the 37% of cases listed in answer D, making that answer incorrect as well.

4. *Answer:* D

Rationale: Increases in the incidence of HIV-positive adults over 50 years of age are attributable to prolonged survival with disease, age-related physiologic changes enhancing risk of transmission, and propensity to engage in unprotected sex. An estimated 1.2 million people in the United States are living with HIV, and one in seven does not know they are infected. Heterosexual contact with HIV-infected individuals accounts for about 83% of new HIV diagnoses in females. Approximately one-third of individuals with HIV infection will die of cancer during their disease trajectory.

5. *Answer:* D

Rationale: B-cell lymphoma is the most frequently diagnosed AIDS-defining malignancy. Other AIDS-defining malignancies include Burkitt lymphoma, non-Hodgkin lymphoma (NHL), Kaposi sarcoma, and cervical cancer. AIDS-defining malignancies are malignancies related specifically to HIV infection and the subsequently altered immune system. Non-AIDS defining malignancies include cancers of the anus, head and neck, kidney, liver and lung, and Hodgkin lymphoma.

6. *Answer:* C

Rationale: HIV-infected women are at an increased risk for cervical dysplasia that rapidly progresses to cervical cancer. AIDS-defining cancers include non-Hodgkin lymphoma (NHL), Burkitt lymphoma, Kaposi sarcoma, and cervical cancer. AIDS-defining malignancies are

more common shortly after initiation of active retroviral therapy, particularly among patients with low CD4 counts. Lung, acute myeloid leukemia, and kidney cancer are all non-AIDS defining cancers.

7. *Answer:* A

Rationale: CAR T-cell therapies and antineoplastic agents may have similar toxicity profiles (i.e. diarrhea, hepatotoxicity, pancreatitis, QT prolongation, etc.) and combination therapy may compound the toxicities when utilizing combination therapy for treatment. Therefore, patients should be monitored for overlapping toxicities when undergoing combination therapy. Steroid use increases the risk of inflammatory response (i.e., IRIS) rather than decreasing inflammation. Vaccines should be modified during or after cancer treatment due to continued immune defect, while antineoplastic therapy should continue to be administered in the setting of low CD4+ counts as these counts are a temporary condition.

8. *Answer:* B

Rationale: An active EBV infection is present in 33% to 67% of HIV lymphomas. In HIV-related lymphoma, the CD4+ count is typically less than 200/mm^3, not 400/mm^3; it lacks the CD20+ marker; and is a late manifestation of HIV infection.

9. *Answer:* C

Rationale: Ocular involvement occurs in 20% of patients diagnosed with primary central nervous system lymphoma; multifocal lesions are common. HIV-infected patients do not have extensive bone marrow involvement, nor do they have other organ/tissue involvement. This patient population also has a low CD4+ count. A pathogenic BCL6 variant is common.

10. *Answer:* C

Rationale: Immune reconstitution syndrome (IRIS) is a brisk inflammatory response when the white blood cell (WBC) count rapidly increases. Manifestations include fever, edema and effusions, weight loss, myalgias, fatigue, hepatomegaly, lymphadenopathy, splenomegaly, respiratory symptoms, mental status changes, diarrhea and gastrointestinal distress, anemia, hypoalbuminemia, thrombocytopenia, and hyponatremia. This most commonly occurs with initial CAR T-cell therapy or with severe inflammatory or infectious reactions. It has occurred with toxoplasmosis, pneumocystis, other opportunistic infections in HIV disease (such as PCP pneumonia), and EBV reactivation. Anaphylaxis to Bactrim would likely occur with the first dose so the patient would not be experiencing symptoms such as altered mental status, fevers, and shortening of breath on Day 2. Superimposing infection or worsening PCP pneumonia would not necessarily be accompanied by altered mental status.

11. *Answer:* D

Rationale: Gastrointestinal lesions or B symptoms (fever, night sweats, unintentional weight loss) shorten the survival in patients diagnosed with Kaposi syndrome. The era of CAR T-cell therapy has increased survival dramatically, and no decrease in survival rates has been reported. Prior or comorbid major opportunistic infections worsen

150

survival, rather than having no impact. The median survival rate is less than 1 year, but not less than 6 months.

12. *Answer:* A

Rationale: The nurse should provide education about the use of latex condoms with a water-based lubricant to reduce risk. A water-based lubricant is recommended because petroleum-based lubricants or cosmetic creams weaken the condom, greater increasing the chance of HIV transmission. To decrease the risk of transmission, a latex condom should be used during every episode of vaginal, rectal, or oral intercourse. Personal hygiene items—such as a toothbrush or a razor—should not be shared, so the best method is to avoid sharing altogether. A solution of 1 part household bleach to 10 parts water (not 1 part water to 5 parts bleach) should be used with gloves during cleanup of emesis or other body fluid spills for protection against the spread of disease.

13. *Answer:* D

Rationale: It is correct that studies of antiretroviral adherence reflect low rates of medication adherence among individuals with low health literacy, linking a low health literacy score with adherence to medication. Low health literacy has a large—not a small—impact on maintaining regular medical care. Only 17% to 40% of patients who have scored low on health literacy scores have maintained regular medical care. Low health literacy is associated with English not being the first language, mental health disorder, and lack of understanding of how to access care and support (and interpreters are not readily available in every place where health care is being provided).

14. *Answer:* B

Rationale: Blood flukes known as schistosomes, can increase the risk for developing bladder cancer. Liver flukes include Opisthorchis viverrini (O. viverrini) and Clonorchis sinensis (Clonorchis). Liver flukes increase the risk of bile duct (Cholangiocarcinoma) due to infection with O. viverrini and Clonorchis and liver cancer due to Clonorchis.

15. *Answer:* D

Rationale: Epstein-Barr virus (EBV) infection is associated with an increased risk of developing head and neck cancers (especially in the nose and throat) and lymphoma.

16. *Answer:* B

Rationale: Infections are estimated to cause 15% of all cancer cases annually. This includes bacterial infections with *H. pylori,* which are associated with gastric cancer. Parasitic infections, which are rare, can increase the risk of developing malignancy. Viral infections that increase the risk of developing cancer include human papilloma virus (HPV), hepatitis B virus (HBV), Epstein-Barr virus (EBV), human herpesvirus type 8 (HHV-8), human T-cell lymphotropic virus type 1 (HTLV-1), and human immunodeficiency virus (HIV).

17. *Answer:* A

Rationale: *H. pylori* irritates gastric and duodenal endothelial cells and increases gastric acid production, reducing the mucosal barrier and increasing inflammation. Chronic inflammation results in carcinogenesis. About 60% of the worldwide population is currently infected with *H. pylori.* Prevention strategies include access to clean water, adequate housing (prevent crowded conditions), and access to sanitation. *H. pylori* is a bacterial infection. Zidovudine is an antiretroviral medication so it will not be effective. There is no recommended screening for gastric cancer in persons of average risk. Colonoscopy is recommended screening for colorectal cancer.

18. *Answer:* C

Rationale: For HPV, vaccination is recommended to start between 11 and 12 years old (can start at 9 years old; recommended to start at 9 if victim of sexual abuse). This is a two dose schedule: if between 9 and 14 years old at start of vaccination, first dose should be followed with second dose within 6 to 12 months. It is a three-dose schedule if 15 years old or older or immunocompromised and between ages 9 and 14 years old; at start of vaccination first dose should be followed with second dose at 1 to 2 months, and third dose at 6 months. For HBV, vaccination is a three-dose schedule. The first dose is recommended at birth; the second dose between 1 and 2 months; and third dose between 6 to 18 months of age. Currently there is no vaccination for prevention of HCV, HIV, EBV, or HHV8.

19. *Answer:* C

Rationale: Universal HCV screening is recommended at least once in an individual's lifetime and with each pregnancy for pregnant females, if community prevalence is greater than 0.1%. There are no routine screening recommendations for EBV, HHV8, or HTLV-1 currently. HBV screening is recommended at the first prenatal visit for pregnant females and for individuals at high risk with no known vaccination history. Universal HIV screening is recommended at least once in an individual's lifetime for those ages 15 to 65. Annual HIV screening is recommended for individuals at higher risk for infection, specifically males who have sex with males.

20. *Answer:* D

Rationale: Tissue damage and chronic inflammation from "long-COVID-19" is a possible mechanism with which COVID-19 infection may result in cancer occurrence, progression, or recurrence. Other mechanisms include elevated cytokines and growth factors, impaired T-cell response, release of chemokines during the acute infection phase, and integration of COVID-19 genetic material into host cells.

CHAPTER 18

1. *Answer:* A

Rationale: Exposure to certain viruses, such as EBV and HTLV-1, is a risk factor for developing ALL. Being of Hispanic descent, not African or Asian, is a risk factor for developing ALL. Having a genetic condition such as Down syndrome, Li-Fraumeni syndrome, Ataxia telangiectasia, Klinefelter syndrome, and Fanconi anemia is a risk factor for developing ALL. A diagnosis of measles is not a known risk factor.

2. *Answer:* A

Rationale: Constitutional symptoms often seen in ALL include fever, night sweats, and weight loss. Other symptoms of ALL include dyspnea, dizziness, infections, and easy bruising or bleeding. In children, the only presenting symptom may be pain in the extremities or joints. 20% of patients may present with lymphadenopathy, splenomegaly, and/or hepatomegaly on physical examination. Chin numbness due to cranial nerve involvement is suggestive of mature B-cell ALL (B-ALL).

3. *Answer:* D

Rationale: Induction therapy for Philadelphia-positive acute lymphoblastic leukemia in patients less than 65 years of age and in adolescents and young adults (AYAs) to achieve a complete remission includes tyrosine kinase inhibitor (TKI)-targeted therapy. TKI therapy using either imatinib, dasatinib, ponatinib, or nilotinib blocks the action of BCR-ABL fusion gene and is given with corticosteroids. Another treatment option is multi-agent chemotherapy that may be given with a TKI, and includes vincristine, pegaspargase, a steroid (prednisone or dexamethasone), and an anthracycline (doxorubicin or daunorubicin). This regimen may also include cyclophosphamide. Central nervous system prophylaxis or treatment with methotrexate or cytarabine is given during a lumbar puncture (intrathecal chemotherapy). Clinical trials are also an option for patients who meet the inclusion criteria. Allogeneic HCT is utilized as consolidation therapy after remission is achieved with induction therapy. Pediatric regimen is used for induction therapy in patients with Philadelphia chromosome negative disease and for those who are less than 65 years of age. Corticosteroids are not used as monotherapy, but in combination with TKI in patients who are less than 65 years of age.

4. *Answer:* D

Rationale: Midostaurin is an oral agent for FLT3 inhibition. Venetoclax is used for CLL. Ibrutinib is indicated for persons with a 17p deletion. Rituximab is a humanized antibody that targets CD20.

5. *Answer:* B

Rationale: ATRA + arsenic trioxide + anthracycline is recommended in high-risk disease in the absence of cardiac disease. ATRA + arsenic trioxide is given with or without anthracycline in low-risk disease. Gemtuzumab ozogamicin is used as a single agent in high-risk, relapse, or inability to tolerate arsenic trioxide due to QT prolongation. Intrathecal chemotherapy is used in consolidation therapy for patients with high-risk APL in combination with ATRA + arsenic trioxide + anthracycline.

6. *Answer:* C

Rationale: CLL is a disease that is diagnosed at a median age of 60 years old and less than 15% of patients are diagnosed under the age of 50. CLL is the most frequent form of leukemia. CLL is slightly more common in men than women. CLL originates from mature B lymphocytes.

7. *Answer:* A

Rationale: Ibrutinib is used for patients with 17p deletion. There is no known targeted therapy for TP53 pathogenic variant. Rituximab is used for patients with CD20 antigen. Alemtuzumab is used for patients with CD52 antigen.

8. *Answer:* D

Rationale: Rai stage III, high-risk disease is noted to have anemia Hgb <11 g/dL and lymphocytosis. The patient may or may not have adenopathy, hepatomegaly, or splenomegaly, and platelets counts are normal. Rai stage I, intermediate-risk disease is noted to have adenopathy and lymphocytosis (no hepatomegaly or splenomegaly, RBC and PLT counts are normal). Rai stage IV, high-risk disease is noted to have thrombocytopenia <100,00 µL and lymphocytosis (with adenopathy, hepatomegaly and splenomegaly, and RBC counts are normal or near normal). Rai stage II, intermediate-risk disease is noted to have splenomegaly and lymphocytosis (may have hepatomegaly, may or may not have adenopathy, and RBC and PLT counts are normal).

9. *Answer:* B

Rationale: One risk factor in developing acute myeloid leukemia (AML) is long-term exposure to benzene. Benzene is a chemical used in heavy industry, including places such as oil refineries, chemical plants, and the gasoline industry. Benzene can also be found in cigarette smoke, and in such common household items such as glue, detergent, and paint. Radiation therapy is not considered a risk factor for AML; however, exposure to high levels of radiation is seen as a risk factor. Those who have been involved in an atomic bomb attack, for instance, or been a survivor of a nuclear accident have an increased risk of developing the disease. Alcohol use and diet are not risk factors, though smoking has been linked to AML. Other risk factors include genetic disorders, such as Fanconi anemia and Down syndrome, family history of AML, as well as treatment with some chemotherapy agents.

10. *Answer:* A

Rationale: Acute lymphocytic leukemia (ALL) is the most common form of leukemia among children and adolescents, representing 20% of all cancers among persons less than 20 years and representing 3000 new cases annually. The risk declines after 5 years of age until the middle twenties and then rises again after the age of 50. In chronic myelogenous leukemia (CML), the average age at diagnosis is greater than 64 years with half of the total cases being over the age of 65. Chronic lymphocytic leukemia (CLL) is the most frequent form of leukemia and originates from mature B lymphocytes. The median age at diagnosis is 60 years, and less than 15% are diagnosed under the age of 50. The lifetime risk of CLL is 1 in 175 and is most commonly diagnosed at 70 years of age. CLL accounts for 25% of all leukemias and is more frequently seen in Caucasians compared with Asians, as well as Hispanics.

11. *Answer:* D

Rationale: The Rai staging system for chronic lymphocytic leukemia defines risk or extent of disease as low, intermediate, or high. There is no medium category. Those with lymphocytosis (lymphoid cells >30%), no lymphadenopathy, splenomegaly, or hepatomegaly are considered low. The intermediate level is defined by lymphocytosis, lymphadenopathy in any site, splenomegaly, or hepatomegaly. In both the low and intermediate levels, red blood cell and platelet counts are near normal. A high level is associated with lymphocytosis; presence of anemia (hemoglobin <11 g/dL) or thrombocytopenia (platelet count less than 100×10^9/L) with or without lymphadenopathy, splenomegaly, or hepatomegaly. M.L.'s lymphocytes are greater than 6000, which indicates more than 30% of the total white blood cell count percentage. He has thrombocytopenia, with the platelet count below 100,000. He has two sites of lymphadenopathy, the groin and axilla area, and he is having early satiety, which is likely caused by splenomegaly.

12. *Answer:* A

Rationale: Chronic myelogenous leukemia (CML) is a clonal disorder that originates from the Philadelphia chromosome translocation of the BCR-ABL oncogene. The translocation between chromosome 9 and 22 fuses together causing tyrosine kinase activity, which results in initiation of leukemia (Philadelphia chromosome). There are three phases of this disorder, which include chronic, accelerated, and blast crisis phase. Inherited pathogenic variants in the ATM (ataxia telangiectasia mutated) gene are associated with increased risk of certain cancers. People who inherit an altered pathogenic copy of the ATM gene from one parent are at increased risk of female breast cancer (up to 52% lifetime risk), and possibly pancreatic, prostate, and other cancers. Persons who inherit two altered pathogenic copies of the ATM gene develop ataxia-telangiectasia syndrome or Louis-Bar syndrome, which is a rare, neurodegenerative, autosomal recessive disease, which causes severe disability. Persons with inherited (germline) tp53 pathogenic variants are at risk for breast, lung, colon, gynecologic, sarcomas, and many other cancers and have a condition known as Li-Fraumeni syndrome. Trisomy 21, also known as Down syndrome, is a human chromosomal disorder caused by having three copies (trisomy) of chromosome 21.

13. *Answer:* D

Rationale: The blast phase is characterized by more than 30% blasts in the blood, bone marrow, or both. The patient may also experience fatigue, shortness of breath, bone and abdominal pain, splenomegaly, bleeding, and infection. An increased leukocyte may be seen in the chronic phase. In the accelerated phase the laboratory report might show 15% to less than 30% myeloblasts in the blood, more than 30% myeloblasts and promyelocytes combined, more than 20% basophils, and less than 100,000 platelets. There is no intermediate phase.

14. *Answer:* A

Rationale: APML is a biologically and clinically distinct variant of acute myeloid leukemia that is characterized by a translocation involving the *RARA* (retinoic acid receptor [RAR] alpha) gene on chromosome 17. Chronic myelogenous leukemia (CML) is a clonal disorder that originates from the Philadelphia chromosome translocation BCR-ABL oncogene. The translocation between chromosomes 9 and 22 fuse together, causing tyrosine kinase activity, which results in initiation of

leukemia (Philadelphia chromosome). An intrachromosomal amplification of chromosome (iAMP21) is associated with B-cell lymphoblastic leukemia/lymphoma. Trisomy 8 is a risk factor for AML.

15. *Answer:* B

Rationale: AML that expresses CD33-positive antigen is treated with FDA-approved gemtuzumab ozogamicin. All-trans retinoic acid (ATRA) plus arsenic trioxide (ATO) is a treatment for low or intermediate risk acute promyelocytic leukemia. Alemtuzumab targets CD 52 in chronic lymphocytic leukemia. Imatinib is a targeted therapy for chronic myelogenous leukemia.

CHAPTER 19

1. *Answer:* A

Rationale: Pancoast syndrome is characteristic of lung cancer arising in the superior sulcus (the apex of the lung) and is manifested by shoulder pain. Other intrathoracic effects of lung cancer include pleural effusions and superior vena cava syndrome. Lower extremity neuropathy and darkening of the skin are not intrathoracic effects of lung cancer. While hypomagnesia does not have an intrathoracic effect due to lung cancer, it can be associated with hypercalcemia, which is a known oncologic emergency seen in persons with lung cancer.

2. *Answer:* B

Rationale: Small cell lung cancer is diagnosed in 0% to 15% of lung cancers and has a more aggressive, rapidly growing course compared to non–small cell lung cancer. Since it is a rapidly growing disease, at the time of diagnosis, small cell lung cancer is likely widely disseminated. Patients with limited disease are often treated with chemotherapy in combination with radiation therapy, which may be followed by PDI immune checkpoint inhibitors. Surgery is not an option for these patients. Small cell lung cancer is associated with a poor prognosis with average overall 5-year survival of 7%.

3. *Answer:* A

Rationale: Current guidelines for lung cancer screening recommend that those individuals who are current or former smokers (>30 pack-years or quit <15 years), asymptomatic, and ages 55 to 74 should have annual screening with low-dose chest CT. The nurse working the local health fair, then, should have provided instructions for answer A. The use of inhaled marijuana and the use of electronic cigarettes have not been established as risk factors in the development of lung cancer.

4. *Answer:* D

Rationale: A VATS (video-assisted thoracic surgery) is a minimally invasive surgical technique and is associated with decreased morbidity. VATS is often done in conjunction with a wedge resection, where a wedge-shaped piece of lung tissue with a small tumor is removed. A pneumonectomy is a surgical procedure to remove the entire lung. Overall morbidity is higher for this type of surgery. Sleeve resection is done if the tumor is in the central area of the lung and growing into the bronchus, and this is not a common surgery.

A thoracotomy is a major surgical procedure done to access the chest cavity with an incision made through the chest wall. A resuscitative thoracotomy is an emergency procedure done for life-threatening emergencies such as chest hemorrhage.

5. *Answer:* A

Rationale: For early-stage NSCLC (stage I or IIa disease), stereotactic body radiation therapy (SBRT) or stereotactic ablative radiotherapy (SABR) is recommended for the patient who is not a surgical candidate or who refuses therapy. Oral chemotherapy is not indicated for treatment for this stage lung cancer. Low energy radiation does not penetrate deeply enough and is used mainly to treat skin cancers, and not NSCLC. Immunotherapy is often used for patients who have failed previous therapies.

6. *Answer:* C

Rationale: Immune checkpoint inhibitor drugs, such as pembrolizumab, nivolumab, and atezolizumab, are anti-PD-1 human monoclonal antibodies and immune checkpoint inhibitors approved for the first-line treatment of NSCLC. Checkpoint proteins, such as PD-L1 found on tumor cells and PD-1 on T cells, help maintain normal immune responses in the body. However, cancer cells are able to downregulate (turn off) the normal immune response of T cells so they don't kill cancer cells that are present. Immune checkpoint inhibitor drugs act to unblock the binding of PD-L1 to PD-1 (take the brakes off the immune response), thus freeing the T cells to kill cancer cells. However, there are immune-related side effects associated with these drugs that can harm normal tissues and cause thyroid dysfunction, rash, type I diabetes, and inflammation of solid organs, including the colon, liver, skin, lung, and thyroid gland. Immune checkpoint inhibitors are widely used in the treatment of NSCLC and SCLC, both as primary therapy and as adjuvant and neoadjuvant therapies, rather than after the patient has progressed on other therapies. Immune checkpoint inhibitor drugs do not harbor molecules that break down cancer cells.

7. *Answer:* A

Rationale: Prophylactic cranial radiation therapy is indicated for individuals with complete response to chemotherapy or radiation therapy to reduce the risk of developing brain metastasis. The overall 5-year relative survival rate is poor at 7%. Alterations in the KRAS oncogene may be seen in non–small cell lung cancers, rather than small cell lung cancer. Surgery is rarely an option for the primary treatment of small cell lung cancer, as the cancer has usually spread by the time it is found.

8. *Answer:* D

Rationale: His potential exposure to asbestos over his long career in home remodeling and demolition could have played a significant role in E.W.'s cancer diagnosis. Those who have been exposed to asbestos have been known to have an increased risk of developing lung cancer (especially mesothelioma). Environmental and occupational factors do increase the risk of developing lung cancer. Other potential factors include exposure to radon gas and air pollution. While it is true that more men (14%) will be newly diagnosed with lung cancer than woman (13%)

and that 53% of all those diagnosed will be between the ages of 53 and 74, his age and gender are not factors in his diagnosis. His weight is also not a factor, though weight is a factor in many cancer cases especially colon, prostate, and breast cancers. Exposure to paint and paint thinners have been linked with limited evidence to bladder cancer.

9. *Answer:* C

Rationale: A.E. will need to be prepared for a thoracentesis. In the presence of pleural effusion, a thoracentesis is performed to determine malignancy. The presence of malignant cells identified in the pleural fluid will alter the stage of lung cancer. Endoscopic ultrasound-guided needle aspiration biopsy is useful to visualize and sample adjacent lymph nodes. Mediastinoscopy is a minor procedure used to obtain samples of all accessible lymph nodes. Bronchoscopy is recommended for a centrally located lung lesion to confirm diagnosis. If negative, further tests are recommended.

10. *Answer*: A

Rationale: The nurse's role is to help manage or decrease the severity of symptoms associated with the disease, treatment, or both. The nurse should assess the patient with lung cancer for the presence of fatigue and weakness. Individuals diagnosed with lung cancer are known to be at high risk for pain and multiple other symptoms such as shortness of breath, fatigue, and weakness. Stomach cramps, diarrhea, or constipation are unlikely to be caused by the disease or the treatment, which are located in the thorax. Night sweats are typically not associated with lung cancer.

CHAPTER 20

1. *Answer:* B

Rationale: Early favorable Hodgkin's lymphoma is a clinical stage I or II without any additional risk factors. The patient has an early favorable stage Hodgkin's lymphoma, which requires a limited amount of chemotherapy (usually two to three cycles) plus involved field radiation therapy. For patients with unfavorable stages, a moderate amount of chemotherapy (four cycles) plus involved field radiation is required. High-dose chemotherapy followed by autologous bone marrow transplant may be required for patients who have relapsed/refractory disease. Combination chemotherapy and radiation is associated with long-term survival in more than 80% of patients. Palliative chemotherapy and radiation therapy are not the correct treatment options for patients who have favorable Hodgkin's lymphoma.

2. *Answer:* B

Rationale: The patient has Stage II diffuse large-B cell lymphoma. Diffuse large-B cell lymphoma is the most common type of non-Hodgkin lymphoma (NHL). Standard treatment options include chemotherapy with or without radiation therapy, and RCHOP. Autologous peripheral blood stem cell transplant is indicated for patients with recurrent NHL. Salvage radiation therapy is not a treatment plan for patients with NHL. Ifosfamide, carboplatin, etoposide (ICE) is a second-line regimen for patients who have relapsed/refractory Hodgkin's lymphoma.

3. *Answer:* A

Rationale: The nurse would expect to see Reed-Sternberg cells reported on the patient's pathology examination as they are present with classic Hodgkin's lymphoma. Bone marrow involvement and lymphadenopathy with extranodal involvement are typically present in NHL. Metastases to the long bones are not diagnostic of Hodgkin's lymphoma.

4. *Answer:* D

Rationale: The Lugano Classification modification of the Ann Arbor Staging system is used to stage lymphoma. Staging is based on the extent of the disease and the presence of systemic symptoms. The Rai staging system is typically used to stage CLL. The Tumor Nodes Metastasis staging is usually used to stage solid cancers; however, the Ann Arbor Staging system is used to stage lymphomas. The Reed-Steenberg pathologic staging system is not a staging system.

5. *Answer:* C

Rationale: A risk factor for the development of mucosa-associated lymphoid tissue (MALT) lymphoma of the stomach is the bacterial infection *Helicobacter pylori* infection (*H. pylori*). Having *H. pylori* does not put a patient at risk for developing inflammatory breast cancer or cancer of the distal colon, but it does increase the risk of developing gastric cancer and should be treated. A risk factor for development of Burkitt lymphoma is Epstein-Barr virus infection.

6. *Answer:* A

Rationale: The majority of patients who have a high-grade, localized non-Hodgkin lymphoma (NHL) who receive radiation plus chemotherapy or combination chemotherapy alone, have an overall survival at 5 years of over 60%. Patients who have aggressive NHL have a cure rate of 50%; however, they can expect to relapse within 2 years after therapy. Those patients with an 80% cure rate are those who are diagnosed with Hodgkin lymphoma and who are treated with combination chemotherapy and/or radiation therapy. High-dose chemotherapy (HDCT) followed by an autologous stem cell transplant is sometimes utilized in Hodgkin lymphoma or NHL, which is refractory or recurrent, but does not ensure a cure.

7. *Answer:* D

Rationale: T.J.'s systemic symptoms—fever, weight loss, fatigue, and night sweats—are considered "B" symptoms of lymphoma. The common clinical presentation of lymphoma is enlarged lymph nodes, spleen, and other immune tissue, with or without the systemic symptoms. Pain in the chest is not a symptom, but some patients do report pain in the nodal site when drinking (though the significance of such pain has not been established). Swelling of the limbs is not symptomatic, and extreme thirst and frequent urination could be signs of many conditions—from dehydration to diabetes—but is not a systemic symptom of lymphoma.

8. *Answer:* A

Rationale: The correct answer is A. A 24-hour urine test is not necessary in staging a non-Hodgkin lymphoma (NHL). The other options are necessary tests to diagnose and stage NHL. A lymph node biopsy is required to determine pathology. If the pathology reveals a CD 20+ tumor, the patient may receive rituximab (Rituxan, a monoclonal antibody specific for CD 20+ cells) as part of his chemotherapy regimen. To complete staging for non-Hodgkin lymphoma, a computed tomography scan of the chest, abdomen, and pelvis must be completed. In addition, a bilateral bone marrow biopsy and aspirate are done to determine whether bone marrow disease is present.

CHAPTER 21

1. *Answer:* B

Rationale: A known risk factor for developing multiple myeloma is a history of monoclonal gammopathy of undetermined significance (MGUS). Additionally, another risk factor includes exposure to the herbicide and defoliant Agent Orange that was used by the U.S. military during deployment in the Vietnam War during the 1960s and early 1970s. Other risk factors include exposures to: ionizing radiation, certain metals (especially nickel), agricultural chemicals, benzene, and petroleum products, aromatic hydrocarbons, and silicone. Multiple myeloma has also been linked to a family history of the disease, obesity, and immunologic issues (patients with AIDS have been associated with developing multiple myeloma). Finally, ethnicity has been shown as a risk factor, with multiple myeloma having twice the incidence in Blacks than in their Caucasian counterparts. Exposure to Epstein-Barr virus is a risk factor for lymphoma but not specific to multiple myeloma. The employment status of a person or female gender are not known risk factors.

2. *Answer*: A

Rationale: In the United States, the highest incidence of multiple myeloma (MM) is seen among Blacks, men, and older adults. MM is twice as common among Blacks in the United States compared to whites and is the leading hematologic malignancy among Blacks. Globally, MM is 1.5 times as common among men. Since 1990, MM incidence has increased by 126% globally and by 40% in the United States. White women, young adults, and diabetic individuals do not have the highest incidence of MM. Most cases of MM are diagnosed between the ages of 65 and 74 with fewer than 14% being diagnosed before age 55.

3. *Answer:* D

Rationale: Multiple myeloma (MM) is a malignancy of the plasma cells (mature B cells) that results in production of a complete or partial monoclonal immunoglobulin protein (M protein), resulting in osteolytic bone lesions, renal disease, anemia, hypercalcemia, and immunodeficiency, a constellation known as CRAB symptoms, that are common presentations of MM. Bence-Jones proteins, the accumulation of monoclonal antibodies, can appear in the urine and lead to kidney damage and ultimately kidney failure. Multiple myeloma is most often associated with hypercalcemia due to osteolytic bone breakdown versus hypocalcemia. Hyperkalemia indicates increased serum potassium levels and is not associated with MM. Polycythemia indicates an excessive amount of red blood cells and is not characteristic of MM.

4. *Answer:* C

Rationale: Bone marrow biopsy is the confirmatory test for establishing the diagnosis of multiple myeloma, which demonstrates the presence of more than 10% clonal plasma cells. Additional tests that might be used to assess the extent of multiple myeloma include serum protein immunoelectrophoresis, urine protein immunoelectrophoresis, serum lactate dehydrogenase, and urinary light chain M proteins (Bence Jones proteins). Multiple myeloma-related organ dysfunction is also evaluated with laboratory assessment for hypercalcemia, renal insufficiency, and anemia, as well as lytic bone lesions. While a bone scan might identify a lytic lesion, it is not diagnostic for multiple myeloma. A renal ultrasound can determine some abnormalities in the kidneys but does not assess for renal insufficiency. A complete blood count will demonstrate anemia, but it is not specific for multiple myeloma.

5. *Answer:* D

Rationale: Lytic bone lesions are the most common source of pain in persons with multiple myeloma. For this reason, supportive care for persons with multiple myeloma often includes treating the lytic lesion with radiation therapy as well as administering medications such as bisphosphonates or denosumab to inhibit bone breakdown. Additionally, neural infiltration of plasma cells and intestinal obstruction are also not common underlying causes of pain in multiple myeloma. Anemia is common in multiple myeloma but symptoms typically include fatigue and possibly shortness of breath, not pain.

6. *Answer:* D

Rationale: The diagnostic criteria for active or symptomatic multiple myeloma requiring therapy is calcium elevation in blood, with a calcium level greater than 11.0 ng/L or >1 mg/dL higher than the upper limit of normal. Fifty percent is the incorrect percentage of clonal bone marrow plasma cells. The correct percentage is 60% or higher. Serum-free light chain ration Kappa: lambda <100 is incorrect. The correct answer is serum-free light chain ration Kappa: lambda >100. Magnetic resonance imaging (MRI) studies with <1 focal lesion (>8 mm in size) is also incorrect. The correct answer is magnetic resonance imaging (MRI) studies with >1 focal lesion (>5 mm in size). Other diagnostic criteria include renal insufficiency (with a serum creatinine level greater than 2 mg/dL), anemia (hemoglobin less than 10 g/dL), bone lytic lesions (detected through a metastatic bone survey, MRI, or positron emission tomography/computed tomography (PET/CT) imaging).

7. *Answer:* D

Rationale: Treatment for this patient is aimed at reduction and control of the disease with a palliative intent. No cure currently exists for MM, but increases in overall survival are due to ongoing development of new therapies and better understanding of the disease. Survival has improved significantly over the last two decades, with an overall 5-year survival in the US of 55.6%. No cure exists for multiple myeloma regardless of trisomy translocations, and surgery is not indicated for treating patients with multiple myeloma.

8. *Answer:* B

Rationale: Primary prevention strategies for multiple myeloma include limiting occupational exposure to chemicals such as pesticides, asbestos, benzene, and other chemicals used in rubber manufacturing, as well as ionizing radiation. There has been no proven link between multiple myeloma and tobacco use or alcohol consumption. Physical activity not shown to be preventative for MM. Consuming a diet rich in fruits and whole grains is recommended, as is maintaining a healthy weight because being overweight or obese increases risk for MM by 12% to 21%.

CHAPTER 22

1. *Answer:* B

Rationale: Myelofibrosis (MF) is a rare, chronic, and progressive blood cancer. It is often grouped together with polycythemia vera (PV) and essential thrombocythemia (ET). The World Health Organization classifies myelofibrosis as a BCR-ABL negative myeloproliferative neoplasm (MPN). A pathogenic variant of a particular gene known as Janus kinase 2 (JAK2) is found in a large proportion of people with types of myeloproliferative neoplasms, such as PV, ET, and MF. These conditions are referred to as JAK2 MPNs.

2. *Answer:* D

Rationale: In this example, M.S.'s age of 66 years is associated with increased risk for developing myelofibrosis. Myelofibrosis is most often diagnosed in persons older than 50 years, with average age at diagnosis of about 65 to 67 years. There are no known additional risks based on lifestyle or environmental factors, gender, race, or ethnicity, so M.S.'s history of cigarette smoking, obesity, and Hispanic ethnicity are not associated with increased risk.

3. *Answer:* A

Rationale: Primary myelofibrosis is characterized by alterations in myeloid stem cells, megakaryocyte hyperplasia, and bone marrow scarring (fibrosis). Pathogenic variants in certain genes, including JAK2, alter normal cell development and the function of multiple cell types deriving from myeloid stem cells including red blood cells, white blood cells, and platelets. Abnormal megakaryocyte production (cells in the bone marrow that produce platelets), referred to as megakaryocyte hyperplasia, is a hallmark of myelofibrosis, and leads to overactivation of inflammatory cytokines and the development of bone marrow fibrosis. Bone marrow fibrosis, or scarring, progressively disrupts normal marrow function and further alters the bone marrow's production of myeloid cells.

4. *Answer:* D

Rationale: Pain localized to the left upper quadrant of the abdomen could indicate the presence of hepatosplenomegaly (enlargement of the liver and spleen). Enlarged spleen is common in primary myelofibrosis.

Recent weight gain, leg cramps during the night, and heart palpitations are not clinical manifestations of myelofibrosis. Symptoms of myelofibrosis may include fatigue, bone pain, early satiety, general abdominal discomfort, itching, night sweats, and difficulty concentrating.

5. *Answer:* C

Rationale: Complete blood count test results from a patient with myelofibrosis would be expected to show anemia and thrombocytopenia. White blood cell count could be elevated (leukocytosis) or decreased (leukopenia). Neutropenia would be expected. Other laboratory test results could reveal elevated lactate dehydrogenase (LDH), elevated uric acid, and elevated or decreased erythropoietin. Polycythemia and decreased LDH would not be present. Neither would high neutrophils and low eosinophils. A peripheral blood smear and bone marrow biopsy would also be performed.

6. *Answer:* B

Rationale: The median overall survival for a patient with secondary myelofibrosis, due to a history of polycythemia vera or essential thrombocythemia, is dependent upon karyotype and ranges from 2 to 6 years. Overall survival for patients with primary myelofibrosis is estimated to be about 7 years from diagnosis. The other options are not accurate.

7. *Answer:* C

Rationale: Management of myelofibrosis is often driven by and adapted to each patient's clinical presentation and risk category as determined by prognostic scoring systems. A 73-year-old patient with chronic medical conditions, such as diabetes and cardiomyopathy, and newly diagnosed intermediate-risk myelofibrosis, would most likely be treated with a Janus kinase (JAK) inhibitor, such as ruxolitinib, as first-line therapy. Low-risk patients may follow a "watch and wait" treatment strategy with diligent clinical observation in favor of systemic therapy. Hematopoietic stem cell transplant (HSCT) is the only curative treatment available for myelofibrosis and should be considered for high-risk patients. However, not all patients are candidates for transplant, and there is significant morbidity and mortality associated with HSCT. Post-transplant survival may be as low as 50%. Clinical trials may be offered to patients who are refractory to treatment with JAK inhibitors. Treatment with radiation therapy is not typical. Supportive care for anemia and thrombocytopenia would consist of transfusions of red blood cells and platelets. Corticosteroids and erythropoietin stimulating agents may also be used as supportive care therapies.

CHAPTER 23

1. *Answer:* A

Rationale: Pediatric tumors are most often malignant and are diagnosed more often than any other type of cancer in pediatrics except for leukemia. More than 4000 primary CNS tumors are diagnosed in children and teens each year.

2. *Answer:* B

Rationale: Points of care where neuro-imaging is indicated are preoperatively, postoperatively, and at follow-up examinations. Preoperatively, imaging is used to identify patterns of cerebral edema or location of lesions. Postoperative imaging with CT or MRI is recommended within 24 hours of surgical resection to assess residual tumor volume and establish new baseline to measure treatment effect. Follow-up examinations ordered every 3 to 4 months is the typical standard practice outside of clinical trials, unless clinically indicated otherwise.

3. *Answer:* A

Rationale: While corticosteroids may be administered preoperatively, and antiepileptic medications may be given perioperatively, they are to control symptoms of the tumor and are not a primary treatment for the tumor. The most important therapy for a primary brain tumor is maximal surgical resection. Chemotherapy is not effective in many types of brain tumors.

4. *Answer:* C

Rationale: Of children and teens diagnosed with a central nervous system tumor, about 75% will be alive more than 5 years after the initial diagnosis. This is important for the oncology nurse to anticipate because of the substantial survivorship issues that these children, teens, and parents must endure.

5. *Answer:* C

Rationale: Each of these drug classes may have one or more of these side effects, but corticosteroids are the only one that has all these risks.

6. *Answer:* B

Rationale: Of all tumor types, lung most frequently metastasizes to the brain. In order of frequency, tumors that most commonly spread to the brain are: lung (18% to 64%), breast (2% to 21%), cancer of unknown primary (1% to 18%), colorectal (2% to 12%), kidney (1% to 8%), and melanoma (20%).

7. *Answer:* A

Rationale: Of all tumor types, leptomeningeal carcinomatosis is more frequently associated with breast tumors (22%), followed by lung tumors (15%), and then prostate (10%); lymphoma (10%); kidney (7%); gastrointestinal tract (5%); melanoma (4%); unknown (4%).

8. *Answer:* C

Rationale: Seizures are the presenting symptom in 15% of primary brain tumors and in 20% of brain metastases. Risk is highest with primary cortical tumors; temporal tumors tend to be most epileptogenic.

9. *Answer:* C

Rationale: Antiepileptic drug (AED) therapy indicated in those with seizures and during the perioperative craniotomy setting; prophylactic use of anticonvulsants is not indicated otherwise. Each of these other options may seem plausible; however, persons with brain cancer treatment require anti-epileptic medication in the perioperative period. Otherwise, anti-epileptic medication is not indicated unless the person has a known seizure disorder. First-line agents include lamotrigine, levetiracetam, pregabalin, or valproic acid.

10. *Answer:* A

Rationale: The World Health Organization (WHO) classification of a central nervous system tumor is universally applicable and prognostically valid. The AJCC TNM classification system is not used to stage primary central nervous system tumors because two of three indicators are not applicable (there are no nodes and extracranial metastases are extraordinarily rare). National Comprehensive Cancer Network (NCNN) does not provide staging/classification of disease criteria.

11. *Answer:* D

Rationale: The section of the brain responsible for personality is the frontal lobe. The frontal lobe is responsible for not only our personality, but a person's movement, reasoning, behavior, memory, planning, decision-making, judgment, initiative, inhibition, and mood. The occipital lobe accounts for our vision. The temporal lobe accounts for language comprehension, behavior, memory, hearing, and emotions, while the parietal lobe gives us the ability to tell right from left, allows us to do mathematical calculations, allows us to feel sensations, and gives us the power of reading and writing.

12. *Answer:* D

Rationale: The most common types of primary spinal tumors are schwannomas, menigngiomas, and ependymomas, which comprise 79% of all spinal tumors. Chordomas are the least common of the spinal tumors. The second most common are sarcomas, followed by astrocytomas, and vascular tumors.

13. *Answer:* D

Rationale: The section of the brain responsible for coordination and balance is the cerebellum. The cerebellum is also responsible for fine muscle control. The temporal lobe accounts for language comprehension, behavior, memory, hearing, and emotions, while the parietal lobe gives us the ability to tell right from left, allows us to do mathematical calculations, allows to feel sensations, and gives us the power of reading and writing. The pituitary gland controls our hormones, growth, and fertility. The brainstem regulates and controls our breathing, blood pressure, heartbeat, and swallowing functionality.

14. *Answer:* C

Rationale: Ionizing radiation (IR) is a known extrinsic risk factor. According to various sources, there is a causal relationship between therapeutic irradiation of doses >2500 cGy and development of brain tumors; risk is higher for nerve sheath tumors and meningiomas than gliomas. Being immunocompromised, including having a diagnosis of HIV/AIDS, taking immunosuppressive medical therapies, and having a congenital immunodeficiency are all examples of situational risk factors. Exposure to pesticides, petrochemicals, electromagnetic fields, inks and solvents, dietary N-nitroso compounds, long-term use of black or brown hair dyes, cell phones, aspartame, and certain viral exposures are unproven risk factors and currently under investigation. Race/ethnicity is an intrinsic risk factor. The most at risk are Caucasian with northern European descent, while meningioma is more common in African American populations.

15. *Answer:* C

Rationale: The most commonly diagnosed primary brain tumor is glioblastoma and anaplastic astrocytomas

(38%), followed by meningiomas and other mesenchymal tumors (27%), pituitary tumors, schwannomas, primary CNS lymphoma, oligodendroglioma, ependymoma low-grade astrocytoma, and medulloblastoma.

16. *Answer:* D

Rationale: Global effects of radiation therapy to the brain include headaches, neurocognitive changes, seizures, and somnolence. Somnolence is also a subacute exacerbation of tumor-related symptoms. Late radiation effects include radiation necrosis, diffuse white matter changes, neurocognitive effects, cerebrovascular events, optic nerve toxicities, endocrine toxicities, and secondary malignancies.

17. *Answer:* B

Rationale: Genetic/inherited risk factors account for 5% to 17% of primary brain tumors. These include: neurofibromatosis 1 (*NF1* gene, 17q11), neurofibromatosis 2 (*NF2* gene, 22q12), Turcot syndrome type 1 (*APC* gene, 3p21, 7p22), Turcot syndrome type 2 (APC gene, 5q21), Gorlin syndrome (*PTCH* gene), tuberous sclerosis (*TSC1,* 9q34, and *TSC2,* 16p13, genes), Li-Fraumeni syndrome (*TP53* gene, 17p13), von-Hippel-Lindau disease (*VHL* gene, 3p25–26), *BRCA1, BRCA2,* and *PALB2* germline mutations, *P14 (ARF)* germline mutations, and Nevoid basal cell carcinoma syndrome (9q22.3).

18. *Answer:* A

Rationale: Whole brain radiation therapy (WBRT) is the mainstay of treatment for brain metastases. Radiation is palliative. If one to three BM, consider stereotactic radiosurgery (SRS) alone (16 to 24 Gy); more than four BM, consider WBRT. Hypofractionated radiosurgery (21 to 25 Gy over three to five fractions) recommended for BM >3 cm due to high risk of radiation necrosis. Systemic chemotherapy or biotherapy is not routine treatment for brain/spine metastasis due to poor penetration through blood–brain barrier. As well, heavily pretreated tumors are less chemosensitive.

CHAPTER 24

1. *Answer:* D

Rationale: HPV vaccination, Pap testing, HPV screening, and addressing risk factors all encourage prevention, early diagnosis, and early treatment of precancerous or cancerous cervical changes, which decreases the risk of death from cervical cancer. Vaccination for HPV types 16, 18, 31, 33, 45, 52, and 58 is recommended for both males and females starting at age 11 to 12. It can be given as early as age 9. Teenage boys and girls who did not get vaccinated when they were younger should be educated about the vaccine and encouraged to get it. The HPV vaccine is recommended for young women through age 26 and young men through age 21 years. There is not a vaccination for hepatitis C. HIV screening is not routinely done in the general population.

2. *Answer:* B

Rationale: Patients with hereditary nonpolyposis colorectal cancer (HNPCC)/Lynch syndrome have a 60% lifetime risk of endometrial cancer due to genetic susceptibility. Increased estrogen is associated with a higher risk of developing endometrial cancer. Modifiable sources of increased estrogen can come from obesity, a high fat diet, or diabetes. Endometrial cancer is hormonally driven, and tamoxifen can work like estrogen in the uterus and increases the risk of endometrial cancer, similarly to unopposed estrogen therapy. Aromatase inhibitors may actually decrease the risk of developing endometrial cancer. Early menarche and late menopause are risk factors for endometrial cancer as they also extend the period of time the uterus is exposed to hormonal drivers over the course of a female patient's life. Late menarche and early menopause would not be considered risk factors.

3. *Answer:* B

Rationale: Known risk factors for ovarian cancer include smoking, nulliparity, older age at first birth, hormone replacement therapy (HRT), pelvic inflammation disease (PID), ovarian stimulation for in vitro fertilization (IVF) (in some cases), as well as genetic risk factors. Although most ovarian cancer is not inherited, this patient meets genetic screening criteria because of the history of ovarian cancer in the patient and breast cancer in her sister. Genetic evaluation in the patient may help determine if her daughter has hereditary risk for developing breast, ovarian, or other cancers. Most new ovarian cancer diagnoses are in patients over age 55, and hormone therapy replacement is a risk factor, not a protective factor, for ovarian cancer. There is no routine screening test for ovarian cancer. Protective factors include a younger age at first pregnancy, use of oral contraception, and breastfeeding.

4. *Answer:* A

Rationale: Patients should wait at least 12 months after completing treatment before conceiving, as (1) it is unsafe to conceive while undergoing or immediately after chemotherapy treatment, and (2) most relapses will occur within as 12-month timeframe. Chemotherapy is effective with good cure rates and has not been shown to decrease fertility after treatment for gestational trophoblastic neoplasia. Levels of human chorionic gonadotrophin reflect a state of nonconception or conception so does not apply to this question.

5. *Answer:* A

Rationale: Diethylstilbestrol (DES) administered to a pregnant woman exposes the developing fetus to DES, and can increase the risk of congenital abnormalities and vaginal cancer in offspring. Breast cancer in a first-degree relative and use of HRT are not known risk factors associated with vaginal, vulvar, or cervical cancer. Asbestos exposure in a parent has not been shown to increase vaginal, vulvar, or cervical cancer risk in offspring.

6. *Answer:* D

Rationale: Testicular cancer most often occurs in males between the ages of 20 and 43. A painless testicular mass or swelling in one testicle is a red flag symptom for testicular cancer. If discovered on self-exam, this finding should be reported by patients to their health care provider for a full diagnostic evaluation. Testicular cancer is less common in African American or Asian/Pacific Islander men. Other risk factors include a personal or family history of germ cell tumor, cryptorchidism, testicular dysgenesis, and Klinefelter syndrome.

7. *Answer:* B

Rationale: Modifiable risk factors for penile cancer include HPV vaccination to prevent HPV infection, prevention of HIV infection, circumcision before puberty, and tobacco cessation. The foreskin should be retracted when cleaning the glans to maintain adequate hygiene in uncircumcised patients. Penile cancer is more common in parts of Asia, Africa, and South America than in North America or Europe. It is a rare cancer in the United States with usual presentation at 50 to 70 years. Infection with HIV/HPV, types 16 or 18 is positive in 60% to 80% of penile cancers and is a modifiable risk factor. Other known risk factors include phimosis, balanitis, chronic inflammation, penile trauma, lack of circumcision, lichen sclerosis, tobacco use, and poor hygiene.

8. *Answer:* A

Rationale: A rising CA125 is a biochemical sign of relapse or recurrence. Possible signs of ovarian cancer recurrence include abdominal bloating, bowel/bladder changes, weight loss, early satiety, nausea, vomiting, and ascites. Vaginal discharge and bleeding is not a common symptom associated with ovarian cancer.

9. *Answer:* B

Rationale: Per National Comprehensive Cancer Network (NCCN) guidelines, the standard of care for endometrial cancer is usually an upfront TAH/BSO, which may or may not be followed by adjuvant treatment. Fertility sparing surgery is not usually recommended and is considered as a treatment only in rare cases with genetic counseling, continuous progestin-based suppression, and hysterectomy after childbearing, or on progression of disease. Hormone therapy is generally reserved for patients who are not surgical candidates and is continued until progression. Assessing for endometrial thickening, or performing a D&C, is a part of the diagnostic, but not treatment process.

10. *Answer:* C

Rationale: Fertility sparing procedures, including conization with cold knife or loop electrosurgical excision (LEEP), or radical trachelectomy are treatments for early-stage (IA1–IA2) cervical cancer. Radical hysterectomy and lymph node evaluation is treatment for select Stage IIA1 disease. For patients with cervical cancer stages IB2, IIA2, or greater, who are nonsurgical candidates, the recommended treatment is definitive chemotherapy and radiation therapy, in combination (chemoradiation), with or without transposition of the ovaries out of the radiation field, if premenopausal, and possibly neoadjuvant chemotherapy followed by resection.

11. *Answer:* D

Rationale: For treatment of metastatic cervical cancer, the recommendation is radiation therapy with or without chemotherapy, palliative systemic agents, and best supportive care. Simple or modified radical hysterectomy with or without lymph node evaluation is a nonfertility

159

sparing option for early-stage disease (IA1–IB1). External beam radiation therapy (EBRT) and neoadjuvant chemotherapy is incorrect. EBRT is used for advanced stage cancers but not in conjunction with neoadjuvant chemotherapy. Neoadjuvant chemotherapy followed by surgical resection, along with definitive chemoradiation (with or without ovarian transposition if premenopausal), is used in IB2, IIA2, or greater nonsurgical candidates: radiation therapy, systemic therapy, local ablation, and surgical resection are treatments for recurrent disease.

12. *Answer:* D

Rationale: Localized testicular cancer has the best 5-year survival rate in the United States at 99.2%. Other 5-year survival rates for testicular cancer in the United States are: regional = 96.1%, distant = 73.2%, unstaged = 76.7%. The overall survival rate is 95.1%.

13. *Answer:* B

Rationale: Sperm banking may be done before or after surgery, but ideally before any radiation therapy or chemotherapy since these treatments may have an adverse effect on male fertility.

14. *Answer:* B

Rationale: Based on her age of 45 years and her symptoms, F.D. is perimenopausal. Following surgery to remove her ovaries, she will become menopausal. Surgery and radiation therapy of the abdomen/pelvis result in sudden loss of estrogen, which can lead to vaginal dryness, pelvic tissue atrophy, hot flashes, mood changes, and osteoporosis. Alternating constipation and diarrhea, as well as change in urinary function, are not common complications following a hysterectomy. Risk of cardiovascular disease is increased in postmenopausal women especially those such as F.D. who are experiencing an early menopause.

15. *Answer:* C

Rationale: Vulvar cancer is most commonly diagnosed in older women aged 55 to 75 years, with most associated deaths occurring over 84 years. Average age in the United States is 68 years. It is the fourth most common gynecologic malignancy in the United States following uterine, ovarian, and cervical cancers and is relatively rare worldwide and in the United States. Vulvar cancer has not been associated with repeated miscarriages.

16. *Answer:* B

Rationale: Risk factors for vulvar cancer include a high number of sexual partners, initiation of sexual intercourse at an early age, previous history of cervical cancer, and Northern European ancestry. Other risk factors include oncogenic HPV infection, types 16 or 18, cigarette smoking, inflammatory conditions of the vulva, and immunodeficiency. Squamous cell skin cancer history, childbirth status, and initiation of menstruation at the relatively late age of 15 years are not known to be associated with vulvar cancer risk.

17. *Answer:* A

Rationale: Hormonal, genetic, and environmental factors play a role in the development of ovarian cancer. As many as 20% of all ovarian cancer cases are due to hereditary factors, which can include pathogenic variants in the BRCA1/BRCA2 genes and the presence of Lynch syndrome. Ovarian cancer is the eighth most common cancer in women worldwide with the highest rates seen in developing countries, except for Japan. Ovarian cancer incidence increases with age, and most women are diagnosed after age 55. Oral contraceptive use can offer long-term risk reduction in ovarian cancer. Reducing ovulation cycles is protective against ovarian cancer, so increased number of pregnancies and lactation can reduce the risk of developing ovarian cancer. It is not true that with each year of ovulation, the risk of ovarian cancer decreases.

18. *Answer:* C

Rationale: Recurrent ovarian cancer is frequently associated with later stages of disease. The nurse should assess for the presence of abdominal bloating, ascites, bowel and bladder changes, weight loss, early satiety, nausea, and vomiting. Neck pain, weight gain, and skin dryness are not symptoms specifically associated with ovarian cancer.

19. *Answer:* A

Rationale: Hydatidiform moles arise from placental tissue and are benign tumors with malignant potential. They do not arise from the cervix, vagina, or ovary. They are relatively uncommon overall and are more common in Asia than Europe or North America. Early detection with hCG level monitoring after molar pregnancies facilitates earlier treatment and better outcomes. Risk factors include very young or geriatric pregnancy (under 16 or over 45). There is some evidence for menarche after age 12, history of light menses, and use of oral contraceptive pills. Autosomal-recessive familial recurrent hydatidiform mole may be responsible

20. *Answer:* D

Rationale: The development of clear cell adenocarcinoma of the vagina is associated with exposure to diethylstilbestrol (DES) in utero. DES was created as the first synthetic estrogen and was prescribed to women from 1938 to 1971 to prevent miscarriages. Female offspring exposed to DES in the womb are called DES Daughters and have a heightened risk of this rare type of vaginal cancer. Excessive alcohol intake, nulliparity, and talcum powder use are not associated with increased risk of clear cell adenocarcinoma of the vagina.

CHAPTER 25

1. *Answer:* A

Rationale: The major risk factor for BCC is exposure to the ultraviolet radiation of sunlight, specifically, intermittent exposure early in life. BCCs develop primarily on sun-exposed skin. They are rarely found on palmoplantar surfaces and never appear on the mucosa. Approximately 80% arise on the head and neck area. They tend to be slow growing and arise without precursor lesions. BCCs can be locally invasive tumors. Family history of skin cancer is associated with increased risk but is not the major cause of BCC. Tobacco smoking and young age are not considered risk factors. Risk increases with older age (>65 years).

2. *Answer:* C

Rationale: The correct answer is actinic keratoses (AKs). Approximately 60% to 65% of SCCs arise from prior AKs. The presence of atypical nevi and multiple moles are associated with increased risk of melanoma. Skin viral infection is associated with Merkel cell carcinoma; 80% of cases are caused by a common virus (Merkel cell polyomavirus).

3. *Answer:* D

Rationale: In a Mohs procedure (called Mohs micrographic surgery), the dermatologist, who has specialized training in this technique, removes tissue in successive thin layers and examines each layer under the microscope to determine the skin depth at which cancer cells are no longer present. In this way, the maximum amount of normal tissue is preserved. The other three types of therapy, cryotherapy with a probe that applies subzero temperature, local chemotherapy injection, and curettage with cautery or electrodessication, are differing techniques used for superficial low-risk skin lesions.

4. *Answer:* B

Rationale: Organ transplant is the correct answer. Transplant recipients of solid organs receive immunosuppressive therapies to prevent organ rejection, increasing their risk of Merkel cell carcinoma. Other factors associated with increased risk are male gender, white European ancestry, and age ≥65 years.

5. *Answer:* C

Rationale: A tendency to bleed is the correct answer. Moles that bleed or itch, or demonstrate changes in shape, size, or color are concerning and require specialized evaluation. Normal moles have a symmetrical shape, regular borders, and are uniformly one color. The ABCDE rule can help reinforce characteristics of melanoma. A refers to asymmetry. B refers to border irregularity or faded borders. C refers to color irregularities or having multiple colors. D refers to diameter more than 5 mm. E refers to evolving.

6. *Answer:* B

Rationale: Immunotherapy is the correct answer. Immunotherapy is considered the standard treatment for metastatic melanoma. Immunotherapy may consist of anti PD-1 monotherapy with pembrolizumab, or nivolumab or combination anti-CTLA-4+ anti-PD-1 with ipilimumab and nivolumab. The other options are not part of standard therapy for metastatic melanoma. Isolated limb perfusion may be used in certain clinical situations, and cranial radiation therapy may be used palliatively for patients with brain metastases.

7. *Answer:* B

Rationale: Merkel cell carcinoma (MCC) presents as papules, plaques, and cyst-like structures or pruritic tumors on the lower extremities. MCC most commonly presents as an erythematous or violaceous, tender, dome-shaped nodule on sun-exposed areas on the head or neck of an elderly white male. Develops primarily on sun-exposed skin and rarely found on palmoplantar surfaces and never appears on the mucosa are characteristics of a basal cell carcinoma (BCC). A BCC can also develop at sites of chemical exposure or chronic trauma. Cutaneous squamous cell carcinoma (cuSCC) often presents as a new or enlarging lesion that may bleed, weep, be tender, or be painful.

8. *Answer:* A

Rationale: A major risk factor in basal cell carcinoma (BCC) is UVR, specifically intermittent exposure early in life. Characteristics of Merkel cell carcinoma (MCC) are that MCCs most commonly present as erythematous or violaceous, tender, dome-shaped nodules on sun-exposed areas on the head or neck of an elderly white male. Most MCC lesions are <2 cm in diameter at the time of diagnosis, and rapid growth is common. Cutaneous squamous cell carcinomas (cuSCC) are typically slow growing; however, those arising in non–sun-exposed sites (i.e., lips, genitalia, perianal areas) are more aggressive with a higher risk of metastases.

9. *Answer:* D

Rationale: The ABCDE rule is an acronym used to help detect early signs of melanoma. E stands for evolving. Normal moles should not change (evolve) in size, shape or color, while melanoma may possess features such as evolving size, shape, color, or concerning symptoms such as itching or bleeding. A stands for asymmetrical. Normal moles are symmetrical in appearance (1/2 of the lesion is a mirror image of the other half) while melanomas tend to be asymmetrical. B stands for border irregularity. Normal moles tend to have even, regular, borders while melanomas tend to have irregular, jagged borders. C stands for color. Normal moles are uniformly one color, while melanomas tend to have color variegation. D stands for diameter. Normal moles tend to be ≤6 mm in size, while melanomas tend to be larger than 6 mm.

10. *Answer:* A

Rationale: Superficial spreading melanoma is the most common type accounting for 60% to 75% of melanomas. It can be found anywhere on the body but is more likely to occur on the trunk in men and lower legs in women, They often have color variation and irregular border and are more likely to harbor BRAF pathogenic variants than other subtypes. Nodular melanomas account for 15% to 30% of melanomas. They often appear as a smooth, dark polypoid nodule, but may also be red or flesh-colored (amelanotic). Nodular melanoma is the most aggressive and more likely to metastasize. The lentigo maligna subtype of melanoma accounts for 4% to 15% of melanoma and are most commonly found in chronically sun-damaged skin in the middle aged and elderly. Acral lentiginous melanomas account for less than 5% of melanomas. They typically appear as a black or brown discoloration under the nails or on the soles of the feet or palms of the hands and occasionally on mucosal surfaces and are the most common subtype among those with Asian or African descent. They are associated with advanced stage and poor prognosis; often misdiagnosed.

11. *Answer:* A

Rationale: Optional components of the histopathology on the pathology report include histologic subtype, cell type, amount of pigmentation, Clark level, tumor growth phase, and tumor-infiltrating lymphocytes. Clark's level refers to the level of tumor invasion through the layers of the skin. The Breslow level refers to depth of tumor invasion into the skin from the surface. Recommended components include size of specimen, tumor thickness/depth (Breslow) reported to the nearest 0.1 mm, ulceration, mitotic rate, microscopic satellites, and status of surgical margins (peripheral & deep).

12. *Answer:* B

Rationale: Cutaneous squamous cell carcinoma (cSCC) high-risk lesions should have at least a 6 mm margin. Low-risk lesions should have at least a 4 mm lesion. Very high–risk lesions should have at least a 10 mm lesion.

13. *Answer:* C

Rationale: These are all immune checkpoint inhibitors. Anti-PD-1 (anti-programmed death-1) antibody agents include pembrolizumab, nivolumab, and cemiplimab. Anti-PD-L1 (anti-programmed death ligand-1) antibody agents include avelumab and atezolizumab. Ipilimumab is an anti-CTLA-4 (anti-cytotoxic lymphocyte 4 [CTLA-4]) antibody, and relatlimab is an anti-LAG-3 antibody.

14. *Answer:* C

Rationale: More than 80% of melanomas possess genetic abnormalities in at least one key node in the MAPK signaling pathway. This occurs most commonly in the BRAF gene (~50%) and is most commonly found in the 600th codon (V600), followed by pathogenic variants in NRAS. Targeted therapy for patients with BRAF V600 pathogenic variant include dabrafenib combined with trametinib, vemurafenib combined with cobimetinib, or encorafenib combined with binimetinib.

15. *Answer:* B

Rationale: Imiquimod is an immune modulator that is a topical treatment used in the treatment of low-risk basal cell skin cancers. MEK inhibitors are targeted therapies directed against the MAPK pathway used in the treatment of melanoma typically in combination with a BRAF inhibitor. HH inhibitors are agents directed against the sonic hedgehog pathway used in the treatment of melanoma.

CHAPTER 26

1. *Answer:* A

Rationale: Prior to surgery, it is important to define the functional importance of the involved organ or structure. It is not an important factor for the nurse to know prior to surgery to determine if a jugular venous catheter will be placed and, if placed, will be communicated to the nurse for postoperative care considerations. Patient placement and wound preparation and irrigation are not principles of cancer surgery that need to be known prior to surgery; this information will be communicated to the nurse postoperatively if important to postoperative care.

2. *Answer:* B

Rationale: A wide excision is the removal of the cancer and adjacent tissues plus or minus any regional lymph nodes. The removal of cancer and large margins of tissue and removal of very small amounts of cancerous tissue with many lymph nodes are not correct definitions of the wide excision. Taking out an entire lesion and a small amount of surrounding tissue is a simple excision often done in an outpatient setting under local anesthesia. En bloc resection is removal of bulky cancer with contiguous

tissues, lymph nodes, and vascular structures required to attain safe margins.

3. *Answer:* C

Rationale: Glycemic control prior to surgery is preferred. Hyperglycemia can lead to volume depletion resulting in electrolyte imbalances, osmotic diuresis, diabetic ketoacidosis, increased surgical site infections, and poor wound healing. The patient is at risk for developing kidney disease due to diabetes, but not as a result of surgery. The patient's blood pressure may be elevated postoperatively but this condition may or may not be due to the diagnosis of diabetes. The patient's blood glucose levels may be high or low after surgery.

4. *Answer:* B

Rationale: Postsurgical radiation (adjuvant radiotherapy) is often done to treat potential microscopic disease that may be present in the breast after conservative surgery, such as lumpectomy, is performed. The action of blocking proteins to prevent the growth of cancer cells is targeted therapy and fighting cancer cells using the patient's own immune system is immunotherapy. Conserving the patient's breast tissue for later reconstruction is not a form of management for breast cancer.

5. *Answer:* C

Rationale: The World Health Organization (WHO) checklist includes ensuring patient confirmation, consent, site marking, a safe environment, and team collaboration through all perioperative phases. The Joint Commission National Patient Safety Goals ensures patient, team, and equipment preparation, site marking, "Universal Protocol" and "Time Out" safety goals. Safety standards to decrease length and cost of surgery are part of the Surgical Care Improvement Project. Completion of a "Pause" to ensure staff are in position and ensuring the proper use and disposal of hazardous drugs are not tools used to ensure safety and caregiving of the patient.

6. *Answer:* C

Rationale: A procedure in which multiple small incisions ("ports'") are made for surgical camera insertion and application of operative tools allowing less tissue manipulation is defined as a laparoscopic surgical approach. An example is a laparoscopic cholecystectomy. A procedure in which surgical tools are passed through an existing orifice (mouth, nares, anus, urethra) without external incision/scar is an endoscopic procedure. An example is a transvaginal cholecystectomy. An open procedure requires an extended, full-thickness incision to allow thorough exploration and manipulation of tissues, while a robotic procedure utilizes remotely controlled instruments allowing for less invasion, improved optics, finer control, and ergonomics to lessen tissue manipulation.

7. *Answer:* C

Rationale: The goal of palliative cancer surgery is to improve comfort when curative resection is not possible; includes surgical debulking or decompression or diversion via stent or ostomy (e.g., gastrojejunostomy, colostomy). Curative surgery removes primary tumor, lymph nodes, adjacent affected organs with negative margins attained via the least invasive means available. Types of this surgery included local excision, wide excision, and en bloc resection. Restorative "oncoplastic" surgery improves function or appearance of a surgical defect. Examples include restoration of a limb, or breast reconstruction after a mastectomy. Surgeries to repair hemorrhaging, organ perforation, or cord compression are procedures to address oncologic emergencies.

8. *Answer:* A

Rationale: In order to avoid the #1 cause of preventable death following surgery (i.e., DVT or pulmonary embolism), perioperative venous thromboembolism prophylaxis is required. This includes early ambulation, compression stockings, intermittent pneumatic compression, and use of antithrombotic medications (low dose fractionated heparin, low molecular weight heparin, factor Xa inhibitors). Hyperglycemic coma and ischemic stroke are unlikely outcomes of surgery. Urinary infection is possible after insertion of Foley catheter but is unlikely to cause death soon after surgery.

CHAPTER 27

1. *Answer:* D

Rationale: An allogeneic hematopoietic stem cell transplantation (HSCT) recipient receives HSCT from a healthy, related, or unrelated donor. Recipients receiving their own procured stem cells after high-dose chemotherapy applies to autologous HSCT. Because patients use their own procured stems cells in autologous HSCT procedures, immunosuppression is not required to prevent graft verse host disease, and neither is HLA matching.

2. *Answer:* A

Rationale: Posttransplant immunosuppression is used to prevent graft versus host disease in which donor T lymphocytes mount an immune response against the tissues of the stem cell recipient. Immunosuppression doesn't prevent relapse of the disease due to a low undetectable level of tumor cells persisting in the infusing cells, nor does it prevent posttransplant infectious complications with viral, bacterial, or fungal organisms. Finally, immunosuppression does not prevent damage to the small sinusoid of the liver from pretransplant conditioning regimen.

3. *Answer:* A

Rationale: Factors significantly affecting the source of donor marrow is the underlining malignancy to be treated, or the nonmalignant hematologic disease. Other factors include the availability of a histocompatible donor, and age and size of the patient. ABO matching is not required. The donor's disease status, physical, and psychosocial status do not affect determining the type of transplant, although they impact whether or not the donor might be suitable.

4. *Answer:* C

Rationale: One of the most common complications of allogeneic hematopoietic stem cell transplantation (HSCT) is graft-versus-host disease (GVHD) and also a major contributor to treatment-related mortality. Prevention and early recognition are some of the key factors in the success of the transplant. Erythematous maculopapular rash involving hands and feet is frequently seen in skin GVHD. Skin desquamation can be seen in severe cases. Hepatic sinusoidal obstruction syndrome is another complication of allogeneic transplant.

5. *Answer:* B

Rationale: Hepatic sinusoidal obstruction syndrome presents with the triad of jaundice, hepatomegaly, and ascites. Monitoring and care includes monitoring for weight gain, monitoring liver function studies, promptly evaluating abdominal pain, using caution when administering drugs that are cleared via hepatic system because increased toxicity may occur, and monitoring renal function.

6. *Answer:* C

Rationale: CMV infection is one of the posttransplant complications often due to viral reactivation in patients with prior exposure to CMV. Foscarnet is one of the medications used to treat CMV infection. Voriconazole and posaconazole are antifungal agents used in fungal infections. Acyclovir is used to treat herpes simplex infections.

7. *Answer:* D

Rationale: Reduced intensity or nonmyeloablative regimens are used in the allogeneic hematopoietic stem cell transplantation setting when the patient has a disease that will benefit from the graft-versus-tumor immunologic effect. Reduced intensity or nonmyeloablative HSCTs are used in the allogeneic transplant setting when the patient is older, has preexisting comorbidities, and has a disease that will benefit from the GVT immunologic effect.

8. *Answer:* B

Rationale: Autologous hematopoietic stem cell transplantation can be effective in treating some autoimmune diseases, even though it is not feasible in patients with a deficiency of their functional marrow, such as aplastic anemia. Allografts are indicated for the diseases such as leukemias that are not amenable to cure with standard treatment.

9. *Answer:* B

Rationale: Infectious and noninfectious pulmonary complications can occur after transplantation. Preventive measures for idiopathic pulmonary interstitial pneumonitis include use of CMV seronegative blood products and use of filtered air system (HEPA). Other measures include antimicrobial therapy with ganciclovir (Cytovene), foscarnet (Foscavir), intravenous immunoglobulin, trimethoprim and sulfamethoxazole, aerosolized or intravenous (IV) pentamidine (NebuPent, Pentacarinat, Pentam 300), azoles (voriconazole, posaconazole), and amphotericin B (Abelcet, AmBisome). High-dose steroids are not used as preventative measures so answer A is incorrect. Tacrolimus is an immunosuppressive therapy.

10. *Answer:* A

Rationale: Ursodiol is used as prophylaxis to protect against sinusoidal obstruction syndrome (SOS). Lovenox is an anticoagulant, which may be used for DVT prophylaxis. Bactrim is used as prophylaxis for pneumocystis jiroveci pneumonia. Pantoprazole is used for gastrointestinal prophylaxis.

11. *Answer:* B

Rationale: Acute graft-versus-host-disease (GVHD) commences during the first 100 days posttransplant. Total bilirubin of 4 mg/dl (liver stage 2) and diarrhea volume greater than 1000 mL/day (GI stage 2) put the patient at GVHD overall Clinical Grade III. The grading scale considers liver function (bilirubin level), amount of skin involvement, and volume of diarrhea to obtain an overall score.

12. *Answer:* C

Rationale: Pretransplantation hepatotoxic drug therapy is a risk factor for the development of hepatic sinusoidal obstruction (SOS) syndrome. Other risk factors include chemotherapy, abdominal radiation, pretransplantation, elevated transaminases before conditioning regimen, HLA mismatched or unrelated allogeneic transplantation, viral hepatitis, metastatic liver disease, Karnofsky score <90% before transplantation (second transplantation), older age recipient, and female gender are risk factors Karnofsky score >90% before transplantation is not a risk factor, nor is the patient undergoing a first transplantation, or 10/10 HLA-matched unrelated allogeneic transplantation.

13. *Answer:* D

Rationale: Immunosuppressant agents such as tacrolimus and cyclosporine have a narrow drug therapeutic window. Monitoring levels is essential to prevent toxicity.

14. *Answer:* B

Rationale: The goals of a pretransplantation conditioning regimen are to eradicate remaining malignancy, to suppress—and not boost—the immune system to allow for marrow engraftment in allografts, and to open spaces within the marrow compartment for newly infused PBSC or marrow to graft.

15. *Answer:* D

Rationale: Evaluating the patient's cyclosporine or tacrolimus levels and notifying the practitioner of significant abnormalities is a nursing implication for managing graft-versus-host disease (GVHD), both acute and chronic. Implement turning, coughing, and deep-breathing routine is a nursing implication for managing idiopathic pulmonary interstitial pneumonitis (infectious and noninfectious). Monitoring liver function and assessing patient's weight gain are nursing measures for managing hepatic sinusoidal obstruction syndrome. Monitoring visual acuity is a major nursing measure in the management of graft-versus-host disease.

16. *Answer:* A

Rationale: Idiopathic pulmonary interstitial pneumonitis (infectious) is most common in patients over the age of 30, with a history of chest irradiation or previous bleomycin therapy. Other characteristics of infection include found in patients with allogeneic transplantation, and CMV-positive with CMV-negative donors. Causative infections include cytomegalovirus, *Aspergillus* species, and *Pneumocystis jiroveci.* Response B describes GVHD. Infection in GVHD results from engraftment of immunocompetent donor T lymphocytes reacting against immunoincompetent recipient tissues (skin, gastrointestinal [GI] tract, liver). GVHD infections occur in 30% to 60% of all allogeneic bone marrow transplant recipients. Idiopathic pulmonary interstitial pneumonitis is less common in those with autologous transplants and in younger patients (men and women) less than 30 years of age.

17. *Answer:* C

Rationale: Aspergillus species is a fungal infection complication that occurs in hematopoietic stem cell transplantation (HSCT) recipients 1 to 4 months after transplantation. This fungal infection commonly occurs in the sinopulmonary site, the central nervous system, and skin. Other fungal infections that occur 1 to 4 months following transplant include *Candida* species, mucormycosis, coccidioidomycosis, and *Cryptococcus neoformans.* Gram-positive organisms are bacterial infections that occur in the sinopulmonary site, the skin, and in venous access devices. The parainfluenza virus is commonly found in the pulmonary system. Finally, the *Pneumocystis jiroveci (carinii)* is a protozoa, and it also strikes the pulmonary system of HSCT recipients.

18. *Answer:* C

Rationale: A bacterial infection complication that occurs in hematopoietic stem cell transplantation (HSCT) recipients 4 to 12 months after transplantation is *Streptococcus pneumoniae.* This bacterial infection is commonly found in the sinopulmonary system and in the blood. Varicella-zoster is a viral infection found in the integumentary and pulmonary systems, as well as in the hepatic and genitourinary sites. *P. jiroveci (carinii)* is a protozoa that is found in the pulmonary system in recipients 4 to 12 months after transplantation. Coccidioidomycosis is a fungal infection commonly found in the sinopulmonary cite of recipients.

19. *Answer:* D

Rationale: A social evaluation during assessment for a potential recipient of a hematopoietic stem cell transplantation (HSCT) is the type, number, and history of support systems in the family and the community available to the recipient. Other social assessments include the previous roles and responsibilities that the recipient had in their family and community, financial status (including employment, insurance coverage, and resources for daily living), and eligibility for community resources. An assessment of the type and effectiveness of coping mechanisms that the recipient used in stressful situations in the past (before transplantation therapy) is an example of a psychological evaluation. Another psychological evaluation is an assessment of the patient's and recipient's feelings about isolation, prolonged hospitalization, creating a living will, use of life-support technology, and potential death or survival. Finally, an assessment of the recipient's understanding of treatment aggressiveness, goals of therapy, and chances of survival is also an example of a psychological evaluation.

20. *Answer:* C

Rationale: CAR T-cells can identify the malignant cells that had previously evaded T-cell destruction.

CAR T-cell therapy is immunotherapy that utilizes a patient's modified autologous lymphocytes to recognize an antigen expressed by the targeted malignant cells.

21. **Answer:** B

Rationale: The FDA requires individuals who prescribe, dispense, and administer CAR T-cell therapy to complete the Risk Evaluation and Mitigation Strategy (REMS) program for approved CAR T-cell therapies. REMS is a safety program to ensure providers are aware of serious side effects and understand the risks and how to mitigate side effects safely. Staff education and training are required prior to the administration of CAR T-cell therapy to ensure safe patient care is provided. Patient and caregiver education must include providing a wallet card listing: date of infusion, provider contact information, and symptoms of cytokine release syndrome (CRS) and immune effector cell-associated neurotoxicity syndrome (ICANS) to monitor and report to the treating provider. Documenting patient comorbidities and performance status is part of the assessment process.

22. **Answer:** A

Rationale: Fever is the hallmark sign of cytokine release syndrome (CRS). Other symptoms of CRS include fever, hypotension, hypoxia, tachycardia, and organ dysfunction. Seizures and hemorrhage are signs of immune effector cell associated neurotoxicity syndrome (ICANS).

CHAPTER 28

1. **Answer:** B

Rationale: In addition to the guidelines of time, distance, and shielding, the oncology nurse should have a full understanding of radiation protection and safety. Inadequate knowledge or fear may lead to suboptimal patient care. Nurses must understand the effects of radiation, the risk of exposure, and the practices required to ensure safety for themselves and patients. A radiation safety officer is responsible for monitoring and reporting exposure results. There is no evidence that a silicone ring protects from radiation exposure. As noted above, time, distance, and shielding should be used to reduce staff exposure to emitted radiation. Alarms and safety mechanisms should be in place to prevent radiation beams from turning on if the room is not secure.

2. **Answer:** A

Rationale: Brachytherapy is defined as optimizing the radiation dose to the tumor and sparing surrounding tissues and organs and allows for high doses directly to the tumor. Radionuclides are used in brachytherapy procedures. These can consist of Cesium-137, Iridium-192, Gold-198, Radium-226, and Tantalum-182. Because of their complexity, brachytherapy requires a radiation safety officer along with the radiation treatment team to implement a very individualized treatment plan. External beam radiation therapy aims beams from outside the body to the tumor using a linear accelerator. Combining the two therapies treats both bulky local disease and improves local control. Side effects for external beam radiation include fatigue, upset stomach, diarrhea, nausea

and vomiting, and skin changes. Side effects for internal radiation (brachytherapy) include vaginal soreness, diarrhea, and bladder problems such as feelings of burning or pain when voiding, frequency, and feelings of the need to urinate shortly after urinating. Combining both types of treatments does not decrease the risk of side effects.

3. **Answer:** D

Rationale: Stereotactic body radiation therapy (SBRT) is a highly effective local therapy that requires accurate targeting, immobilization, and tumor motion management, to deliver a large dose of radiation therapy in fewer fractions. Stereotactic radiosurgery (SRS) and stereotactic body radiation therapy (SBRT) are precise methods of delivering high doses of radiation to well-defined target volumes that are not possible with conventional techniques.

4. **Answer:** A

Rationale: Xerostomia or dry mouth may be a permanent side effect. While the patient may experience secondary thyroid gland toxicity, secondary cancers such as AML are not a chronic side effect. Moist desquamation is an acute side effect. Neurological effects are frequently a consequence of brain radiation.

5. **Answer:** B

Rationale: Three-dimensional conformal radiation therapy (3DCRT) shapes the distribution of radiation dose to conform as closely as possible to the volume of the target, while minimizing the radiation dose to healthy tissue surrounding the target. Cobalt is not used as the radiation source. 3DCRT is delivered with photon and electron beams and involves the use of multileaf collimators or blocks to shape the treatment field. This helps to achieve uniform dosing at the prescribed treatment depth. Stereotactic radiosurgery is delivered in a single fraction of radiation and is used primarily to treat brain lesions using multiple beams. Image-guided radiation therapy (IGRT) uses imaging to assess and modify target treatments based on variations in patient setup and anatomy and to synchronize treatment with patient movement during therapy.

6. **Answer:** B

Rationale: The guidelines for radiation safety include time, distance, and shielding. Shielding provides a barrier between the individual with the radioactive source and others who enter the room to provide care, preventing primary exposure through direct contact or secondary exposure through scatter radiation. Gloves may be worn in providing care but radioisotopes will not be excreted through body fluids because the brachytherapy is delivered in a sealed source and not systemically. Fluid-resistant materials are often worn to cool the body during hot weather. Radiation does not emit fumes or odors and respiratory equipment is not necessary.

7. **Answer:** B

Rationale: Radiation therapy dosing depends on the distance from the radiation source to the skin. Density of the bone type to be penetrated is incorrect; the density of the tissue type to be penetrated is what is important. Radiation treatment dosing is dependent on the size of the field on the skin surface, depth below the point of beam entry, tissue density, distance from the source of radiation to the skin, and energy and penetration of the radiation beam. The size of the beam is not what is measured. Instead, what is measured is the energy and the penetrating power of the beam.

8. *Answer:* B

Rationale: The 5 R's of radiobiology provide the rationale for delivering radiation therapy in individual fractions. The 5 R's of ionizing radiation therapy are repair, reassortment, repopulation, reoxygenation, and radiosensitivity. Repair: Refers to DNA repair lethal radiation damage. Treatment fractionization allows for repair of normal tissue. Reassortment: Following a fraction of radiation, there is redistribution of cells into a radiosensitive phase of the cell cycle. Repopulation: During radiation, tumor cell proliferation can occur during radiation. During the prolonged duration of radiation therapy treatment, this can be problematic. Reoxygenation: Tumors consist of both oxygenated and hypoxic cells. Oxygenation of hypoxic cells following a radiation treatment refers to the process of reoxygenation. Oxygenation of hypoxic cells increases the sensitivity of tumor cells to radiation therapy. Radiosensitivity: Refers to the differences in cell metabolism, maturity, and microenvironment of cells. This explains the differences in sensitivities of different tissues.

9. *Answer:* D

Rationale: A buildup of toxins in the body can cause other issues but does not directly influence the biologic response to radiation. The level of DNA damage determines the biologic effect of the radiation therapy on tissues. Other factors include the oxygen effect and sensitivity of the cell to radiation. Well-oxygenated tumors tend to show a greater response, and certain tumors are more sensitive, while others are more resistant.

10. *Answer:* B

Rationale: Fractionation allows for recovery of surrounding normal tissues and redistribution of cells into a radiosensitive phase of the cell cycle. As tumor cells are damaged or destroyed by radiation therapy, remaining hypoxic malignant cells become oxygenated and thus more sensitive to the damaging effects radiation therapy. Delivery of the same total dose is possible by other methods, not just brachytherapy. But fractionation with smaller doses allows for repair and repopulation of surrounding healthy tissues, decreasing toxicity. Time between fractions also allows for recruitment of the malignant cells into the cell cycle, making these cells more radiosensitive. The presence of oxygen (not the process of deoxygenation) enhances the effects of ionizing radiation.

CHAPTER 29

1. *Answer:* A

Rationale: During the synthesis phase the cell is preparing for DNA division. Cellular DNA is replicated in preparation for DNA division. Protein and ribonucleic acid (RNA) synthesis occurs in the Gap 1 (G1) phase. Enzymes for deoxyribonucleic acid (DNA) synthesis are also produced in G1 in preparation for entry into the following synthesis phase. Cells are ready for division or mitosis in the G2 phase. Cells in G0 are in a resting phase and are not dividing. The five phases of cellular division occur during mitosis (the shortest phase of the cell cycle) and include prophase, prometaphase, metaphase, anaphase, and telophase.

2. *Answer:* B

Rationale: The cell cycle time is the amount of time required for a cell to move from one mitosis to the next mitosis. Tumor burden is the volume of cancer present. Growth fraction is the percentage of cells actively dividing at a given point in time. The cell cycle phase is a highly regulated five-stage process of reproduction that occurs in both normal and malignant cells.

3. *Answer:* A

Rationale: Approaches to chemotherapy can vary depending on the tumor type and disease stage. Single agents may be used in certain situations, but frequently, different agents are used in combination. This treatment method is called combination chemotherapy. If cells are in different cell cycle phases, combination therapy will increase the number of cells exposed to cytotoxic effects. With combination chemotherapy, two or more antineoplastic agents with differing mechanisms of action are used together to produce additive or synergistic results against tumor cells. The likelihood of drug resistance also decreases. Single agent chemotherapy is most commonly used in the recurrent setting. Single agent chemotherapy is more likely to be given sequentially, one agent at a time. Combination therapy is not limited to the adjuvant or recurrent cancer setting.

4. *Answer:* D

Rationale: Radiosensitizers make cells more vulnerable to the cell-killing effects of radiation. Protein-bound paclitaxel is not used as a radiosensitizer. Cisplatin is a radiosensitizer used to treat cervical cancer. 5-Fluorouracil is a radiosensitizer used to treat rectal cancer. Mitomycin is a radiosensitizer used to treat bladder cancer.

5. *Answer:* B

Rationale: Regional chemotherapy is delivered directly to the liver, bladder, peritoneal cavity, central nervous system, or pleural space, while reducing the intensity of systemic toxicity. Systemic therapy is chemotherapy that is distributed through the bloodstream to exert effects widely throughout body. High-dose chemotherapy is a more intense dose of chemotherapy administered with supportive therapy or with an antidote to diminish toxicity. Dose-dense chemotherapy regimens drugs are given with less time between treatments. Dose-dense chemotherapy aims to achieve maximum tumor kill by increasing the rate of chemotherapy delivery, not by increasing dosage by administering the same doses of chemotherapy previously given every 3 weeks on an every 2 week schedule instead, the chemotherapy interrupts the rapid growth phase of the tumor cells.

6. *Answer:* A

Rationale: Chemotherapy drugs are classified according to whether or not they exert their toxic effects on cancer cells during specific phases of cell division. Drugs that are most effective in treating actively dividing cells as they pass through different phases of reproduction are called cell cycle–specific agents. Gemcitabine is a pyrimidine antagonist and is cell cycle specific. Cyclophosphamide is an alkylating agent and is cell cycle nonspecific. Busulfan is an alkylating agent and is cell cycle nonspecific. Cisplatin is an alkylating agent and is cell cycle nonspecific. With cell-specific agents, major cytotoxic effects are exerted on actively dividing cells at specific phases throughout the cell cycle. Agents are schedule dependent and most effective if administered in divided doses or by continuous infusion. Continuous infusion and multiple frequent doses of a cell cycle–specific agent results in exposure of a greater number of cells and in a higher cell kill in tumors with short cell cycle times. Cell cycle–specific drugs include antimetabolites and plant alkaloids.

7. *Answer:* B

Rationale: Carboplatin is an alkylating agent and is cell cycle nonspecific. Faslodex is hormonal therapy and works as an estrogen receptor downregulator. Goserelin is used to suppress production of the sex hormones (testosterone and estrogen), particularly in the treatment of breast and prostate cancer. It is an injectable gonadotropin-releasing hormone agonist. Paclitaxel is a plant alkaloid and is cell cycle specific.

8. *Answer:* C

Rationale: Fluorouracil is an antimetabolite. Antimetabolites interfere with the normal metabolic processes within cells, typically by combining with enzymes. Nitrogen mustards, nitrosoureas, and platinum compounds are alkylating agents. Alkylating agents interfere with DNA replication through cross-linking of DNA strands, DNA strand breakage, and abnormal base pairing of proteins; all of these mechanisms interfere with normal DNA replication. The seven major subgroups of alkylating agents are nitrogen mustards, aziridines, alkyl sulfonates, DNA methylating agents, nitrosoureas, platinum compounds, and triazine compounds.

9. *Answer:* B

Rationale: Aromatase inhibitors inhibit synthesis of estrogen by preventing conversion of estrogen precursors to estrogen and are a type of hormonal therapy. Differentiating agents cause cancer cells to become more like normal cells and to grow and spread more slowly. Alkylating agents interfere with normal DNA replication. Immunotherapy uses the immune system to fight cancer.

10. *Answer:* B

Rationale: Side effects of hormonal therapy can include hot flashes, headache, thromboembolic risk, vaginal discharge, menstrual irregularities, endometrial thickening, endometrial cancer, osteoporosis, decreased libido, mood change, and weight gain. Increased libido is not a common side effect of hormonal therapy.

11. *Answer:* A

Rationale: Reactions to paclitaxel and docetaxel occur most often in the first or second infusion. Oxaliplatin reactions most likely occur with the fifth infusion.

12. *Answer:* B

Rationale: Chemotherapy is excreted in bodily fluids for the first 48 hours following chemotherapy administration. Precautions remain in effect for 48 hours after chemotherapy administration is complete for most agents. In the home setting, patients should wear gloves when handling soiled linen. Patients should be instructed to place their soiled clothes in a pillowcase and washing twice in hot water using regular detergent. It is important to keep soiled clothing separate from other laundry. Patients should flush the toilet twice with the lid down to prevent particles from splashing. When a lid is not present, cover the toilet bowl with a plastic-backed pad. Some chemotherapies may contain metabolites present in urine or feces for up to a week and require personal protection for a week. These precautions apply to the chemotherapy agents carmustine, cisplatin, docetaxel, doxorubicin, etoposide, gemcitabine, methotrexate, mitoxantrone, teniposide, vincristine, and vinorelbine.

13. *Answer:* C

Rationale: Mesna protects against bladder toxicity from ifosfamide. Dexrazoxane is used to protect against cardiotoxicity in patients who require more than 300 mg/m^2 of doxorubicin treatment and for anthracycline extravasation. Amifostine protects against renal toxicity from cisplatin therapy. Leucovorin protects against mucositis from methotrexate.

14. *Answer:* B

Rationale:. Recommendations to avoid extravasation include administering vesicants in larger veins of the arm, above the wrist, and below the elbow. Also avoid areas of flexion such as the antecubital area to prevent accidental dislodgement of the catheter, avoid areas where there is increased risk to damage tendons and/or nerves, and areas with minimal overlying tissue. Selected peripheral IV sites should not be older than 24 hours. The nurse should always check for blood return prior to, during, and after administration of a vesicant.

15. *Answer:* D

Rationale: Only physicians can administer drugs via the intrapleural route. Nurses may administer chemotherapy intravenously, intraperitoneally, and subcutaneously. Chemotherapy administration should be limited to knowledgeable, clinically competent staff as defined per institutional policy. Competence is based on didactic education and clinical experience.

16. *Answer:* B

Rationale: Hyaluronidase may be used to treat vinca alkaloid extravasations. Warm, not cold, compresses are used to treat extravasations of vinca alkaloids. Sodium thiosulfate is used to treat cisplatin and mechlorethamine extravasations. Dexrazoxane is used to treat anthracycline extravasations.

17. *Answer:* A

Rationale: A skin rash is more commonly associated with EGFR-targeted therapies. Common side effects of cisplatin include peripheral neuropathy, ototoxicity, and renal toxicity. Interventions to reduce renal toxicity include to monitor creatinine, blood urea nitrogen (BUN),

167

and urinary output, avoid use of other nephrotoxic agents, and provide adequate hydration or diuresis. Interventions to reduce ototoxicity include to teach patient to report tinnitus and refer patient for audiography, if indicated. Interventions to deal with peripheral neuropathy include to monitor for sensory and motor nerve changes and stocking-glove distribution of dysesthesia as peripheral neuropathy appears in the distal extremities of hands and feet and progresses proximally. Nurses should anticipate that dose modifications or delays may be utilized to minimize neuropathy. Nurses should assess for and report loss of sense of proprioception, vibration, pain, temperature, and touch.

18. *Answer:* B

Rationale: Cyclophosphamide can cause nasopharyngitis, which is sometimes referred to as "wasabi nose." Etoposide is associated with hypersensitivity reactions and hypotension. Carboplatin is associated with hypersensitivity and peripheral neuropathy. Doxorubicin is associated with hypersensitivity and cardiotoxicity.

19. *Answer:* D

Rationale: Oxaliplatin can lead to peripheral neuropathy and other neurotoxicity. Oxaliplatin is also associated with cold, not heat, sensitivity. Hypersensitivity is commonly seen after the fifth dose. Cardiotoxicity is a known side effect of doxorubicin.

20. *Answer:* B

Rationale: Trastuzumab is a monoclonal antibody used for treating HER2-positive breast cancer. It has cardiotoxic properties that are increased when it is used in combination with anthracycline drugs, such as doxorubicin, which is often used in the treatment of breast cancer. Assessment of cardiac function with echocardiograms is required before, during, and after therapy with these agents. Patients receiving these agents should be assessed for signs of cardiotoxicity, including ECG changes, weight gain, pedal edema, chest pain, heart rate (irregular, too fast or too slow), shortness of breath, left ventricular ejection fraction (LVEF), and jugular vein distention.

21. *Answer:* A

Rationale: As a tumor grows in size and the tumor burden increases, the growth rate slows, and the number of cells actively dividing decreases. As active growth diminishes, the number of cells undergoing mitosis decreases, leading to a decreased cellular growth rate. Cells within a tumor mass develop differing characteristics as the tumor continues to grow. The is called cellular heterogeneity. The higher the tumor burden, the greater the heterogeneity of cells within the tumor. This property of tumor development increases the likelihood that clones of tumor cells will arise within the tumor that are resistant to drugs that destroy the other cells and will continue to proliferate.

22. *Answer:* B

Rationale: Chemotherapy administered prior to surgery in order to shrink the size of the tumor mass to be removed is called neoadjuvant chemotherapy. Adjuvant chemotherapy is given after the known cancer has been surgically removed or irradiated. Consolidation chemotherapy is given after cancer has gone into remission following the initial therapy, usually in treating the acute leukemias. Concurrent chemotherapy is delivered to the patient at the same time as radiation therapy so that the chemotherapy sensitizes the tumor cells to radiation.

23. *Answer:* A

Rationale: Doxorubicin is an anthracycline drug that should not be given above a maximal cumulative dose to avoid increased drug toxicity. As a class, anthracycline drugs, such as doxorubicin, are associated with an increased risk of cardiotoxicity. Patients need to be monitored for a maximum cumulative dose of doxorubicin, which is 550 mg/m². Higher doses significantly increase the risk for cardiotoxicity. Hemorrhagic cystitis is a toxicity associated with use of cyclophosphamide and ifosfamide. Ototoxicity can occur with the use of the platinum drugs—carboplatin, cisplatin, and oxaliplatin. Neurotoxicity is not associated with doxorubicin, but with a wide variety of chemotherapy agents and can affect mentation (central neurotoxicity) or cause changes in sensory, motor, and bowel function (peripheral neurotoxicity).

24. *Answer:* B

Rationale: Aromatase inhibitors (AIs) inhibit the synthesis of estrogen in body tissues by preventing the conversion of estrogen precursors to estrogen. AIs are used in the treatment of postmenopausal women with breast cancer and in premenopausal women whose ovarian function has been suppressed or ablated. Selective estrogen receptor modulators (SERMs) act as estrogen antagonists in breast tissue by blocking estrogen from binding with estrogen receptors. In other tissues, such as the endometrial lining of the uterus, SERMs serve as estrogen agonists, and mimic the effects of estrogen on these tissues. SERMs are used in both postmenopausal and premenopausal women with hormone receptor-positive breast cancer. Gonadotropin-releasing hormone (GnRH) agonists act on the pituitary gland to suppress secretion of gonadotropins, resulting in diminished production of estrogen by the female gonads (ovaries). Adrenocorticoids are used in treatment regiments for lymphoma, leukemia, and multiple myeloma.

25. *Answer:* D

Rationale: Hot flashes are a frequent side effects of hormonal therapy in both women with breast cancer and men with prostate cancer. Other side effects of hormonal therapy that can occur in both women and men include decreased libido, hyperglycemia, and weight gain.

26. *Answer:* B

Rationale: An advantage of oral administration of antineoplastic agents is the ease of administration and the fact that taking oral agents gives patients a sense of control and independence. Another advantage in oral administration of antineoplastic agents is that oral administration decreases the time that patients spend in health care facilities or infusion centers. Requiring adequate muscle mass and tissue for absorption is a disadvantage of subcutaneous or intramuscular administration, while ease of administration and rapid absorption is an advantage of subcutaneous or intramuscular administration. Providing an increased dose to the tumor with decreased systemic side effects is an advantage of intra-arterial administration of antineoplastic agents.

27. *Answer:* C

Rationale: A disadvantage of intrapleural administration of antineoplastic agents is that this type of administration methods requires insertion of a thoracotomy tube, and the Nurse Practice Act may not allow the nurse to administer the drug through intrapleural administration as only physicians may administer the drug through this method. A disadvantage of intraperitoneal administration is the requirement of placing a Tenckhoff catheter or intraperitoneal port. Another disadvantage of this type of administration is that only patients with minimal diseases are candidates. A disadvantage of intravesicular administration is that this type of administration requires insertion of an indwelling catheter. Intrathecal or intraventricular administration is disadvantageous because this method requires lumbar puncture or surgical placement of reservoir or implanted pump.

28. *Answer:* A

Rationale: A nursing consideration for subcutaneous or intramuscular administration of antineoplastic agents is to evaluate the patient's platelet count before administration as needed and use the smallest gauge needle possible. Additional nursing considerations include preparing the injection site with an antiseptic solution, accessing the injection site for signs and symptoms of infection, and rotating injection sites. In addition, nurses are recommended not to massage or use heat or ice packs on the injection site. Nurses are recommended to wear PPE. Monitoring for signs and symptoms of bleeding and occlusion is a nursing recommendation for intra-arterial administration of antineoplastic agents. Nursing recommendations for intravenous administration of antineoplastic agents include using the smallest catheter available and avoiding areas of flection, the lower extremities, and arms where lymph nodes have been removed. An additional recommendation for intravenous administration is that the peripheral IV site should not be older than 24 hours.

29. *Answer:* D

Rationale: A nursing consideration for intraperitoneal administration of antineoplastic agents is the requirement to rotate the patient side to side every 15 min for 1 hour post infusion. The patient should be placed in a semi-Fowler's position, and the antineoplastic agent should be administered at room temperature (unless using heated intraperitoneal chemotherapy "HIPEC," which is administered in the operating room).The patency of catheter should be checked but there will not be blood return.

30. *Answer*: C

Rationale: Medication adherence refers to the extent to which a person follows their health care provider's pharmaceutical recommendations. Demographics favorable for oral drug nonadherence include a high school education or less, low socioeconomic status, and living in an area with limited access to health care. A patient who has an advanced college degree will be able to read and comprehend pertinent educational materials and prescription instructions. In addition, health care access in proximity to affluent communities is much more likely than in rural or poorer communities. Treatment-related challenges to oral adherence includes experiencing toxicities, side effects, and adverse reactions to the drugs taken at home. This is the main reason for nonadherence. In addition, the drug regimen may be complicated, consisting of multiple daily doses, or noncontinuous cycles (i.e., 14 days on, 7 days off). Patients may forget to take their medications, forget to pick up their prescriptions, or forget provider instructions. Both younger and older patients are at risk for nonadherence. The high cost of medications, high co-pays, and lack of insurance may all lead to nonadherence.

CHAPTER 30

1. *Answer:* A

Rationale: The same targeted treatment does not work on every tumor due to different targets the tumor may possess. Companion diagnostic testing—such as KRAS and EGFR—are designed to be paired with a specific drug. Companion diagnostics evaluate molecular, genetic, and chemical characteristics of the tumor for appropriate application of targeted therapy. The development of both the drug and the test requires close collaboration with the FDA. Not all targeted therapies for cancer require a companion diagnostic test. Companion testing can be used to predict outcomes. Companion tests that measure biomarkers allow oncologists to select effective therapies that can benefit patients and improve outcomes.

2. *Answer:* B

Rationale: Crizotinib is an oral tyrosine kinase inhibitor that specifically blocks ALK or ROS1. The drug is a small molecule inhibitor that blocks the growth and spread of non–small cell lung cancer by interfering with these molecular targets. Most standard chemotherapies act on all rapidly dividing normal and cancerous cells. Side effects can still occur with targeted therapies, but potentially there are fewer collateral side effects to off-target cells.

3. *Answer:* C

Rationale: Hypertension is a class effect of angiogenesis inhibitors such as bevacizumab and other agents that target VEGF or the VEGF receptor due to the rarefication of blood vessels. The monoclonal antibody bevacizumab is a VEGF inhibitor (not mTOR). Risk factors for hypertension in patients receiving bevacizumab include age over 60, smoking, obesity, and a sedentary lifestyle. Signs or symptoms may or may not be present. Hypertension can be managed through pharmacological (e.g., ACE inhibitors) and nonpharmacological methods (e.g., healthy lifestyle, healthy weight, dietary modification). Seizures are not side effects of bevacizumab.

4. *Answer:* C

Rationale: Inhibition or binding of the aberrant protein prevents the transmission of molecular "messages" down the cell signaling pathway. Doing so effectively

169

shuts down the aberrant cell signaling pathway. Binding and inhibiting excessive circulating growth factors present in cancer can block those cancer proliferation pathways. Deregulation of cell signaling pathways leads to oncogene activation that results in excessive growth of cancer cells. Targeted therapies do not block but can affect proteins involved with apoptosis resulting in death of cancer cells.

5. *Answer:* A

Rationale: Gemtuzumab ozogamicin is a type of antibody drug conjugate. It is a conjugated monoclonal antibody chemically linked to a chemotherapy agent. Chimeric antibodies have "ximab" in the substem. Humanized have "zumab" in the substem. Monoclonal antibodies bind to only one specific target.

6. *Answer:* D

Rationale: Monoclonal antibodies bind to a specific antigen with exceptional specificity to block signaling and can initiate antibody-dependent cell-mediated cytotoxicity and complement-dependent cytotoxicity. Accessible targets are generally outside the cell or on the cell surface.

7. *Answer:* A

Rationale: Olaparib is a PARP inhibitor used in the treatment of epithelial ovarian cancer with a BRCA pathogenic variant. PARP repairs single-strand DNA breaks, not the inhibitor, which is why choice B is incorrect. Cyclin-dependent kinase inhibitors are used to treat estrogen receptor positive (not negative) breast cancers. Proteasome inhibitors block the ubiquitin-proteasome pathway and are used primarily in the treatment of multiple myeloma.

8. *Answer:* B

Rationale: Low baseline left ventricular ejection fraction (LVEF), hypertension, and older age are all risk factors for cardiotoxicity that are associated with pertuzumab and trastuzumab. The lab values of liver enzymes showing an AST of 35 U/L and ALT of 40 U/L, hemoglobin A1c (HbA1c) at 5.0%, and creatinine clearance at 100 mL/min are all normal readings.

9. *Answer:* C

Rationale: Use of rituximab can lead to reactivation of the hepatitis B virus. Although the other comorbidities—hypertension, type 2 diabetes, and basal cell carcinomas—should be assessed and monitored during and after treatment, screening for hepatitis B prior to starting treatment and monitoring for symptoms of hepatitis B during and after treatment with rituximab should be done. Rituximab generally results in hypotension.

10. *Answer:* D

Rationale: Patients should be instructed to use broad-spectrum physical sunscreen with SPF of at least 30; wear protective clothing, including a wide-brimmed hat. Zinc oxide or titanium dioxide–containing sunscreens are preferred. Agents such as benzoyl peroxide are known to dry out the skin and can aggravate the rash as can taking hot showers. Oral hydration should be maintained. Not all patients develop a rash when on an EGFR inhibitor and rash does not necessarily correlate with efficacy.

11. *Answer:* A

Rationale: Hypertension is a class effect of VEGF inhibitors such as bevacizumab. It is most important to monitor the patient's blood pressure and educate the patient on symptoms of hypertension as antihypertensive agents should be prescribed immediately upon detection of hypertension in patients receiving VEGF inhibitors. Treatment is provided in intravenous form and should not be initiated until 4 weeks after surgery.

12. *Answer:* B

Rationale: Loperamide can help to decrease the passage of stool through the intestines. A low-fat, low-fiber diet is appropriate as are isotonic solutions of 1 to 1.5 L/day. The patient should limit hypotonic fluids (tea, water, fruit juice) to 0.5 L/day. Fever should be reported. Signs and symptoms of dehydration include orthostatic hypotension, dry mouth, excessive thirst, dizziness, feelings of weakness, decreased urination, and weight loss. There is no evidence for the use of probiotics in the management of EGFR inhibitor–related diarrhea.

13. *Answer:* A

Rationale: A common and serious class side effect of mTOR inhibitors such as everolimus includes noninfectious pneumonitis, metabolic disorders, and mucosal toxicity. Only a steroid-based mouthwash has the potential to prevent stomatitis.

14. *Answer:* C

Rationale: Immune system memory refers to the ability to recall previous encounters with an antigen. Memory cells include activated T and B cells. Once treated with immunotherapy, memory cells can more rapidly respond to tumor recurrence due to the ability to recall previous encounters with a tumor antigen. The use of antibodies to direct activity against tumors, the ability of the immune system to distinguish between healthy tissue and tumor, and immune-mediated cytotoxicity against cancer cells are all qualities and characteristics of immunotherapy, but do not address immunotherapy's ability for potential effectiveness after treatment has concluded.

15. *Answer:* A

Rationale: Checkpoints keep the immune system from attacking normal cells. Checkpoint inhibitors release the "brakes" and restore the T-cell's ability to recognize cancer cells. Monoclonal antibody treatment tags a protein produced by the tumor to allow the immune system to recognize the protein and destroy it, leading to tumor cell death. Oncolytic virus immunotherapy using viruses to directly infect tumor cells. Adoptive cellular therapy enhances the patient's own immune cells to be able to fight cancer cells.

16. *Answer:* B

Rationale: Immunotherapy activates memory function of immune cells and adverse events may be prolonged and unpredictable. Cytotoxic therapy results in "off-target" cytotoxicity, whereas immunotherapy has "on-target, off-tumor" adverse events from immune activity fighting against normal tissues that also express the target antigen.

17. *Answer:* D

Rationale: Symptoms of cytokine release syndrome associated with CAR T-cell therapy include fever, tachycardia, fatigue, and hypotension that can progress to capillary leak syndrome and cardiac arrhythmias. Pseudoprogression is the appearance of T-cells at the tumor site that may appear as though the tumor is growing but reflects T-cell infiltration. Fever is generally not a symptom of CNS metastases.

18. *Answer:* A

Rationale: Corticosteroids are the backbone of treatment for immunotherapy-related adverse events. Resumption of the checkpoint inhibitor can be considered when the adverse event is a Grade 1 or less. Permanent discontinuation of the checkpoint inhibitor is generally done with Grade 3 and Grade 4 adverse events.

19. *Answer:* D

Rationale: Patients should report any symptom or change in their health to the health care provider who is managing their PD-1 therapy. Minor changes may indicate early signs of an adverse event.

20. *Answer:* A

Rationale: Many primary care physicians are unaware of the long-term effects and symptoms of immunotherapy adverse events. Adverse events may occur long after the immunotherapy has been completed, which is why C is incorrect. Most adverse events can be managed by the treating physicians, but some will require a multidisciplinary team, especially if they are a Grade 3 or a Grade 4. Some adverse events are long term.

21. *Answer:* A

Rationale: Genomic instability is a typical characteristic of tumor cells. To maintain genomic integrity, tumor cells have multiple mechanisms to repair DNA, including the poly (ADP-ribose) polymerase enzyme that binds to damaged DNA and catalyzes the repair. PARP inhibitors block the PARP enzyme in cells, thus blocking repair of damaged DNA at single-strand DNA breaks. If single-strand DNA damage is unrepaired, double-strand breaks in DNA may occur, leading to death of the cell. The addition of PARP inhibitors increases the single-strand breaks that cannot be repaired and may sensitize tumor cells to the effects of DNA-damaging chemotherapy. PARP inhibitors may trap PARP on DNA, preventing PARP release from the site of damage. BRCA-mutated cells are sensitive to PARP inhibition. PARP inhibitors are used primarily in the management of patients with epithelial ovarian cancer who have known mutations (germline or somatic) in BRCA. Olaparib and rucaparib are both used in BRCA-mutated epithelial ovarian cancer. Niraparib is also a PARP inhibitor. Ceritinib and erlotinib are tyrosine kinase inhibitors. Alectinib blocks certain proteins made by the ALK gene.

22. *Answer:* B

Rationale: Monoclonal antibodies are engineered proteins that bind to only one specific target substance with exceptional specificity, thereby interfering with the action of that target substance. Intracellular enzymes that control DNA repair and cellular apoptosis include proteasome inhibitors and PARP inhibitors. Circulating growth factors in serum that stimulate growth include agents such as vascular endothelial growth factor. Tyrosine kinase inhibitors block the binding site the intracellular portion of a receptor.

23. *Answer:* B

Rationale: Companion diagnostics evaluate molecular, genetic (somatic pathogenic variants), and chemical characteristics of the tumor for appropriate application of targeted therapy. These tests are developed in parallel to the drug and have clinical utility after a drug's approval; they are included in the labeling instructions for both the therapeutic product and the corresponding diagnostic test. A companion assay can be used both to predict outcome and to monitor response. The FDA specifies three areas where a companion diagnostic is essential, which include the identification of patients most likely to benefit from a therapeutic product, the identification of patients likely to be at increased risk of serious adverse reactions as a result of treatment with a particular therapeutic product, and monitoring response to treatment by adjusting treatment (e.g. schedule, dose, discontinuation) to achieve improved efficacy or effectiveness. Companion tests may include germline testing such as BRCA1/2, but that is not the primary reason for ordering the test. They do not determine dosing of an agent or facilitate staging of the tumor.

24. *Answer:* C

Rationale: The suffix -ximab refers to a chimeric human-mouse monoclonal antibody such as cetuximab. The suffix -zumab refers to a humanized mouse antibody such as Bevacizumab. The suffix -(m)umab refers to a fully human such as Pantitumumab. The suffix -momab refers to a mouse (murine) monoclonal antibody such as britumomab.

25. *Answer:* D

Rationale: Monoclonal antibodies are associated with infusion reactions, including hypersensitivity reactions and cytokine release syndromes. EGFR-targeted therapies are frequently associated with cutaneous reactions such as rash, hair, and nail changes, as well as diarrhea resulting from EGFR therapy impact on intestinal mucosa. Left ventricular ejection fraction decreases can result from anti-HER2 therapies binding of the EGFR-1 tyrosine kinase, which plays a role in cardiac development and physiology and is also observed in VEGFR therapies. Hypertension is frequently observed with anti-VEGFR therapies due to the rarefication of blood vessels, an on-target, off-tumor response. Fluid retention (i.e., peripheral edema, pulmonary edema) is often observed in patients treated with BCR-ABl agents. Mucositis is commonly observed with mTOR, oral EGFR, and oral VEGFR inhibitors. Diarrhea is commonly observed with anti-EGFR monoclonal antibodies.

26. *Answer:* A

Rationale: Antibody–drug conjugates facilitate highly specific delivery of cytotoxic agents to the intended cancer cell target (monoclonal antibodies [MoABs] conjugated to radioisotopes or toxins or chemotherapy) in addition to actions of unconjugated MoABs. Not all body cells are affected, only cells with the specific target of the MoABs. Cytotoxic agents conjugated with the MoABs can be radioisotopes or toxins as well as chemotherapy drugs. ADCs do not act to suppress immune checkpoints.

Immune checkpoint inhibitor drugs are used for this purpose. They act to prevent regulatory checkpoint molecules from binding with their partner proteins, thus "releasing the brakes" on normal T-cell immune function allowing for T-cell recognition of the cancer cells.

27. *Answer:* C

Rationale: Adoptive T-cell therapies are highly individualized treatments wherein the patient's own T cells are extracted, enhanced in a laboratory, then reinfused back to the patient to destroy tumor. Adoptive T-cell therapies can recognize tumor cells without the interaction of antigen-presenting cells, which is required by native, nonmodified T cells. Adoptive T-cell therapies include all of the necessary elements for intracellular signaling and activation of helper and cytotoxic T lymphocytes. This type of therapy delivers a larger volume of activated T lymphocytes than the volume naturally produced in situ.

28. *Answer:* A

Rationale: CAR T-cell therapy recognizes one specific antigen. CAR T-cell therapy is a type of adoptive T-cell therapy and is associated with serious adverse events, including cytokine release syndrome, neurotoxicity, and decreased B-cells (B-cell aplasia). CAR T-cell therapy adverse events require intensive supportive care. Autoimmune endocrine disease is not treated with CAR T-cell therapy but may occur as an immune response adverse event (irAE).

29. *Answer:* B

Rationale: Biotherapy refers to a broad range of treatments made from living organisms that mimic or augment the signals that normally control cell functions to reverse the deleterious effects of tumor genes. These substances may occur naturally in the body or may be made in the laboratory. They are not cytotoxic.

30. *Answer:* C

Rationale: Biotherapies that interfere with specific molecules or pathways involved with tumor growth and progression are referred to as targeted therapies. Examples include lapatinib and trastuzumab, which both target human epidermal growth factor receptor 2 (HER/EGFR-2) implicated in tumor growth and metastases. These agents are not cytotoxic and do not lead to release of cytokines.

31. *Answer:* D

Rationale: Biotherapies that use, stimulate, augment, or suppress the immune system are referred to as immunotherapy or biological response modifier therapy. They include monoclonal antibodies (MoAbs), checkpoint inhibitors (CPIs), cytokines, vaccines, and T-cell transfer therapy. Biotherapies that interfere with specific molecules or pathways involved with tumor growth and progression are referred to as targeted therapies.

32. *Answer:* C

Rationale: Biosimilars are Food & Drug Administration (FDA) approved agents that are highly similar to existing FDA-approved drugs and have no clinically meaningful difference in safety, purity, and potency from the FDA reference product. Although identical generic versions of small molecules can be chemically synthesized, it is not possible to create identical versions of biologic medicines, due to their complexity.

33. *Answer:* B

Rationale: Targeted therapies act on specific molecular targets while most standard chemotherapies act on rapidly dividing normal and cancerous cells. Targeted therapies are deliberately chosen or designed to interact with their target, whereas many standard chemotherapies were identified because they kill cells. Targeted therapies are cytostatic, meaning they block tumor cell development and metabolism, whereas standard chemotherapy agents are cytotoxic, meaning they destroy already developed tumor cells. Targeted therapies are designed to enhance activity towards cancer cells while reducing their systemic toxicity profile. They do not augment tumor metabolism.

34. *Answer:* C

Rationale: Engineered MoAbs bind with target molecules either outside the cell or on the cell surface as they are relatively large and generally cannot enter cells. Small-molecule inhibitors are typically developed for targets located inside of the cell. MoAbs can be classified as both a targeted therapy and as an immunotherapy.

35. *Answer:* C

Rationale: Small-molecule inhibitors are generally orally available synthetic chemicals of smaller molecular size and weight than MoAbs. They are typically developed for targets that are located inside the cell. Small molecule–targeted therapies have a higher rate of cell entry relative to MoAbs and are designed to interfere with intracellular signaling molecules. They may interact with multiple targets simultaneously or act on a single target. Multiple-target inhibitors increase the risk of toxicity. Unlike MoAbs, small-molecule inhibitors do not stimulate immune response.

36. *Answer:* B

Rationale: Specificity refers to the ability to distinguish between molecules that characterize "self " and "nonself "tissues. Memory refers to the ability to recall previous encounters with an antigen. Memory T-cells and B-cells can more rapidly respond to tumor recurrence, leading to more lasting results. Specificity and memory are important concepts in immunotherapy. Immunotherapy is the use of immunologic cells and pathways to directly attack tumors, or to engage the immune system to fight cancer. Immunotherapy utilizes antibodies, T-cells, cytokines, and engineered viruses to orchestrate immune-mediated cytotoxicity against the tumor. Immunotherapy capitalizes on the immune system's unique specificity and memory abilities.

37. *Answer:* D

Rationale: Immunotherapy is used to overcome a variety of tumor escape mechanisms. Tumor escape occurs when the immune system fails to recognize an in situ tumor, resulting from either deficient host immunity (from age- or disease-related alterations) or suppressive tumor microenvironments The tumor microenvironment suppresses natural immune response by upregulating checkpoint molecules, manipulating T-cell activity, manipulating cytokine control, and increasing pro-tumor vasculature. T-cell (not B-cell) exhaustion is the fading of cytotoxic and memory functions resulting from prolonged exposure to a specific antigen leading to tumor escape.

38. *Answer:* B

Rationale: Dabrafenib works on the RAF tyrosine kinase RAF/RAS/MEK pathway. Bortezomib and erlotinib are tyrosine kinase inhibitors. Olaparib is a PARP inhibitor.

39. *Answer:* D

Rationale: According to the nomenclature used for monoclonal antibody targeted therapies, a humanized mouse derived monoclonal antibody ends in -zumab. -ximab refers to a chimeric human-mouse derived monoclonal antibody. A fully human derived monoclonal antibody ends in -(m)umab and a mouse derived monoclonal antibody ends in -momab.

40. *Answer:* A

Rationale: A new naming system has been adopted for monoclonal antibodies that eliminates the stem "mAb" and replaces it with one of four stems classifying the construction of the immunoglobulin. The stem -bart is used to indicate an artificial engineered monospecific immunoglobulin. Other stems are -mig for bispecific or multispecific immunoglobulins, -tug for unmodified monospecific immunoglobulins, -mig for bispecific or multispecific immunoglobulins, and -ment for fragments of immunoglobulins.

41. *Answer:* D

Rationale: Immune-related AEs (irAEs) are common (80%) with immunotherapy. Onset of irAEs can occur or recur any time after treatment initiation or after treatment has stopped. Because irAEs can present at any time after initiation of drug and persist after cessation, nurses should assure that primary care providers are informed of long-term risk and associated signs of immune dysfunction. It is accurate that multiple organ systems can be affected simultaneously by the immunotherapy, that autoimmune disorders can result from immune system activation from immunotherapy, and that organs that share the same antigen as the target may be affected by immunotherapy.

42. *Answer:* B

Rationale: Moderate or Grade 2 AEs will generally require dose interruption or delay until symptoms resolve. In general, patients experiencing Grade 1 AEs should be carefully monitored during treatment. Severe or Grade 3 and higher AEs generally require treatment cessation and intensive long-term management to prevent deleterious autoimmune sequelae. Assume a high level of suspicion that symptoms are treatment related unless definitive evidence supports an alternative cause.

43. *Answer:* D

Rationale: Immune-related adverse events (irAEs) can affect almost any organ with varying frequencies and severities; however, cutaneous, pulmonary, and hepatic irAEs are the most common.

44. *Answer:* A

Rationale: EGFR is highly expressed in normal skin and gastrointestinal cells. Introduction of anti-EGFR therapies will block normal EGFR-based cell signaling in those organs, resulting in dermatologic and gastrointestinal toxicity. Early identification and management are preferable to early dose reduction or treatment discontinuation

45. *Answer:* C

Rationale: B-cell lymphoma 2 (BCL-2) inhibitors: The BCL-2 family of proteins consists of more than 20 members that regulate the intrinsic apoptosis pathway. Dysregulation of the apoptosis pathway is common in hematological malignancies especially. Venetoclax was the first selective BCL-2 inhibitor. Olaparib was the first approved PARP inhibitor. Palbociclib is an inhibitor of cyclin-dependent kinases (CDK) 4 and CDK 6. Bevacizumab is a monoclonal antibody targeting vascular endothelial growth factor that is found in circulation.

46. *Answer:* B

Rationale: Cardiomyopathy in trastuzumab-treated patients results from "on-target, off-tumor" attachment on myocytes that express HER2-neu. Decrease in left ventricular end-diastolic fraction (LVEF) can result from anti-HER2 therapy (i.e., trastuzumab) that binds the HER2 protein that is physiologically expressed on myocytes. The exact mechanism of trastuzumab-induced cardiotoxicity is still unknown. The other organ systems are not affected.

47. *Answer:* C

Rationale: Selected targeted therapy AEs are biomarkers of efficacy. Patients who develop hypertension while being treated with bevacizumab generally have had better outcomes. Acneiform rash is associated with EGFRD therapy. Shortness of breath and diarrhea are not AEs associated with bevacizumab.

48. *Answer:* A

Rationale: Vaccine therapy is an active form of immunotherapy that conditions the host's immune system to generate its own sustained response to current and future tumor growth. Prostate cancer vaccines are dendritic cell vaccines (i.e., sipuleucel-T) that are personalized therapies based on a patient's own extracted antigen-presenting cells (dendritic cells) engineered to recognize tumor-associated antigen (TAA). Oncolytic viral therapy is the injection of an attenuated virus into tumor, resulting in tumor lysis and presentation of TAA to circulating T cells and B cells. Cytokines are immunomodulators that orchestrate host immune cells communicating inflammatory, stimulatory, or suppressive chemical signals. Monoclonal antibodies interrupt the binding between tumor-related growth factors in the serum (ligands) and tyrosine kinase receptors on the cell surface, thereby restoring apoptosis and halting intracellular proliferation, migration, and invasion signaling pathways.

49. *Answer:* D

Rationale: Bispecific antibodies (bsAbs) combine at least two distinct antigen binding regions, allowing them to bind to different target molecules simultaneously. Bispecific T-cell engagers (BiTEs) are one type of bsAbs that bind to tumor antigen on one binding site and simultaneously bind to effector T cells on the other binding

173

site. The BiTE connects the tumor and the T-cell bringing the T-cell into close proximity with the tumor cell and activating the T-cell to release enzymes destroying nearby tumor. Checkpoint inhibitor drugs are monoclonal antibodies that target regulatory checkpoint molecules. Antibody–drug conjugates are formed when a monoclonal antibody binds with either chemotherapy agents or radionuclide molecules. There are no genders associated with bsAbs.

CHAPTER 31

1. **Answer:** D

Rationale: Leukocyte-reduced platelets are the initial products used for febrile platelet transfusion reaction. The filtering process eliminates leukocytes that could produce febrile reactions. Leukocyte-reduced platelets reduce alloimmunization. HLA-matched platelets are used for poor response to prior platelet transfusion because of alloimmunization. Single-donor platelets reduce risk of alloimmunization and lower infection risk due to one donor; however, febrile reactions could occur. Pooled platelets are typically used for patients who are bleeding or during operative procedures and carries a risk for febrile reactions.

2. **Answer:** C

Rationale: Autologous blood is self-donated blood usually collected before elective surgery. Blood can also be salvaged during surgery by an automated "cell saver" device. Whole blood is rarely used except in extreme emergency of blood loss. Homologous blood is collected from screened donors for transfusion to another individual. Directly donated blood component is collected from another donor to a specific recipient.

3. **Answer:** B

Rationale: Transfusion of platelets should correct thrombocytopenia and decrease signs of bleeding. RBC transfusion corrects anemia and decreases symptoms of fatigue, shortness of breath, and tachycardia. Serum immune globulin (IgG) transfusion corrects IgG deficiency and provides passive immunity protection. Plasma transfusion corrects clotting factor deficiencies and expands blood volume.

4. **Answer:** A

Rationale: Febrile nonhemolytic reaction is an acute reaction that manifests during the initial infusion with fever, chills, rigors, nausea, vomiting, and general discomfort. Hemolytic reaction can be acute or delayed occurring up to 10 days after transfusion. The most common reason for hemolytic reaction is due to ABO incompatibility. Symptoms include low grade fever, chills, rigors, and abdominal and back pain. TRALI is an acute reaction occurring within 6 hours of the transfusion causing acute respiratory symptoms such as dyspnea, hypoxia, hypotension, fever, and tachycardia. Iron overload is a delayed reaction occurring from frequent RBC transfusions.

5. **Answer:** C

Rationale: According to the guidelines, red blood cells are administered when the hemoglobin is less than 7 g/dL or when the patient becomes symptomatic. Platelets are administered if the platelet count is less than 10,000/mm³ with or without bleeding or less than 20,000/mm³ with active bleeding. Neutrophils are administered when an infection is unresponsive to antibiotic therapy and neutrophils less than 500/mm³. Immunoglobulins are administered when immunoglobulin G level is decreased to provide passive immunity.

6. **Answer:** A

Rationale: Acetaminophen and diphenhydramine are commonly administered as premedication prior to transfusions, especially for a history of a previous reaction. Meperidine is administered for uncontrolled rigors. Hydrocortisone is available for severe reactions and may be added as a premedication for a history of severe transfusion reaction. Diuretics are administered for fluid overload or to reduce intravascular volume.

7. **Answer:** C

Rationale: Appropriate filter or blood component set should be attached to the blood product prior to transfusion. Leukocyte reduction filter reduces the number of leukocytes transfused in a unit of red blood cells. Medications or IV fluids should not be added to blood products. Restrict transfusions to those who have clear indications for therapy and only transfuse the minimum number of units necessary. It is recommended to monitor patients for approximately 2 hours after transfusion.

8. **Answer:** C

Rationale: Autologous blood is collected from the intended recipient prior to the elective surgery or during surgery by the use of an automated "cell saver" device. HLA matched is used for platelet transfusions when alloimmunization has occurred, resulting in a poor response to platelet transfusions Blood collected at a blood drive is a homologous blood component from a screened donor. Directly donated blood is collected from a donor and designated to a recipient.

9. **Answer:** D

Rationale: Platelets will be transfused with the patient presenting with active bleeding. Guidelines stipulate transfusion of red blood cells when hemoglobin is less than 7 g/dL or symptomatic. Plasma is transfused to correct clotting factor deficiencies or to expand blood volume.

10. **Answer:** B

Rationale: Administer iron component therapy for iron deficiency. Use of vitamin supplementation such as folic acid, vitamin B, and vitamin K may be beneficial in decreasing need for blood components. Minimize routine blood testing. Proton pump inhibitors are used to minimize gastrointestinal bleeding, not histamine-2 antagonist. Use pediatric small volume blood collection tubes to minimize blood collected.

11. **Answer:** D

Rationale: The initial step in a suspected reaction is to stop the transfusion and keep the intravenous line open with normal saline. The provider should be notified and orders obtained if standing orders are not available. Diphenhydramine and meperidine could be ordered to control symptoms. Blood bank should be notified of the potential reaction after the transfusion is stopped.

12. *Answer:* D

Rationale: The PICC can remain inserted for up to 12 months; however, evidence supports longer duration if the device is functioning without complication. PICCs are inserted into a central vein at the antecubital fossa. PICCs are available with single, double, or triple lumens.

13. *Answer:* C

Rationale: Chest x-ray, fluoroscopy, or ultrasound (used during placement) can be used to confirm placement of the catheter tip. CT scan is not used to confirm placement. Blood return on aspiration and ease of fluid administration can be used to evaluate the catheter after catheter tip placement is confirmed post initial placement.

14. *Answer:* B

Rationale: Bundle care includes frequent hand washing before and after use, optimal catheter site selection, maximal sterile barrier precautions on device insertion, use of alcohol hub decontamination prior to each access, and daily reviewing line necessity with prompt removal if no longer necessary. Incorporating this care has been shown to decrease the risk of line infection. Bundle care does not decrease the risk of bleeding, catheter dislodgement, or catheter migration.

15. *Answer:* C

Rationale: The most common cause for a partial occlusion is a fibrin sheath causing a one-way valve effect allowing infusion of IV fluids into the catheter but causing withdrawal occlusion. Deep vein thrombus can cause a partial occlusion with a presentation of edema. Intraluminal blood clot and precipitation are not as common and cause complete obstruction.

16. *Answer:* D

Rationale: Elastomeric pumps do not have audible alarms. Peristaltic and syringe pumps are available with audible alarms to alert the patient and/or caregiver of an occlusion, kinked tubing, or pump malfunction. Smart pump is technology equipped in peristaltic and syringe pumps to minimize the risk of incorrect dosing.

17. *Answer:* A

Rationale: Intraventricular catheter is implanted directly into the lateral ventricle of the brain, providing direct access to the cerebral spinal fluid. Peritoneal catheter provides direct access to the peritoneal cavity. Epidural catheters provide access to the epidural space used for delivery of opioids or anesthetics. Intrapleural catheters give direct access to the pleura cavity.

18. *Answer:* A

Rationale: Maintaining a flushing routine and flushing with pulsatile (push-pause) method to cause swirling action in device are preventative measures for occlusion. Changing the intrathoracic pressures with a recommendation of having the patient inhale fully and hold his or her breath or exhale fully and hold his or her breath is a restoration of the problem of occlusion. Surgical removal, as indicated, to avoid a fracture, is a restoration of the problem of "pinch-off syndrome." Finally, removing the needle and re-accessing the port using a noncoring needle

is an example of restoring the dislodgement of the port access needle.

19. *Answer:* B

Rationale: The best management strategy for catheter migration is to refer the problem to a physician for repositioning the catheter using fluoroscopy. In order to prevent catheter migration, the recommendation is to monitor the length of the catheter (tunnel, midline, PICC) to ensure placement is intact. Other recommendations for prevention of catheter migration include protecting the device from potential trauma and anchoring the device appropriately with a securement device. Avoidance of placing the port at the sites of actual or potential tissue damage (in radiation field) is a recommendation for prevention of erosion of the port through the subcutaneous tissue. High-pressure infusions or flushing with 1 or 3 mL is a prevention technique for complications arising from port-catheter separation.

20. *Answer:* D

Rationale: A characteristic of a short-term or intermediate-term peripheral catheter is the capability to infuse fluids, medications, blood products, and peripheral total parenteral nutrition (TPN) and to obtain blood specimens. Short-term or intermediate-term peripheral catheters are single lumen or multi-lumen catheters. Insertion is done peripherally in the forearm or antecubital fossa into the cephalic, basilic, or median cubital vein. Nontunneled catheters are inserted centrally into the jugular vein, subclavian vein, superior vena cava (SVC), or inferior vena cava. Nontunneled venous short-term catheters are available in single or multi-lumen and offer immediate access. Long-term venous catheters are available with a pressure-activated safety valve (PASV) located in the catheter hub and are designed to permit fluid infusion and decrease risk of blood reflux. Also, in long-term venous catheters the tip must be confirmed before initial use by ultrasound (during placement if used), fluoroscopy, or chest x-ray.

21. *Answer:* A

Rationale: Blood component therapy (BCT) exposes the patient to components that are foreign to the individual's system and can lead to allergic reactions, as well as the destruction of blood cells (hemolysis). Although fluid volume overload may occur, and the nurse should monitor the patient closely, deep vein thrombosis is not a common reaction. Other coagulation problems are not seen as acute reactions to blood component therapy. Blood components can contain hematopoietic stem cells, and there have been cases of graft-versus-host disease in individuals with impaired immune system function. However, this condition is not seen as an acute reaction. Protocols will indicate when a patient may require irradiated blood products to decrease this risk.

22. *Answer:* D

Rationale: Two licensed health care professionals must verify that the blood component therapy product is correctly labeled and dated, and that it matches the information on the patient's blood identification band, usually worn as a bracelet. The patient's name must be spelled correctly, and the blood group and blood type must be identified on both the product and the patient identifiers. Using a gravity flow infusion line is not the priority intervention to maximize patient safety. Gravity infusions, although not the preferred method, may be used if controlled infusion pumps are not available. Slowly adding medications through the Y-port is incorrect. Medications must never be added to blood component therapy (BCT) infusions. Intravenous therapy guidelines recommend larger catheters be used for viscous infusions, such as BCT products. BCT products must be infused within 4 hours, maximum time, to prevent degradation of the components.

23. *Answer:* D

Rationale: Although most individuals can be taught to care for commonly used access devices, those who are not good candidates should be considered for an implanted device, as these devices require less self-care. Demonstration of the ability to care for the device is critical for all external devices. The need for chemotherapy infusions and blood samples is a clinical indication for all types of access devices. The patient expressing concerns about the implication is an indication for the nurse to provide additional education.

24. *Answer:* B

Rationale: The patient should be able to assess the system to determine that the power is on and the infusion is occurring. The line should be flushed, not with water, but with normal saline. Flushing is unnecessary while infusion is ongoing. Flushing the line with sterile water every 12 hours is incorrect. Normal saline solution would be used, and when the infusion is ongoing, there is no need to flush the line. These systems should be used only for their intended purpose, and only a trained nurse should access the system and determine whether a second line is appropriate. Doses are programmed on the ambulatory infusion pumps with a sequence intended to prevent accidental or uninformed alteration by lay individuals. Changes in dose need to be made by the nurse when an order is changed or when the infusion is complete.

25. *Answer:* C

Rationale: The use of blood component therapy has increased in the oncology setting due to the use of more aggressive single-modality and multimodality cancer therapies that result in bone marrow suppression. In addition the development of donor programs, advances in hemapheresis technology, and hematopoietic stem cell transplantation therapies all serve to increase the available range of blood component therapies. There is also less use of erythropoietin to stimulate red blood cell production due to potential for disease progression. Delay in initiating antineoplastic therapies and in providing hematopoietic stem cell transplantation therapies are not associated with need for blood transfusions.

26. *Answer:* A

Rationale: Transfusion of 1 unit of packed red blood cells is expected to increase hemoglobin by 1 g/dL or the hematocrit by 3% with each unit. Packed red blood cells are not used to increase the platelet count. Transfused platelets are used to correct thrombocytopenia. One unit

of apheresis platelets (from one donor) would increase the platelet level 35 to 40 uL. Pooled platelets come from four to six donors.

27. *Answer:* D

Rationale: Fresh frozen plasma (FFP) transfusions are given to correct clotting factor deficiencies, expand blood volume, or provide osmotic diuresis. All coagulation factors should be present, and plasma compatibility with the recipient is preferred. When thawed, FFP must be transfused within 24 hours. The recipient must be watched for fluid overload. Serum immune globulin is used to provide passive immunity protection (e.g., against cytomegalovirus) or treat hypogammaglobulinemia. IgG transfusion is used to maintain antibody levels, prevent infection, or confer passive immunity. White blood cell transfusion is used to increase the WBC count and prevent and/or treat infections in neutropenic patients.

28. *Answer:* D

Rationale: Recipients of a blood product transfusion must be monitored carefully to detect the development of acute reactions that occur within 24 hours of the transfusion. Allergic reactions indicate hypersensitivity reaction to donor plasma proteins. Delayed transfusion reaction develops after 24 hours, months, or (rarely) years later depending on the time of onset relative to the inciting transfusion. Hemolysis and iron overload are delayed transfusion reactions. Hemorrhage may be treated with blood component therapy; it is not an acute event of a plasma transfusion.

29. *Answer:* A

Rationale: Posttransfusion purpura is a delayed reaction in which transfused antibodies destroy platelets in the transfused blood as well as the patient's own platelets. Transfusion-related acute lung injury (TRALI) is an acute reaction caused by WBC antibodies in the transfused product reacting with the patient's own WBCs. Hemolytic reactions causing immune destruction of transfused RBCs, which are attacked by the recipient's antibodies, is an acute transfusion reaction. Alloimmunization is a delayed reaction after blood component transfusion in which the recipient develops alloantibodies against the donor's antigens.

30. *Answer:* B

Rationale: Guidelines for blood component therapy include transfusion of red blood cells when the hemoglobin level is less than 7 g/dL or the patient is symptomatic. Neutrophils are transfused when there are less than 500/mm^3, with an infection unresponsive to antibiotic therapy. Platelet count transfusion guidelines include: transfuse for less than 10,000/mm^3, with or without bleeding; less than 20,000/mm^3, with active bleeding; less than 50,000/mm^3 to 75,000/mm^3 and scheduled for surgical procedure per institution guidelines. International normalized ratio (INR) greater than 1.69 and prolonged partial thromboplastin time (PTT) and prothrombin time (PT) require blood component transfusion.

31. *Answer:* D

Rationale: Transfusion complications may be indicated by the presence of a variety of signs/symptoms

(S/S). General: flank/back pain, fever, chills, muscle aches and pain, back pain, chest pain, headache. Respiratory: shortness of breath, tachypnea, apnea, cough, wheezing, rales, air embolism; of a transfusion. Cardiovascular: bradycardia or tachycardia, hypotension or hypertension, facial flushing, cyanosis of extremities, cool clammy skin, distended neck veins, and edema. Gastrointestinal: nausea, vomiting, abdominal cramping, and pain. Renal: dark, concentrated, red- to brown-colored urine.

32. *Answer:* A

Rationale: Techniques to diminish blood loss in patients who refuse blood component therapy include: Minimize routine blood testing, use small pediatric blood collection tubes, suppress menstrual cycles in patients with thrombocytopenia, minimize GI bleeding with proton pump inhibitors and bowel management, and avoid anticoagulation, including heparin flushes or alteplase use, and use vitamin supplementation such as folic acid, vitamin B, and vitamin K.

33. *Answer:* C

Rationale: Intra-arterial chemotherapy is delivered through an arterial catheter that is directly threaded into the artery that feeds the tumor. This type of catheter is inserted in the Interventional Radiology or surgery suite. The catheter is inserted into the artery for perfusion, usually into the hepatic artery, similar to venous placement; hypogastric, femoral, and brachial arteries are also used. The nontunneled catheter and the midline catheter are inserted into veins, not arteries. An intrathecal catheter is inserted below the dura where cerebrospinal fluid (CSF) circulates. Intrathecal catheters are used for the administration of opioid analgesics and anesthetic mediations, chemotherapy, CSF sampling, and antispasmodic agents intrathecally.

34. *Answer:* B

Rationale: There are several advantages of using arterial catheters for short- or long-term chemotherapy administration, as listed. B does not pertain to arterial catheters. Catheters that are nontunneled for short-term use or tunneled for long-term use are typically venous or subcutaneous catheters.

35. *Answer:* C

Rationale: An allogeneic blood component is blood collected from screened donors for transfusion to another individual. Autologous blood is blood collected from the intended recipient either as a self-donation usually made before elective surgery or as a red blood cell (RBC) salvage during surgery using an automated "cell saver" device or manual suction equipment. Directly donated blood is a blood component collected from a donor designated by the intended recipient.

36. *Answer:* D

Rationale: Cryoprecipitate corrects dilution of clotting factors secondary to massive hemorrhage, extensive transfusion, liver failure, or consumption coagulopathy secondary to disseminated intravascular coagulation (DIC) by raising fibrinogen level by 5 to 10 mg/dL. Plasma corrects clotting factor deficiencies, expands blood volume, and provides osmotic diuresis.

HLA platelets are used for the correction of thrombocytopenia. Red blood cells are used for the correction of anemia.

37. *Answer:* C

Rationale: Hemophilia A is an inherited condition in which the individual does not clot because of a deficiency of factor VIII. Factor IX is used to correct clotting in hemophilia B. Platelets correct thrombocytopenia. Plasma corrects clotting factor deficiencies, expands blood volume, and provides osmotic diuresis. HLA platelets are used for the correction of thrombocytopenia.

38. *Answer:* A

Rationale: Pooled platelets are indicated to control or prevent bleeding; platelet count <10,000 to 20,000/mm^3 or patient is bleeding or preoperative. There are a few RBCs present, but ABO compatibility is not required. Single donor platelets are used for the reduction of alloimmunization and lower risk of infection with exposure to one donor. Single donor platelets are indicated when there is an inadequate increase in platelet count or a history of platelet additive solution (PAS) reactions. Leukocyte reduced platelets are indicated when there is a prior febrile reaction to platelets; they are associated with a reduction of alloimmunization. HLA-matched platelets are used when there is a poor response to prior platelet transfusion because of alloimmunization.

39. *Answer:* C

Rationale: Access device infections are managed if possible with antibiotics. Vancomycin is recommended for empiric therapy until organism is identified. Adjustment of antibiotics can be made based on culture results when available. Some consider the use of antibiotic lock therapy in patients diagnosed with catheter-related infection, or at a high risk of infection. Indications to remove the access device include complicated infection, tunnel, or port pocket infection, endocarditis, osteomyelitis, or septic thrombosis, septic shock, or recurrent line infection despite adequate antibiotic therapy. Acetaminophen is not a treatment for infection.

CHAPTER 32

1. *Answer:* A

Rationale: Fever may be the earliest and/or only warning sign of infection in a neutropenic patient. Patients with a single oral temperature of 38.3°C (101°F) should be considered to have an infection. The nurse should anticipate orders to obtain cultures and initiate empiric antimicrobial therapy.

2. *Answer:* C

Rationale: Ganciclovir is an antiviral agent that provides coverage for CMV treatment. Levofloxacin and fluconazole do not provide coverage against viruses. Acyclovir is indicated for herpes simplex virus (HSV) and varicella zoster (VZV), not CMV. Valganciclovir is preemptive therapy for CMV.

3. *Answer:* A

Rationale: Fever is often the first and only sign of infection in neutropenic patients. Antipyretics, including acetaminophen, aspirin, and nonsteroidal antiinflammatory agents, should be avoided in high-risk individuals as they may mask fever.

4. *Answer:* D

Rationale: Vancomycin should not be routinely included in empiric therapy, except in select clinical situations. The routine use of vancomycin can lead to the occurrence of vancomycin-resistant organisms (VRE). Vancomycin is indicated for gram-positive bacterial coverage, and dose adjustments are required to prevent renal toxicity.

5. *Answer:* A

Rationale: Amphotericin B adverse effects include nephrotoxicity, electrolyte wasting, and infusion reaction. Prehydration and premedications are needed to prevent complications.

6. *Answer:* C

Rationale: Stewardship tasks performed by the nurse include reviewing culture results and reporting positive results to the provider in a timely manner. Overuse of antibiotics should be avoided to prevent organism resistance.

7. *Answer:* B

Rationale: Influenza is an inactivated virus and safe for patients receiving cancer treatment. Inactivated viruses can be administered 2 weeks prior to chemotherapy or in between cycles. CD34 markers do not need to be used as a means of timing his vaccination schedule since he is not a stem cell transplant patient.

8. *Answer:* B

Rationale: Antiinflammatory agents work by decreasing the adverse effects of inflammation. Their mechanism of action inhibits cyclooxygenase, which leads to decreased prostaglandin production and decreased inflammation. Antiinflammatory agents should be avoided in individuals at risk for infection and/or neutropenia as they may mask fever, which is a side effect. Another side effect is decreased platelet function and increased risk for bleeding.

9. *Answer:* B

Rationale: The antiplatelet effects of NSAIDs require that caution be taken when prescribing patients other anticoagulation or antiplatelet medications like clopidogrel. Taking these medications together can increase the risk of adverse reactions and/or potentiate toxicities.

10. *Answer:* D

Rationale: Corticosteroids can cause muscle weakness/wasting. The oncology nurse should monitor the patient with cancer's muscle strength, encourage regular exercise, and implement safety measures to prevent fall or injury. Other side effects include hyperglycemia, hypernatremia, hypokalemia, and hypocalcemia, leading to edema, hypertension, diabetes, and osteoporosis.

11. *Answer:* A

Rationale: Ondansetron and granisetron are 5-HT3 antagonists, blocking the action of serotonin along nerve pathways. Dopamine is a D2 antagonist. Histamine is an H1 antagonist. Neurokinin is an NK1 antagonist.

12. *Answer:* B

Rationale: The general principle of breakthrough chemotherapy-induced nausea and vomiting (CINV) treatment is to introduce one agent from a different drug class to the current regimen. If palonosetron is given prior to chemotherapy, the use of another 5HT3 antagonist is not warranted for the management of breakthrough CINV.

13. *Answer:* B

Rationale: Metoclopramide has a black box warning for sudden death related to prolonged QT intervals. This medication should not be administered if QTc is >500 msec. If the patient experiences shortness of breath or palpitations while receiving this medication, they should immediately notify their health care provider. Extrapyramidal side effects may occur.

14. *Answer:* A

Rationale: Chronic pain lasts longer than 3 months and can be a source of background pain for patients with cancer. Chronic pain is commonly associated with breakthrough pain. Analgesic medication management should be prescribed to provide pain control for a 24-hour period. If opioids are used, patients should have long-acting and breakthrough options available when pain is constant. Prophylaxis for constipation with a stool softener and bowel stimulant should be considered for all patients who are started on opioid analgesics, and the regimen should be optimized to assure regular bowel movements. Tolerance occurs in patients who take opioids regularly; that is, they require higher doses to achieve the same amount of analgesia.

15. *Answer:* D

Rationale: Abrupt discontinuation of opioids can lead to withdrawal. Symptoms of withdrawal include nausea, vomiting, perspiration, chills, tachycardia, anxiety, and insomnia. Addiction is a psychological sign where the patient craves the drug despite knowing the harm. An assessment for pain and GI is needed to determine adequate pain control and monitor for signs of constipation.

16. *Answer:* A

Rationale: Methylphenidate (Ritalin) may be helpful for somnolence or mental clouding from opioids. Metoclopramide is used as an antiemetic. Micafungin is an antifungal agent. Mithramycin is a chemotherapy agent.

17. *Answer:* B

Rationale: Opioids can cause nausea and vomiting. Patients should be taught to take medication with food to prevent GI upset.

18. *Answer:* A

Rationale: Anxiolytics can be used to reduce anxiety associated with diagnosis and treatment of cancer, to manage anticipatory nausea, reduce pain associated with anxiety, and manage alcohol or narcotic withdrawal.

19. *Answer:* D

Rationale: Lexapro is an SSRI. Effects may not be seen for the first 2 to 4 weeks. To prevent withdrawal, patients should slowly taper off the medication so they do not experience side effects.

20. *Answer:* C

Rationale: Zolpidem (Ambien) is a nonbenzodiazepine receptor agonist indicated for sleep latency and midnight awakenings. Linezolid is used to treat gram-positive bacterial infections. Posaconazole is used to treat fungal infections. Temozolomide is a chemotherapy agent.

21. *Answer:* B

Rationale: Antidepressant therapeutic effect can take up to 3 weeks. Patients with major depressive disorder may have suicidal thoughts and should be routinely screened for suicidal ideation or emotional changes until a therapeutic response is achieved. A and C are appropriate assessment questions, but suicide prevention is an important safety issue.

22. *Answer:* D

Rationale: Amitriptyline is a tricyclic antidepressant (TCA). TCAs are associated with anticholinergic effects and have a 4+ toxicity comparison. Fluoxetine, sertraline, and citalopram are SSRIs and do not have anticholinergic toxicities.

23. *Answer:* C

Rationale: Carmustine is a chemotherapy drug that has the potential to lower seizure threshold.

24. *Answer:* A

Rationale: Somnolence is a side effect associated with levetiracetam. The agent may also be associated with dizziness and rash and occasionally psychosis.

25. *Answer:* A

Rationale: Anticonvulsants are enzyme inducers, which causes an increase in metabolism and decreased exposure to the medication. Enzyme inhibitors decrease metabolism, causing exposure of the medication to be increased. A substrate for an enzyme is vulnerable to changes in enzyme activity. If an oncology nurse has concerns about drug–drug interactions while caring for a patient, consider consulting with a pharmacist.

26. *Answer:* B

Rationale: Filgrastim is a myeloid growth factor used after autologous stem cell transplant and cord blood transplantation to support neutrophil engraftment.

27. *Answer:* A

Rationale: Myeloid growth factors are biological agents that stimulate the proliferation and maturity of neutrophils and macrophages.

28. *Answer:* B

Rationale: The oncology nurse should understand the increased risk for thrombotic events when administering erythropoietin. Patients and their families should be taught to monitor for signs of swelling or redness in the lower extremities and to notify their provider should this occur.

29. *Answer:* C

Rationale: Splenectomy and functional asplenia may increase the risk of infection where antimicrobials would be warranted. A lobectomy is a surgery to remove one of the lobes of the lungs; an appendectomy removes the appendix, and a cholecystectomy is surgery to remove the gallbladder. These surgeries do not impact immune suppression.

30. *Answer:* D

Rationale: Serotonin selective reuptake inhibitors (SSRI) may induce anxiety symptoms, not relieve them, early in therapy. SSRIs are started at a low dose, not a high dose, and then increased to an optimal dose. The effect of SSRIs may not be seen for the first 2 to 4 weeks. Abrupt discontinuation may precipitate withdrawal syndromes.

31. *Answer:* B

Rationale: Major depressive disorder is characterized by recurrent thoughts of dying, and depressive symptoms lasting most of the day, every day, for at least 2 weeks. Major depressive disorder occurs in about 25% of patients with cancer, leading to poor quality of life and functional status, higher use of health care services, and nonadherence with treatment.

32. *Answer:* D

Rationale: Dietary modifications to avoid tyramine-containing foods are critical for patients on monoamine oxidase inhibitors (MAOIs). Tyramine does not impact serotonin selective reuptake inhibitors (SSRIs), serotonin and norepinephrine reuptake inhibitors (SNRIs), or tricyclic antidepressants (TCAs).

33. *Answer:* A

Rationale: Therapy should continue for 6 months following improvement in symptoms to avoid relapse of depression. Taking antidepressants as scheduled and allowing the time necessary for a therapeutic response to the medications is required. There is a potential for withdrawal effects with abrupt cessation; therefore, gradual taper of dose should occur at discontinuation.

34. *Answer:* B

Rationale: Risk of neutropenia is increased in select patients, including those who have recent surgery or open wounds, prior chemotherapy or radiation therapy, persistent neutropenia, bone marrow involvement of the tumor, liver dysfunction, renal dysfunction, and age greater than 56 years.

35. *Answer:* C

Rationale: EPO is associated with an increased risk of venous thromboembolism. Patients who are iron deficient will not respond to EPO. EPO should not be given in patients with hemoglobin greater than 10 g/dL. EPO decreases, not increases, the number of RBC transfusions required to treat anemia.

36. *Answer:* D

Rationale: The cell nadir occurs 7 to 14 days after the chemotherapy treatment. Neutropenia occurs when the absolute neutrophil count (ANC) is less than 500/mm^3.

37. *Answer:* A

Rationale: Central obesity, moon face, buffalo hump, easy bruising, acne, hirsutism, striae, and skin atrophy occur with use of corticosteroids and would warrant the assessment of the patient's body image and concerns. The oncology nurse should provide the opportunity for the patient with cancer to share concerns and discuss coping strategies and educate the patient regarding care of skin and safety precautions. NSAIDS, Cox-2 selective agents, salicylates, and aminoglycosides do not cause a significant degree, if any, of body image concerns.

38. *Answer:* B

Rationale: The onset of effect for oral morphine is 30 minutes and morphine IV is 5 to 10 minutes. Morphine 10 mg IV has equivalent potency as morphine 30 mg orally. The peak effect is 10 to 15 minutes with morphine IV and 60 minutes for morphine oral. Morphine IV and oral both have a duration of effect of 3 to 4 hours.

39. *Answer:* C

Rationale: For accurate results, axillary temperature should be avoided. Rectal temperatures should be avoided to prevent potential injury to the rectal mucosa. Temperature threshold for the neutropenic patient should be defined as a sustained oral temperature of 38°C (100.4°F) over 1 hour or a single oral temperature of 38.3°C (101°F).

40. *Answer:* D

Rationale: The gold standard for diagnosis in this patient population is to draw one set peripherally and one from central lines when the patient has a central venous catheter. Two peripheral cultures should be drawn if no central venous catheter is in place. Cultures would be obtained before 48 hours, so medication can be administered for symptom relief.

41. *Answer:* A

Rationale: Human immunodeficiency virus (HIV) and respiratory syncytial virus (RSV) are viruses, but only herpes simplex virus (HSV) would routinely warrant antimicrobial prophylaxis. Pseudomonas infections are diseases caused by a bacterium from the genus Pseudomonas, which is found widely in the environment, such as in soil, water, and plants; this is not a virus.

42. *Answer:* B

Rationale: In low-risk patients who are clinically stable with negative cultures and an ANC remaining less than 500, consider discontinuation of antibiotics after a total of 5 to 7 days. Continuing beyond this amount of time may unnecessarily cause additional antimicrobial side effects.

43. *Answer:* D

Rationale: Stevens-Johnson syndrome is a severe skin reaction with one of the primary symptoms being the presence of blisters. The infection can spread to the mucous membranes, which could cause blisters to form inside the body, making eating and drinking painful. If left untreated, Stevens-Johnson syndrome can spread to other organs and be life threatening. The impact is on dermatologic area, and not the liver, heart, or gastrointestinal.

44. *Answer:* C

Rationale: Live virus vaccines use the weakened (attenuated) form of the virus. The measles, mumps, and rubella (MMR) vaccine and the varicella (chickenpox) vaccine are examples. Inactivated vaccines may be administered >2 weeks prior to chemotherapy; live virus vaccines should be given >4 weeks prior to chemotherapy.

45. *Answer:* B

Rationale: CD34 is the most commonly used marker for hematopoietic stem/progenitor cells in clinical hematology. Clinicians even use this marker as a quality criterion for the hematopoietic graft. Human leukocyte antigen-DR and vascular endothelial growth factor receptor (VEGFR) are associated markers. A complete blood count (CBC) would not be used alone for timing vaccines.

46. *Answer:* A

Rationale: Patients at risk for toxicities with NSAIDs are age 65 or older with a history of GI ulcers, renal insufficiency, cardiovascular disease, concurrent aspirin or anticoagulant use, or a history of ulcerative colitis. Anticonvulsants, acetaminophen, or corticosteroids would be less toxic with the history presented.

47. *Answer:* D

Rationale: Highly emetogenic intravenous chemotherapy would warrant medications such as NK1 RA + 5-HT3 RA + dexamethasone prior to chemotherapy followed by NK1 RA (if needed) and dexamethasone. Agents for breakthrough nausea and vomiting include cannabis (medical marijuana) in addition to dopamine antagonists such as prochlorperazine, droperidol, promethazine, dexamethasone, lorazepam, ondansetron, metoclopramide, and cannabinoids such as dronabinol and nabilone. Legalization of marijuana for medical use is growing in a number of states, but not legal in every state. Cannabis may have long- and short-term side effects but may still be prescribed for breakthrough nausea and vomiting.

48. *Answer:* B

Rationale: Absorption and onset of pain medications vary with patients with any route including buccal, rectal, and subcutaneous. Fat-to-lean body ratio impacts transdermal preparations and is not recommended in cachectic patients and takes a longer time to onset in obese patients.

49. *Answer:* A

Rationale: Amphotericin B and fluconazole are antifungals that are indicated for a fungal infection such as *Candida*. Caspofungin (Cancidas) is an antifungal, but ciprofloxacin is an antimicrobial for gram-negative bacteria. Voriconazole (Vfend) is used for *Candida* infection, but imipenem is for gram-positive infections. Cidofovir is an antiviral agent.

50. *Answer:* D

Rationale: Fluid hydration is necessary if high doses of acyclovir are used. Doses are based on ideal, not actual, body weight. Ganciclovir, not acyclovir, is the antiviral regarded as being effective preemptive therapy for cytomegalovirus in high-risk patients with cancer. Probenecid is given to patients to prevent renal reabsorption of cidofovir.

51. *Answer:* D

Rationale: The serotonin (5 HT3 antagonists) include ondansetron (Zofran). Prochlorperazine is a D2 antagonist. Aprepitant is an NK-1 antagonist.

52. *Answer:* B

Rationale: Major neurotransmitter targets and agents are as follows: cannabinoid agonist, e.g., dronabinol, serotonin (5HT3 antagonists, e.g., ondansetron), neurokinin (NK-1 antagonist, e.g., aprepitant), dopamine (D-2 antagonist, e.g., prochlorperazine), histamine (H-1 antagonist, e.g., promethazine), and acetylcholine (muscarinic, e.g., scopolamine).

53. *Answer:* C

Rationale: The majority of the serotonin reuptake agents can contribute to sexual dysfunction. The other options—hot flashes, neuropathy, and increased appetite—are not expected side effects.

54. *Answer:* D

Rationale: Bone pain is the main side effect of filgrastim. Bone pain occurs as a result of expansion of granulocytic precursors in the patient's bone marrow. Often, a patient's peripheral white blood count will be correspondingly high. Sedation is not a side effect of filgrastim and the other options of liver dysfunction and constipation are not expected side effects.

55. *Answer:* B

Rationale: Fluoroquinolones are broad-spectrum antibiotics, and include ciprofloxacin, levofloxacin, and moxifloxacin. As a class, fluoroquinolones can cause long-lasting, disabling, and potential permanent side effects involving tendons, muscles, and joints. Their use is not associated with increased risk of glaucoma, constipation, or hypertension.

56. *Answer:* C

Rationale: Acetaminophen is an analgesic and antipyretic (i.e., reduces fever) but does not have antiinflammatory effects.

CHAPTER 33

1. *Answer:* B

Rationale: Complementary and alternative medicine, or CAM, describes the entire domain of therapies that fall outside of conventional medicine. Integrative therapy combines conventional treatment with evidence-based complementary therapy, but integrative therapy is not the domain. Allopathic therapy enhances conventional therapy but is not the domain. Mind body is a complementary therapy but is not the domain.

2. *Answer:* D

Rationale: Natural products as well as mind and body practices are the two subgroups defined by the National Center for Complementary and Integrative Health (NCCIH). Massage and acupuncture are therapies within the mind and body group. Tai chi and healing touch are therapies within the mind and body group. Chiropractic and osteopathic manipulation are therapies within the mind and body group.

3. *Answer:* D

Rationale: Herbal and botanical medicine can interact with prescribed medication. Herbal/botanical medicine can pose significant risks to the patient due to interactions with conventionally prescribed medications. Herbal/botanical medicine is not FDA approved and is not well-regulated in the United States as in other countries. Herbal/botanical medicine safety and efficacy is not guaranteed.

4. *Answer:* A

Rationale: Mind body modalities include art and color therapy, music therapy, guided imagery, meditation, yoga, and T'ai chi. Whole medical systems are therapeutic approaches that include chiropractic medicine, homeopathic, and osteopathic medicine. Biologically based therapies use substances found in nature to promote wellness and treat illness, such as biofeedback, hydrotherapy, and energy work. Manipulative and body-based practices include acupuncture, acupressure, dance therapy, and traditional Chinese medicine.

5. *Answer:* C

Rationale: Patient values and preferences, which include cultural and religious practices, are part of a comprehensive complementary and alternative medicine (CAM) assessment. Relevant clinical information is incorporated into the assessment and includes items such as comorbidities, allergies, and all medications, including CAM. A comprehensive patient assessment of CAM is done at first visit and ongoing through their cancer care. Biologically based therapies, such as biofeedback, herbal therapy, and energy work, are a part of the CAM assessment.

6. *Answer:* B

Rationale: Docetaxel is noted to have interactions with allium sativum, echinacea purpurea, and hypericum perforatum. Adriamycin, Lupron, and Bleomycin are not known to have specific interactions with natural products.

7. *Answer:* C

Rationale: Patients with peripheral neuropathy Grade 3 or less may receive massage over the affected area. Massage is contraindicated in a patient diagnosed with thrombocytopenia with a platelet count of less than 50,000 due to the risk of bleeding. Patients with suspected or known bone metastasis should not receive pressure or jostling over the affected areas. Patients with severe neutropenia and WBC below 1500 should not receive massage therapy.

8. *Answer:* B

Rationale: With the mind–body modality of neuro-linguistic programming (NLP), the patient focuses on positive aspects of his or her life to promote a positive outlook over time. An example of this modality is having a patient record daily entries in a "gratitude journal." The entries focus on recalling positive aspects of his or her life to promote a positive outlook over time. The overriding principle behind NLP is that an individual gets more of whatever that person is focusing on. The modality that has a meditative component that brings harmony to body, mind, and spirit is yoga. Practices within the modality of meditation share characteristics and often involve focused breathing and a relaxed yet alert state that promotes control over thoughts and feelings. Guided imagery is a modality with a structured process that uses live or recorded readings describing different scenarios or detailed images to guide the patient through a certain process.

9. *Answer:* C

Rationale: A technique in guided imagery is to lead the patient through progressive muscle relaxation or visualization of a treatment process (e.g., visualization of chemotherapy entering the body and seeking out cancer cells to remove them from the body). Tai chi is a modality that enhances coordination and balance and promotes physical, emotional, and spiritual well-being. Mindfulness-based stress reduction (MBSR) is a technique whereby patients are trained to develop awareness of experiences moment by moment and in the context of all senses. This technique falls under the larger category of meditation. A psychotherapy technique based on the concept that distressing events are associated with specific rapid eye movements is eye movement desensitization and reprocessing (EMDR).

10. *Answer:* D

Rationale: The manipulative and body-based practice of acupressure is defined as the use of finger or hand pressure over specific points on the body to relieve symptoms or to influence specific organ function. Acupuncture is an ancient Oriental technique associated with traditional Chinese medicine (TCM), used to restore or promote health and well-being using fine-gauge needles inserted into specific points on the body to stimulate or disperse the flow of energy. The use of manual pressure and strokes on muscle tissue is the definition of massage. Conflicting evidence currently exists as to the effectiveness of massage therapy in patients with cancer. The use of vigorous massage to stimulate flow of lymphatic fluid is the definition of lymphatic therapy.

11. *Answer:* A

Rationale: There are currently no standards of practice or processing regulations for aromatherapy since essential oils have a wide range of quality levels. Aromatherapy targets physical imbalances, as well as psychological and spiritual issues. Although individuals can develop an allergy to the transporting vehicle, allergies are not a major safety concern.

12. *Answer:* C

Rationale: Feldenkrais refers to a method that teaches movement and manipulation to increase body awareness. Gentle manipulation of the skull to reestablish natural configuration and movement is the definition for cranial osteopathy. Lymphatic therapy is the use of vigorous massage to stimulate flow of lymphatic fluid. The technique that uses movement and touch to restore balance to the body is called the Alexander technique and is not a part of the Feldenkrais method.

13. *Answer:* D

Rationale: In Reiki, the practitioner directs the flow of energy by placement of the hands on the body in specific patterns (without applying deep pressure) to redirect or restore energy flow. Therapeutic touch is described in A, while B refers to healing touch, and C describes magnetic therapy.

14. *Answer:* C

Rationale: Acupuncture needles applied in one part of the body can affect the pain sensation in another part of the body when impulses stimulate the nerve fibers in the dorsal horn of the spinal cord. Acupuncture treatments could create a placebo effect and could help patients to refocus their concentration, but these are not the primary actions of the therapy. Acupressure, not acupuncture, uses pressure applied to skin surface with the finger and thumb. Acupressure is similar to acupuncture, but without the needles.

15. *Answer:* B

Rationale: Qi gong is Chinese meditative practice that combines physical postures with focused intention and breathing techniques to release, cleanse, strengthen, and circulate energy. It is used for stress reduction and to enhance the body's natural healing abilities, may increase vitality and awareness of internal energy that furthers the mind–body connection, and can be performed in a standing or sitting position. Shiatsu is a Japanese form of acupuncture. Homeopathy is not necessarily an Eastern practice and is based on the precept of healing through the administration of specific substances. The Alexander technique is movement and touch to restore balance in the body and neuromuscular function, thus allowing the body to regain a relaxed, healthy posture.

CHAPTER 34

1. *Answer:* D

Rationale: A lymph node dissection is related to treatment with surgery and is a treatment-related risk factor for developing lymphedema. An elevated BMI, not a lowered BMI, would be a nonmalignant-related risk factor. Tumor invasion is a cancer diagnosis–related risk factor, not a treatment-related risk factor. Prolonged immobilization is a cancer diagnosis–related risk factor, not a treatment-related risk factor.

2. *Answer:* A

Rationale: Treatment of suspected infection by prescribing an antibiotic early will prevent further potentially life-threatening complications, including serious bacterial infections of the skin (cellulitis) or an infection of the lymph vessels (lymphangitis). Weight management is important to reduce skin changes and potential infection but occurs over time, not as an urgent, acute management strategy. An exercise program is important but will also be over time, not as acute intervention. Axillary reverse mapping (ARM) using blue dye facilitates identification and avoidance of arm lymphatics within the axilla during surgery and its use may reduce lymphedema. It is not an urgent priority; it is a prevention strategy.

3. *Answer:* D

Rationale: Complete decongestive therapy is the standard of care in the management of lymphedema. Wearing a compression garment is recommended for practice in persons with lymphedema. Exercise would not be restricted but would be encouraged. The patient should be taught to elevate the affected extremity, not dangle it. Extreme heat may worsen the swelling.

4. *Answer:* C

Rationale: Maintenance of healthy weight is encouraged since obesity is a risk factor for worsening of lymphedema. Loose, not tight-fitting, clothes should be worn. The diet should be low sodium and high fiber. Lifelong, not short-term, follow-up will be necessary in persons with lymphedema.

5. *Answer:* B

Rationale: Increased capillary permeability can occur with treatment with interleukin-2 or vascular endothelial growth factors. Increased, not decreased, capillary pressure would lead to edema when the volume of blood is expanded or with obstruction. Decreased, not increased, plasma oncotic pressure results in increased fluid in the tissues. When albumin is decreased, fluid leaks into interstitial spaces. Raised, not lowered, hydrostatic pressure drives fluid from the capillaries into the interstitial spaces.

6. *Answer:* D

Rationale: Iatrogenic causes of edema occur from plasma expanders, intravenous fluid overload, and blood components. Medications associated with edema may include treatment with hormones, calcium channel blockers, and steroids. An allergic response would be from histamine release. Systemic conditions include diagnoses such as heart failure, nephrotic syndrome, and liver failure.

7. *Answer:* C

Rationale: Long distance travel is a known risk factor. Decreased, not increased, mobility is a risk factor. A prior history of edema is a risk factor. Hypertension, not hypotension, is a risk factor.

8. *Answer:* A

Rationale: The treatment of the underlying cause of edema is the primary and most effective medical intervention. This includes treatment of congestive heart failure, nephrotic syndrome, liver failure/cirrhosis, thrombophlebitis, lymphedema, and deep vein thrombosis. Beta blockers may be indicated, not restricted, but would be after the underlying cause is determined. Dietary sodium intake should be decreased, not increased. Fluid restriction, not increasing fluid intake, is recommended.

9. *Answer:* B

Rationale: Mesothelioma is the most common diagnosis associated with malignant pericardial effusion. Melanoma, not basal cell, may be associated with malignant pericardial effusion if metastatic. Brain tumor is not a common cause of malignant pericardial effusion. Amyloidosis is not a common cause of malignant pericardial effusion.

10. *Answer:* D

Rationale: Radiation targeted to more than 33% of the heart with more than 300 cGy/day is a risk factor. Fraction doses of 300 cGy/day are tolerated by the heart; however, the iliac crest would not be in the field of treatment. Hormones do not cause capillary permeability. Coexisting cardiac disease, lupus, or endocarditis would increase risk. Renal infection is not associated with malignant pericardial effusion.

11. *Answer:* B

Rationale: Dyspnea is the most common symptom with malignancy-related pericardial disease. The onset is sudden, not gradual. The cough is nonproductive, not productive. Distention may cause dyspnea but is not related to pericardial disease. Tachycardia, hypotension (not hypertension), jugular vein distention, and decreased peripheral pulses are also seen in malignancy-related pericardial disease.

12. *Answer:* A

Rationale: Rapidly developing effusions may be symptomatic at 50 to 80 mL. Normal pericardial fluid volume is 15 to 50 mL.

13. *Answer:* B

Rationale: Pulse pressure is the difference between systolic and diastolic pressure and "narrowing" if less than 40 mmHg. This occurs with pericardial effusions. There are not sufficient data with vital signs alone to indicate stroke, and the diagnosis needs physical assessment. Widening pulse pressure may be suggestive of valve regurgitation, aortic stenosis, or hyperthyroidism. Pulsus paradoxus refers to a decrease in blood pressure with inspiration and may be associated with a pulmonary embolism or hypovolemic shock.

14. *Answer:* C

Rationale: Antimetabolites, such as 5FU, capecitabine, and gemcitabine, can cause coronary artery spasm resulting in angina, arrhythmia, myocardial infarction, cardiac arrest, and sudden death. Alkylating agents, such as cyclophosphamide, can cause acute myopericarditis, pericardial effusions, and arrhythmias. Anthracyclines, such as doxorubicin, daunorubicin, and epirubicin, can cause toxicity from injury of free radicals that result in myocardial cell loss. Angiogenesis inhibitors, such as thalidomide and lenalidomide, can cause bradycardia, thromboembolism, and hypertension.

15. *Answer:* C

Rationale: An acute reaction is reversible. Acute reactions are infrequent, occur within 24 hours of drug administration, are usually self-limiting, and cease when the drug is stopped. They may not require discontinuation of the drug.

16. *Answer:* D

Rationale: Nurses should document the total cumulative dose of chemotherapy. This is the only nursing intervention and prevention strategy listed. Doxorubicin maximum cumulative dose is 550 mg/m^2, cumulative dose; mitoxantrone is 160 mg/m^2 and high-dose cyclophosphamide is 144 mg/kg for 4 days, and the nurse should document cumulative dose with each administration and know the maximum cumulative dose. Treating hyperlipidemia is a medical intervention and is used to treat cardiotoxicity, not prevent the complication. Prescription of a beta blocker is a medical intervention and is used to treat cardiotoxicity, not prevent the problem. Prescription of an ACE inhibitor and calcium channel blockers are used to treat hypertension.

17. *Answer:* A

Rationale: Risk factors for a thrombotic event include stomach, brain, pancreas, and bladder cancers, advanced stage, lymphadenopathy, infection, renal disease, poor performance status, prolonged immobilization, and older age. Risk factors for lymphedema include advanced disease, infection, immobilization, or traumatic injury to an affected extremity. Risk factors for malignant pericardial effusion include mesothelioma direct tumor invasion of the myocardium, obstruction of mediastinal lymph nodes by tumor, infection, and fibrosis secondary to radiation therapy. Risk factors for cardiovascular toxicity include many classes of chemotherapy drugs.

18. *Answer:* B

Rationale: Characteristics of an arterial embolus are severe pain in the involved extremity, extremity coolness, pallor, and absent or decreased pulse. Characteristics of venous occlusion would include tenderness over involved vein and unilateral edema of involved extremity. Characteristics of pulmonary embolus would include chest pain, dyspnea, sudden onset of anxiety, and decreased pulse oximetry. Valvular abnormality with S3 or S4 murmurs are characteristic of cardiovascular toxicity, not an embolus.

19. *Answer:* B

Rationale: Stage 1 pitting edema is mild, spontaneously reversible, and presents with slight heaviness of the extremity with smooth skin texture. Pain and erythema may be present with stage 1. There is no stage 0; begins with stage 1. Stage 2 characteristics would be moderate, irreversible, with possible tissue fibrosis. The skin is stretched, shiny with nonpitting edema. Characteristics of stage 3 would be severe with lymphostatic elephantiasis, and is irreversible. The skin is discolored, stretched, and firm.

20. *Answer:* C

Rationale: In Grade 3 the limb starts to look disfigured, interferes with ADLs, and there is more than 30% difference in size at greatest point or mass of limbs. In Grade 1 there is swelling, pitting edema, and a 5% to 10% difference in size at greatest point of limbs. In Grade 2 there is obvious obstruction, taut skin, and a 10% to 30% difference in size at greatest point of limbs. Grade 4 often progresses to malignancy is disabling and may need removal of affected extremity.

21. *Answer:* A

Rationale: Anthracyclines may cause toxicity from injury of free radicals that result in myocardial cell loss, fibrosis, and loss of contractility, resulting in left ventricular dysfunction, heart failure, and myopericarditis. Agents in this classification include doxorubicin, daunorubicin, epirubicin, idarubicin, and mitoxantrone. Alkylating agents are associated with acute myopericarditis, pericardial effusions, arrhythmias, HTN, thromboembolism, and heart failure. An agent in this classification is cyclophosphamide. Angiogenesis inhibitors are associated with bradycardia, thromboembolism, and HTN may be seen, and agents in this classification include thalidomide, lenalidomide, and pomalidomide. Antimetabolites can cause coronary artery spasm resulting in angina, arrhythmia, myocardial infarction, cardiac arrest, and sudden death. Agents in this classification include 5FU, capecitabine, and gemcitabine.

22. *Answer:* D

Rationale: Ambulating frequently, and implementing leg exercises, if the patient is bedridden, are techniques that are recommended for oncology nurses to use for the prevention of thrombotic events in high-risk patients. Elevating the patient's foot with their knee flexed is a recommended nursing management technique for prevention. Elevating the patient's foot with their knee extended and elevating the patient's knee with their foot extended are

incorrect and not recommended. Finally, employing A constant pneumatic compression device is not a recommendation. The recommendation is for the nurse to apply intermittent pressure.

23. *Answer:* D

Rationale: Regular measurement of extremities facilitates early recognition of changes. Another action in nursing management for treatment and prevention of lymphedema is the use of elastic sleeves and grading wraps, which serve to facilitate movement of lymph out of the arm. The use of the sterile technique with antineoplastic agents is always indicated and is not specific to patients with lymphedema. Carefully applied massage therapy has been shown to be beneficial, but vigorous weightlifting with the affected limb is not indicated. Moderate use limits risk, while allowing lymphatic fluid to drain normally. Extreme heat, such as use of hot tubs, is to be avoided.

24. *Answer:* B

Rationale: Lymphedema may occur initially years after the surgical procedure has been completed, even if the patient has reported no previous problems. Less invasive breast surgery still requires some lymph node dissection for staging. Sentinel node mapping does not eliminate the need for sentinel node dissection for biopsy, which can contribute to future lymphedema. Although less extensive node disruption with breast conservation and radiation therapy may well decrease the risk of lymphedema, those treatments do not eliminate the risk.

25. *Answer:* B

Rationale: Hypoproteinemia contributes to edema by fluid leaks into the interstitial space. When albumin levels are decreased, fluid leaks into interstitial spaces (i.e., proteinuria, hepatic failure, malabsorption, protein malnutrition). An S2 heart sound is normal. Blood pressure and pulse readings usually increase with edema, while peripheral pulses usually diminish as a result of poor cardiac output.

CHAPTER 35

1. *Answer:* A

Rationale: Cognitive impairment is a functional decline in one or more cognitive domains, including executive functioning. Posttraumatic stress is a mental disorder that can occur after a traumatic event. Delirium is associated with a disturbance in the level of an individual's attention and awareness. Decreased confidence is related to belief in one's own abilities.

2. *Answer:* D

Rationale: Either a CT or an MRI can be ordered to rule out structural abnormalities in patients with focal neurological deficits or who are at high risk for recurrence or metastatic central nervous system disease. A bone scan is more useful to evaluate the presence of an infection, fracture, or bone metastases. Laboratory tests are done to rule out more general causes of cognitive impairment, such as electrolytes for metabolic disturbances, or LFTs for liver dysfunction.

3. *Answer:* A

Rationale: Cognitive training is an intervention that is likely to be effective in improving cognitive skills, such as attention or memory. Cognitive training often includes structured repetitive tasks aimed at improving a specific cognitive skill, such as memory or attention. Although the National Comprehensive Cancer Network (NCCN) guidelines suggest that a trial of psychostimulants be considered if nonpharmacological interventions are not effective, effectiveness of acetylcholinesterase inhibitors, N-methyl-D-aspartate receptors, or psychostimulants has not been established for management of cancer treatment-related cognitive impairment. Mindfulness stress reduction is typically utilized to decrease symptoms such as stress, anxiety, or pain.

4. *Answer:* B

Rationale: While changes in other cognitive domains (e.g., motor function, attention/concentration, and memory) may occur, an acute onset of hypervigilance or sedation is the classic symptom of delirium.

5. *Answer:* C

Rationale: Treatment toxicities and tumor effects leading to metabolic abnormalities (e.g., calcium, glucose, sodium) may put patients at a higher risk for delirium. Individual characteristics such as advanced age and sensory impairments (e.g., visual, hearing) may contribute to both cognitive impairment and delirium. Dose intensity, cumulative effect, and/or multimodality therapy are risk factors for cognitive impairment. Genetic polymorphisms (e.g., APOE E4 allele) are associated with cancer-related cognitive impairment as well as dementia, but not delirium.

6. *Answer:* A

Rationale: The best initial step would be to identify any risk factors for delirium, including medications known to cause delirium or have high anticholinergic potential. A CBC might identify anemia or sepsis, which can contribute to delirium. An MRI of the brain would detect a traumatic brain injury or brain tumor. Lumbar puncture would only be done if etiology is not obvious.

7. *Answer:* D

Rationale: Low-dose antipsychotics may be used to manage severe agitation. Low-dose antipsychotics may cause drowsiness, but they do not typically affect sleep patterns or treat sleep problems. Metabolic imbalances may be due to dehydration or electrolyte loss and will require hydration and electrolyte replacement. Sensory deficits such as hearing impairment or visual problems should be corrected whenever possible.

8. *Answer:* D

Rationale: A nursing management technique for cancer- and cancer treatment–related cognitive impairment is to reinforce cognitive and exercise training plans. Cognitive training and exercise include having the patient participate in structured, repetitive tasks aimed at improving a specific cognitive skill, such as attention or memory. Exercise training may include aerobics, tai chi, or yoga. Avoiding excessive sensory stimulation and/or restraints, incorporating environmental strategies such as having a visible clock or calendar available and keeping a room well-lit and surrounded by familiar objects, and providing frequent reorientation and reassurance are all nursing management techniques for patients with delirium.

9. *Answer:* C

Rationale: The use of assistive devices, such as eyeglasses or hearing aids, will decrease the distortion of sights and sounds, while decreasing the client's anxiety, and reducing delirium. The remaining choices—removing calendars, not putting up photos of loved ones, and exposing the patient to environmental noises that might be discomforting and unfamiliar—all serve to increase, and not decrease, the patient's delirium.

CHAPTER 36

1. *Answer:* D

Rationale: Cortisol is the correct answer. Cortisol is a glucocorticoid steroid hormone produced by the adrenal gland. Antidiuretic hormone is produced by the pituitary gland, as is luteinizing hormone. Thyroxine is secreted by the thyroid gland in response to a thyroid stimulating hormone released by the pituitary gland.

2. *Answer:* A

Rationale: The presentation of hypothyroidism includes weakness, depression, constipation, and intolerance to cold temperatures. Although weakness and depression may be seen with the other conditions, the presence of cold intolerance differentiates hypothyroidism from the other options. Patients with hyperthyroidism have heat intolerance.

3. *Answer:* A

Rationale: Methylprednisolone is the correct answer. Patients being treated with immune checkpoint inhibitors can develop hyperthyroidism. Those who do, and are also at high risk for cardiovascular events, such as patients with a history of coronary artery disease, receive methylprednisolone 1 to 2 mg/kg daily until thyroid function returns to baseline. Dexamethasone is used as a long-acting glucocorticoid for patients with adrenal insufficiency. Levothyroxine is used as thyroid hormone replacement for hypothyroid patients. Cinacalcet may be used to treat patients with hyperparathyroidism.

4. *Answer:* B

Rationale: It takes 4 to 6 weeks for TSH and T4 levels to reach steady state concentration, at which point the levothyroxine dose may be adjusted. Therefore, TSH and T4 levels are monitored every 4 to 6 weeks; after a steady state is reached, TSH and T4 levels are monitored every 6 months. The other options are inaccurate.

5. *Answer:* C

Rationale: Option C, a low calcium, high phosphate diet, is the correct answer. Patients with primary hyperparathyroidism have elevated levels of serum calcium (hypercalcemia). They may be advised to avoid calcium-rich foods and to include foods high in phosphorus in their diet. The reason is because calcium and phosphorus levels are regulated in inverse proportion to each other so factors that increase one level will decrease the other. Thiazide diuretics would not be recommended because they can increase the level of calcium in the blood. In addition, dehydration is to be avoided as it aggravates hypercalcemia, and fluid intake should be increased. Phosphate binding drugs would not be used because usage of these agents would decrease serum phosphate levels, causing calcium levels to increase.

6. *Answer:* D

Rationale: Serum calcium levels are regulated by parathyroid hormone (PTH) released by the parathyroid glands. When these glands are removed, serum calcium levels decrease to below normal. Calcium replacement is needed at a dose dependent on the level of corrected serum calcium. The other electrolytes—potassium, chloride, and sodium—are not regulated by the parathyroid glands.

7. *Answer:* B

Rationale: Diabetes insipidus is the correct answer. Radiation therapy delivered to the head has caused pituitary gland dysfunction resulting in hypopituitarism (hypophysitis) and central type 1 diabetes insipidus. The other options are not caused by alterations in pituitary gland function.

8. *Answer:* A

Rationale: The correct answer is A. The patient should wear an alert bracelet indicating steroid stress doses. The alert bracelet should include the patient's condition (adrenal insufficiency) and necessary treatment in the case of an emergency (i.e., the need for stress dose steroids). Prior to surgical procedures, the patient may require increased steroid doses rather than decreased. During "minor sick day" periods, such as for a head cold, the patient may need to increase their usual steroid dose two to three times. A fivefold dose increase would be unlikely. Steroid dosing does not change on a weekly basis, but as needed to meet the patient's needs for dose adjustments.

9. *Answer:* A

Rationale: Patients presenting with symptoms of anxiety, agitation, weakness, and heat intolerance, with a physical examination showing the patient has weight loss and hyperactivity, denotes a diagnosis of hyperthyroidism/thyrotoxicosis. Other indications of this condition include tremor, rapid speech, lid lag, hair thinning, tachycardia, an irregular pulse, hyperreflexia, and proximal muscle weakness. A patient presenting with bone pain, fatigue, weakness, and anorexia, with a physical examination revealing hypertension and bradycardia, is showing signs of hyperparathyroidism. Patients with hypoparathyroidism present with fatigue, anxiety, depression, and irritability. The patient's physical examination might reveal chronic skeletal abnormalities. The patient presenting with visual changes, headache, and myalgias has indications of hypopituitarism and hypophysitis. A physical examination shows the patient has experienced weight loss and is showing signs of hypotension.

10. *Answer:* A

Rationale: Medications affecting levothyroxine absorption include sucralfate, aluminum hydroxide, ferrous sulfate, antacids, proton pump inhibitors, H2 receptor antagonists, laxatives, calcium carbonate and soy supplements, coffee, grapefruit juice, and dietary fibers. Metabolic clearance of levothyroxine is increased with rifampicin carbamazepine, phenobarbital, and phenytoin. Drugs that block t4 to T3 conversion include amiodarone, glucocorticoids, beta-blockers, and selenium deficiency. Other drugs that interfere with levothyroxine absorption include estrogens, sertraline, and chloroquine tyrosine kinase inhibitors imatinib, motesanib, and sorafenib.

CHAPTER 37

1. *Answer:* C

Rationale: Elevated rather than lower levels of proinflammatory cytokines, interleukins, and tumor necrosis factor are all underlying mechanisms of fatigue along with 5-hydroxytryptophan dysregulation and circadian rhythm disturbances. Some patients have circadian rhythms that align with morning or evening preference, but no studies suggest this is a risk for cancer-related fatigue.

2. *Answer:* C

Rationale: All ages and both sexes are susceptible to cancer-related fatigue. Some of the greatest risks include patients receiving opioids during treatment, those with poor performance status, weight loss >5% in 6 months, and those receiving concurrent chemoradiation. Immobilization, anxiety, pain, and infection are additional risk factors. Therefore, answer C, low performance status, is the best answer.

3. *Answer:* B

Rationale: Patient-reported outcomes are those reported directly by the patient. Patient report is considered as the gold standard for fatigue assessment. Onset, intensity, duration, patterns, exacerbating factors, impact on quality of life, and function comprise a comprehensive fatigue assessment. C includes physiologic assessments that are not patient-reported outcomes. A and D include caregiver insight, which is not a patient-reported outcome.

4. *Answer:* A

Rationale: Several laboratory analyses can suggest contributing factors of fatigue. These include low thyroid function; electrolyte disturbances; low levels of iron, vitamin B12, folate, and ferritin; low hemoglobin/hematocrit, low hormone levels (e.g., testosterone), and low vitamin D levels. Therefore, answer A is the best choice. SPEP and tumor marker elevations can suggest disease progression, but this may or may not be associated with fatigue as patients can sometimes be asymptomatic. A low platelet count may indicate treatment toxicity or disease but is not always suggestive of fatigue.

5. *Answer:* A

Rationale: Answer A is the best choice, as blood transfusions can correct anemia and improve fatigue. While erythropoiesis-stimulating agents (ESAs) may benefit patients with severe fatigue, they should be avoided in patients with myeloid malignancies because they may stimulate cancer cell growth. Low-dose dexamethasone rather than high dose is sometimes used for severe fatigue. Benzodiazepines often compound the fatigue experience as sedation is a major adverse event.

6. *Answer:* D

Rationale: While answers A, B, and C may reduce fatigue, exercise and physical activity have the strongest evidence in the management of cancer-related fatigue. With cancer, resting and napping do not alleviate fatigue properly. Exercise is shown to be superior to any medical or alternative interventions. Moderate exercise routines lasting 30 minutes per day, 3 days a week for at least 12 weeks show the greatest benefit. The exercise should be tailored according to patient's ability. The type of exercise does not appear to influence fatigue outcomes.

7. *Answer:* B

Rationale: Answer B is the best choice as depression and fatigue can both present with feeling of exhaustion. Screening for depression is important for all patients with cancer, and differentiating between depression and fatigue is essential, although often both may be present. Exercise should be employed as tolerated. No evidence exists that vigorous exercise is more effective in managing fatigue. High-intensity exercise can worsen fatigue if the patient is not ready to tolerate this regimen. Too much stimulation can increase fatigue in some patients; therefore, decreasing environmental stimuli should be considered to alleviate fatigue. While some patients' fatigue resolves over time, fatigue can be long term in many patients.

8. *Answer:* D

Rationale: Symptoms in patients with cancer that have been known to cluster with fatigue are sleep disturbances, pain, and distress. Anxiety, depression, stress, and cognitive changes are not known symptoms to cluster with fatigue in patients with cancer.

CHAPTER 38

1. *Answer:* A

Rationale: During the initiation phase of mucositis, DNA damage occurs, as well as a primary damage response, which includes transcription factors upregulating an innate immune response and activation of gene expression and multiple pathways, leading to production of cytokines and modulators, which are associated with the progression of mucositis. Secondary infection occurs in the ulcerative phase as a result of loss of mucosal integrity, painful lesions, and submucosal breach with bacterial colonization. The development of small nodules due to the absence of angiogenesis and the development of mucositis due to interferons and TNF cell proliferation are not part of the pathogenesis of mucositis.

2. *Answer:* C

Rationale: Impaired renal function (high serum creatinine – 2.7 is elevated) may increase the risk for mucositis. A BMI of <18.5 and persistent smoking and alcohol

use puts the patient at risk for mucositis. The use of non-alcohol-based mouthwashes does not put the patient at risk for mucositis.

3. *Answer:* D

Rationale: Palifermin is a keratinocyte growth factor and is FDA approved for patients with hematological malignancies receiving high-dose chemotherapy and total body irradiation followed by autologous HSCT prior to and post conditioning regimen to reduce the incidence and severity of oral mucositis. Palifermin is not used to alleviate nausea and vomiting or cramping during treatment. Palifermin is also not used to increase blood counts after transplant.

4. *Answer:* A

Rationale: Emetogenic chemotherapy damages the gastrointestinal mucosal cells and releases serotonin (5HT) from enterochromaffin cells. 5HT binds to and activates 5HT3 receptors on the vagus nerve, initiating emetic signal and acute chemotherapy-induced nausea and vomiting (CINV) during the first 24 hours after chemotherapy. Emetic stimuli cause substance P (SP) binding at neurokin-1 (NK1) receptors in the chemotherapy trigger zone, amplifying the emetic message—particularly during *delayed CINV* that may persist for a few to many days. Small intestine and abdominal contraction do not lead to acute CINV.

5. *Answer:* D

Rationale: No or low history of significant alcohol consumption puts the patient at risk for nausea and vomiting. History of smoking, GERD, and use of NSAIDS do not put the patient at risk for chemotherapy-induced nausea and vomiting (CINV). Other risk factors for CINV include being of the female gender, being between the ages 5 and 60 years, a history of motion sickness, and a history of hyperemesis with pregnancy.

6. *Answer:* A

Rationale: CINV/RINV standard of care antiemetics include 5HT3 antagonists, NK1 drugs, a corticosteroid such as dexamethasone, and olanzapine. Dopamine is a rescue antiemetic, and benzodiazepines are typically used for anticipatory nausea/vomiting to decrease anxiety. Antisecretory drugs are not emetics and are not used for standard of care.

7. *Answer:* C

Rationale: Some tumors seed malignant cells within the peritoneal cavity (carcinomatosis), and these are known to increase osmotic pressure leading to malignant ascites. Other causes include cancer cells lining the peritoneum that produce inflammatory cytokines, causing large molecules to amass and exert osmotic pressure with subsequent malignant ascites. Another cause is tumor expressed VEGF that induces angiogenesis and alters vascular and peritoneal membrane permeability, leading to increased malignant ascites accumulation. Increased drainage from the malignant tumor and lymphatic cell drainage are not causes of malignant ascites. Too much fluid moving from the intravascular to interstitial space is third-spacing.

8. *Answer:* D

Rationale: Paracentesis is safe and well-tolerated with 80% to 90% of patients stating symptom relief such as decreased abdominal distension and discomfort, dyspnea, nausea, anorexia, fatigue, and mobility. The procedure for paracentesis does not have a risk for bowel obstruction or cardiac effects, but rather there is a low complication risk for bowel perforation. The procedure is done under ultrasound guidance and does not require deep sedation.

9. *Answer:* A

Rationale: Metabolic causes, such as dehydration, hyponatremia, hypokalemia, hypercalcemia, hypothyroidism, uremia, and diabetes, may cause constipation. Dietary causes could include insufficient fluid intake. However, the patient's diabetes and uremia make the possibility of metabolic cause more likely. Both kidney stones and a urinary fistula are not the causes of constipation.

10. *Answer:* B

Rationale: Rectally administered agents, such as suppositories and enemas, are the preferred method for rapid and predictable evacuation of stool from the rectum and distal colon, such as for patients with fecal impaction. Liquids in enemas do not form fiber and do not soften the stool. Oral stool softeners are ineffective for established constipation and opioid-induced constipation. Oral bulking agents may worsen slow-transit opioid- or anticholinergic-related constipation. Some oral agents are ineffective for established constipation and are better used as first-line laxatives to prevent constipation. Water taken along with oral medications will not induce cramping and bloating.

11. *Answer:* C

Rationale: Drugs that commonly are the cause of diarrhea include methotrexate, 5FU, irinotecan, capecitabine, gemcitabine, cyclophosphamide, cisplatin, oxaliplatin, carboplatin, doxorubicin, paclitaxel, docetaxel, cabazitaxel, and thalidomide. Fecal impaction can lead to overflow diarrhea. Other causes of diarrhea include C-difficile, viral enteritis, and enteral tube feedings.

12. *Answer:* D

Rationale: The patient should eat a low-fat, high-potassium diet, with six to eight small meals and snacks per day. The patient should also drink room temperature clear liquids. Dietary modifications to decrease diarrhea include avoiding spicy, fatty, greasy food, as well as those high in fiber (cereals), high in sugar, and stone fruits, such as peaches and nectarines. Beverages that may worsen diarrhea include caffeine, alcohol, fruit juices, lactose-containing dairy products, and hot liquids.

13. *Answer:* B

Rationale: Pilocarpine is contraindicated in patients with chronic cardiovascular or pulmonary disease, uncontrolled asthma, narrow-angle glaucoma, or taking β-blockers. Medications that may be considered are cevimeline (Evoxac), Aquoral, Xero-Lube, Biotene mouthwash, Moi-Stir, NeutraSal, SalivaMAX, and Salivart.

14. *Answer:* C

Rationale: The appropriate grading is Grade 3. According to the National Cancer Institute, Common Terminology Criteria for Adverse Events (NCI-CTCAE) for Gastrointestinal symptoms, tube feeding, TPN, or hospitalization is indicated. For Grade 1, intervention is not indicated. Grade 2 indicates outpatient IV hydration and medical intervention. Grade 4 includes life-threatening complications, and treatment is urgent. Grade 5 is death.

15. *Answer:* A

Rationale: Oropharyngeal dysphagia (OD) occurs at the start of swallowing and is a symptom of a problem in the mouth or in the pharynx. Usually, this condition causes reflexive coughing and a sense of choking with swallowing. Other possible symptoms include symptoms such as voice change, frequent throat clearing, and earache. Mechanical dysphagia may occur postsurgery from inflammation and edema. The onset of mechanical dysphagia may precede the diagnosis of large (T3–T4) base of tongue, supraglottic, or pharyngeal tumors. Esophageal dysphagia (ED) is caused by esophageal disease. ED is relatively uncommon, and the patient feels like food is sticking in their neck or upper chest a few seconds after they start to swallow. Radiation therapy is an effective part of treatment for many cancers that arise in the head and neck. However, following radiation for these cancers, some patients develop difficulty swallowing because the radiation caused the muscles and mucosal lining of the mouth, throat, and esophagus to become stiff and deformed. Swallowing becomes effortful and painful.

16. *Answer:* B

Rationale: In addition to caffeinated beverage consumption, lifestyle factors include tobacco use, alcohol use, dehydration, heavy snoring, and mouth breathing. Use of an antihistamine and an anticholinergic agent are drug-related causes. Secondary Sjögren syndrome is a disease-related cause.

17. *Answer:* D

Rationale: Sialometry is a test to measure saliva flow. The test is performed after an overnight fast or after a 2 hour fast. The patient is sitting upright for the procedure. Results of the test for normal salivary flow rate stimulated is 1.5 to 2.0 mL/min and unstimulated is 0.3 to 0.4 mL/min; less than 0.12 to 0.16 mL/min is abnormal. The evaluation is not done at normal bedtime, but upon waking, and the test is also not done after a full meal. The test is not a measure of regurgitation, but of saliva flow.

18. *Answer:* D

Rationale: Reminding the patient to have a pretreatment dental examination and providing them with instructions (both written and oral) for implementing an oral hygiene regimen is an example of a preventative nursing management measure. Reminding patients to avoid spicy foods, hot drinks, or foods with too hot temperatures is not a preventative measure but a dietary instruction when the patient is experiencing painful oral mucositis. To ease pain when eating or drinking, patients should eat soft or moistened foods. Instructing patients to use topical protective or coating agents is not a preventative nursing management instruction, but, instead, a tip to provide some temporary relief from oral mucositis pain. Patients can use such agents as benzocaine (Orabase, Oratect Gel, Hurricaine), plus an analgesic such as viscous lidocaine.

Finally, the instruction to use a solution of normal saline, salt, and baking soda is also not a preventative tip but a way for the patient to reduce pain. The formula for the solution is 0.5 teaspoon each in 1 cup of warm water.

19. *Answer:* B

Rationale: Xerostomia is a drying of the oral mucosa, resulting in a loss of saliva caused by damage that occurs to the salivary glands subsequent to radiation therapy. Dysphagia, mucositis, and trismus do not result in dry mouth. Dysphagia is an inability to swallow or difficulty in swallowing. Mucositis is defined by inflammatory lesions of the mucous membranes and may include the intestine. Trismus is a contraction of the muscles of mastication.

20. *Answer:* B

Rationale: Sucking ice cubes or sugarless popsicles wets the mouth and numbs the mucosa and is an intervention that may provide moisture to the oral mucosa. Decreasing intake of liquids will cause less moisture to be present. The other two answers—encouraging the patient to eat dry and spicy foods and having the patient rinse with a commercial mouthwash—may irritate the mouth and cause excessive burning.

21. *Answer:* B

Rationale: Ascites is associated with various tumors, mainly intra-abdominal malignancies. Ovarian cancer accounts for 38% of ascites.

22. *Answer:* C

Rationale: Constipation lasting for 3 days or more is unusual for this patient and suggests a need for immediate relief. Use of a stimulant laxative until a bowel movement occurs should be recommended. Then evaluation, as needed, for daily stool softeners or lubricant laxatives. At 10 days after chemotherapy, patients are at nadir and susceptible to infection. Rectal medications or treatments should be avoided. Opioids can increase the risk for constipation. Bulk-forming laxatives can take longer to provide relief than oral stimulant laxatives.

23. *Answer:* B

Rationale: Diet can affect radiation-induced diarrhea. The patient should consume solid foods that contain low residue and high protein. A low-residue diet will decrease irritation of the gastrointestinal tract; a high-fiber diet will increase irritation of the gastrointestinal tract. Foods to avoid include stone fruits (e.g., apricots, cherries, peaches). Beverages that can worsen diarrhea should be avoided and include fruit juices, caffeinated drinks, alcohol, high-osmolar dietary supplements, lactose-containing dairy products, and hot liquids. In addition, decreasing spicy, fried, and fatty foods may help relieve diarrhea.

24. *Answer:* A

Rationale: Paracentesis is the first-line interventional management for refractory ascites. A fine is tube inserted into the peritoneum under ultrasound guidance, then connected to a collection bag into which the ascites fluid freely drains, and then the catheter is removed.

It is a safe, well-tolerated procedure that provides 90% symptom relief and has a low risk of complications.

Nontunneled catheters should be avoided due to a higher complication rate (cellulitis, blockage, leakage, and infection) but may be used in patients with very limited life expectancy. A peritoneovenous shunt is not as effective as other measures and has more complications. Intraperitoneal surgery is only considered for very selected patients with longer expected survival.

25. *Answer:* C

Rationale: The patient has a history of breast cancer that is associated with increased risk for hypercalcemia of malignancy. Gastrointestinal changes, including constipation, are common manifestations of increased serum calcium levels. Changes in the other electrolytes listed—bicarbonate, sodium, and chloride—would not lead to constipation.

CHAPTER 39

1. *Answer:* D

Rationale: Stress incontinence is the involuntary loss of urine that occurs with increased abdominal pressure associated with laughing, coughing, sneezing, and other physical activities, such as heavy lifting. Stress incontinence is not associated with psychological distress. It is not caused by neurologic changes that cause urinary sphincter dysfunction or impair reflexes for emptying of the bladder. Urge incontinence is the involuntary loss of urine with an abrupt and strong desire to void. Reflex incontinence is the involuntary loss of urine with no sensation of urge or bladder fullness. Functional incontinence is the state in which an individual experiences incontinence because of difficulty in reaching or inability to reach the toilet before urination. Total incontinence is the continuous loss of urine without distention or awareness of bladder fullness.

2. *Answer:* A

Rationale: Treatment-induced bladder inflammation is the correct answer. Radiation therapy to the bladder is associated with an inflammatory reaction within the bladder that increases the risk for urinary incontinence. Reduced size of the bladder tumor is not a risk factor for incontinence. Advanced patient age is not the most likely explanation for urinary incontinence in this patient whose age is not specified. Radiation to renal structures may lead to permanent fibrosis and atrophy but not kidney stones. Kidney stone development is more likely to be associated with tumor lysis syndrome.

3. *Answer:* A

Rationale: Tests to determine the amount of residual urine after voiding provides important information about how completely the bladder empties with voiding. Gathering information about a patient's usual voiding habits and reviewing a patient's bladder diary may be useful but are not diagnostic tests. Colonoscopy is used to visualize changes within the colon.

4. *Answer:* B

Rationale: Behavioral techniques, such as voiding at the same time every day, help the patient establish the habit of voiding according to a schedule and gain control

189

of urination. Suggesting that the patient stay shut in the house as much as possible is not therapeutic. Increasing daily fluid intake is more likely to increase uncontrolled loss of urine. Learning bladder self-catheterization is appropriate for patients who are unable to urinate voluntarily.

5. *Answer:* C

Rationale: Catheterization of urine will be done every 4 to 6 hours is the correct answer. This type of continent diversion involves creating an internal reservoir for urine from the ileum or large intestine with a stoma brought out to the skin. Urine is removed via catheterization through the stoma several times per day. The other choices are incorrect. A continent diversion does not require an external collection device, and thus is not associated with dribbling of urine, nor with the need to empty a pouch.

6. *Answer:* D

Rationale: Emptying the collection pouch when it is half-full is the correct answer. With an ileal conduit, urine collects almost continuously into an external collection pouch, which should be emptied whenever it is one-third to one-half full. The pouch should also be emptied prior to chemotherapy. There are no recommendations to avoid certain foods, such as cruciferous vegetables. The peristomal skin should be cleansed with water rather than alcohol, which causes drying. There is no need to catheterize the stoma because urine is collected externally in the pouch.

7. *Answer:* C

Rationale: Hypercalcemia of malignancy is the correct answer. Hypercalcemia of malignancy more commonly occurs in patients with metastatic breast cancer and causes renal dysfunction. When hypercalcemia of malignancy is present, the kidneys become unable to concentrate urine, resulting in diuresis of large amounts of diluted urine. Decreased blood flow to the kidneys would most likely lead to decreased urine output. Breast cancer commonly metastasizes to bone rather than to lymph nodes in the pelvis; obstruction of these lymph nodes would not lead to increased output of urine. Radiation therapy directed to the leg would not cause nephrotoxicity. Radiation therapy is a local treatment and would have no effect on the kidneys if they are not in the radiation treatment field.

8. *Answer:* D

Rationale: The nurse realizes that what the patient has been experiencing is most likely urge incontinence. Urge incontinence is when an individual has the involuntary loss of urine, with an abrupt and strong desire to void. Stress incontinence is the involuntary loss of urine during such activities as laughing, coughing, sneezing, or heavy lifting. These activities place increased pressure on the abdomen and cause the release of urine. Reflex incontinence is the involuntary loss of urine with no sensation of urge to void or fullness of the bladder. Finally, functional incontinence occurs when a person has a strong desire to void and experiences incontinence because they have difficulty reaching or cannot reach the toilet in enough time before urination occurs.

9. *Answer:* B

Rationale: The medical management of renal dysfunction for a patient with cancer as a pharmacologic intervention is treatment with amifostine and sodium thiosulfate for cisplatin nephrotoxicity. Other pharmacologic interventions include saline hydration with appropriate diuretics and oral or intravenous (IV) sodium bicarbonate to maintain alkaline urine. Other pharmacologic interventions include replacing electrolytes and administering diuretics, as needed. Anticholinergics, tricyclic antidepressants, and potassium channel openers are all examples of medical management for urinary incontinence.

10. *Answer:* D

Rationale: Electrostimulation is a medical management treatment for urinary incontinence. Other medical management strategies include anticholinergics, tricyclic antidepressants, potassium channel openers, and a consultation with a urologist. Answers A, B, and C—saline hydration with appropriate diuretic, oral, or intravenous (IV) sodium bicarbonate to maintain alkaline urine, and replacement of electrolytes—are all examples of pharmacologic interventions for patients with cancer diagnosed with renal dysfunction.

11. *Answer:* A

Rationale: A neobladder is a urinary reconstructive procedure in which a surgically constructed bladder is created from the intestine and attached to the urethra. Thus, patients with any intestinal or urethral issues are not appropriate candidates for the surgery. Factors that exclude creation of a neobladder include cancer extending into the urethra, a past history of inflammatory bowel disease, radiation, or short gut syndrome from previous bowel resection. Patients with a history of benign prostatic hypertrophy and urinary incontinence may be appropriate candidates for the surgery.

CHAPTER 40

1. *Answer:* C

Rationale: Granulocytes are myeloid cells and include monocytes, neutrophils, eosinophils, and basophils. Red blood cells and platelets are myeloid cells but are not granulocytes. Lymphocytes arise from lymphoid progenitor cells.

2. *Answer:* B

Rationale: An absolute neutrophil count (ANC) below 1500/mm³ places the patient at increased risk of infection and sepsis. An ANC of 2500/mm³ is within the normal range. A white blood cell count of 4.3×10^9/L is within the normal range. An increased absolute basophil count can be a sign of chronic inflammation.

3. *Answer:* A

Rationale: Febrile neutropenia is present when a patient has a sustained temperature of ≥38°C (100.4°F) that lasts for more than 1 hour. An ANC <1000/mm³ and a single temperature of >38.3°C (101°F) also indicates febrile neutropenia. The other options—thrombocytopenia, hypercalcemia, and hemolytic anemia—are not associated with elevated temperatures.

4. *Answer:* D

Rationale: One of the most common adverse events associated with G-CSF agents is bone pain. Others are myalgia, arthralgia, and fever. The other options, eye inflammation, acne-like rash, and lung fibrosis, are all associated with use of epidermal growth factor receptor (EGFR) inhibitor agents.

5. *Answer:* A

Rationale: Radiation to bone marrow-producing regions, such as the pelvis, ischium, and long bones (e.g., femur), can cause prolonged bone marrow suppression. The other options of peripheral neuropathy, wet desquamation, and urinary retention are unlikely to occur.

6. *Answer:* D

Rationale: Fresh flowers are not allowed to be delivered to the room of a patient who is at risk of immunosuppression. This is an intervention to minimize the occurrence of infection. The other options are not correct. Recommended interventions include meticulous personal hygiene, including daily baths, and attention to oral and perineal care. So, avoid frequent bathing as it is drying to the skin would be inaccurate. Standing water in pitchers should be changed daily and not every 4 hours. Visits from family members who do not have communicable illness are allowed, so not every visit from a family member would be prohibited.

7. *Answer:* B

Rationale: Sore throat can indicate infection. Other signs and symptoms of infection might be the presence of temperature higher than 100.5°F (38.1°C), a productive cough, and painful urination. Therefore, the other options, including the symptoms of a dry mouth, a temperature of 99.8°, and urinary hesitancy, are not correct.

8. *Answer:* C

Rationale: Chronic blood loss from the gastrointestinal tract can result in anemia. Iron deficiency, rather than iron overload, can also result in anemia. Alterations in platelet function and estrogen levels are not contributing factors for anemia.

9. *Answer:* A

Rationale: Patients with anemia are at an increased risk of fatigue, dyspnea, and tachycardia. These manifestations are not typically seen together in the other conditions of neutropenia, lymphocytopenia, and thrombocytopenia.

10. *Answer:* A

Rationale: The target value when transfusing packed red blood cells (PRBCs) is to maintain a hemoglobin level greater than 10 g/dL. The other options, although all are in the normal range, are not taken into consideration when determining the need to transfuse PRBCs.

11. *Answer:* C

Rationale: Patients receiving cytotoxic chemotherapy can develop coagulation abnormalities, such as disseminated intravascular coagulation (DIC), a condition in which massive clotting causes platelets (and clotting factors) to be consumed. Results of red blood cell count and hemoglobin and ferritin levels are not as important as results indicating the presence of thrombocytopenia.

12. *Answer:* A

Rationale: Safety measures should be taught to decrease the occurrence of bleeding, which includes fall prevention. Invasive procedures such as enemas are to be avoided, as is shaving with a straight-edge razor. Ice packs are applied to areas of bleeding rather than warm packs.

13. *Answer:* A

Rationale: Blood pressure of 86/50 and respiratory rate (RR) of 26 is the correct answer as the presence of hypotension (i.e., 86/50) or tachypnea (RR >24) portend high risk for clinical deterioration. Therefore, a blood pressure of 155/90 (hypertension) and respiratory rate of 20 (normal RR) is not correct. A heart rate of 80 and sleepiness are normal signs. A temperature of 100.1°F is not considered indicative of febrile neutropenia (i.e., a single temperature of 101°F or a sustained temperature of 100.4°F for more than 1 hour), and depression can be a normal response to a cancer diagnosis.

14. *Answer:* C

Rationale: Hemorrhage is the correct answer. Signs of hemorrhage include weak or irregular pulse, pale skin, and cold or moist skin. In addition, patients with leukemia, especially nonlymphocytic leukemia, are at increased risk of hemorrhage as a result of a paraneoplastic process. Anemia and thrombocytopenia can result from hemorrhage.

15. *Answer:* B

Rationale: Giving the patient tepid sponge baths is the correct answer. Slow cooling of the skin and mucous membranes is recommended for patients experiencing fever and chills. Therefore, heating blankets or immersion in an ice bath are contraindicated. Fluid intake should be increased to prevent dehydration.

16. *Answer:* D

Rationale: Dose intensity is a disease and treatment-related risk factor associated with chemotherapy-induced myeloid toxicity. How a patient reacts to a dosage level can affect the risk for myeloid toxicity. Disease-related risk factors include the prevalence of high tumor burden and the bone marrow involvement of a tumor. Decreased immune function is related to the patient and how the host can fend off toxicities, based on treatment, or symptoms of the disease. Recently completed surgery or open wounds is another risk factor associated with the host, as is the example of drug–drug interactions.

17. *Answer:* D

Rationale: D is the only correct answer. Prophylactic use of G-CSF is recommended in patients with Grade 3 and 4 chemotherapy-induced neutropenia and a high risk of febrile neutropenia. If the chemotherapy dose is reduced and will not compromise the goal of cancer treatment, growth factor is not recommended. However, if the chemotherapy dose cannot be reduced, growth factor may be prescribed. Colony-stimulating growth factors for neutrophils are not prescribed for anemia or patients with cancer undergoing radiation.

18. *Answer:* B

Rationale: Lymphopenia, a reduction in the number of B or T lymphocytes, places the patient at risk for

191

opportunities infections. The other answers are incorrect. Thrombocytopenia increases risk of bleeding and anemia is associated with fatigue. Myalgia is a common adverse event associated with G-CSF agents. Myalgia can also be a symptom of cytokine storm and cytokine release syndrome.

19. *Answer:* C

Rationale: Circulating neutrophils are comprised of segmented neutrophils (segs) and bands and are important to fighting infection. If a patient has a decreased number of circulating neutrophils in the blood, the risk of infection is increased. It is important for nurses to know how to calculate an absolute neutrophil count (ANC). The ANC is calculated by taking the % neutrophils (% segs + % bands) multiplied by WBC.

20. *Answer:* C

Rationale: Platelets arise from the myeloid stem cells. Lymphoid stem cells produce lymphocytes. Megakaryocyte stem cells are immature platelets. Epithelial stem cells produce skin cells.

21. *Answer:* A

Rationale: Granulocytes include basophils, eosinophils, monocytes, and neutrophils.

22. *Answer:* C

Rationale: Neutrophils and lymphocytes are part of the white blood cell components and fight infection. Erythrocytes are red blood cell components. Levels of platelets below 20,000/mm³ increase the patient's risk for severe bleeding.

23. *Answer:* C

Rationale: Nadir refers to the lowest point—not the highest point—blood cells reach after a cancer treatment. Nadir occasionally happens after biotherapy administration, but this is not a regular occurrence.

24. *Answer:* A

Rationale: When the platelet levels drop below 100,000 mm³, the client has thrombocytopenia. WBCs and neutrophils help fight infection. A drop in RBCs is associated with anemia.

25. *Answer:* C

Rationale: Grade 1 of cytokine release syndrome is associated with a fever of ≥38°C, with hypotension or hypoxia. Grade 2 is associated with a fever of ≥38°C, is responsive to fluids and low flow nasal cannula oxygen. Grade 3 is associated with a fever of ≥38°C and receiving a vasoactive agent and high flow nasal cannula oxygen, face mask, nonrebreather, or Venturi mask. Grade 4 is associated with a fever of ≥38.3°C and receiving more than one vasoactive agent and positive pressure ventilation, intubation with mechanical ventilation.

26. *Answer:* C

Rationale: Neutropenia is characterized by grade. Grade 1 is an ANC < lower limit of normal—1500/mm³. Grade 2 is an ANC <1500 to 1000/mm³. Grade 3 is an ANC <1000 to 500/mm³. Grade 4 is an ANC <500/mm³.

27. *Answer:* B

Rationale: Factors associated with poor prognosis neutropenia include hypotension (systolic BP less than 9 mm Hg), tachypnea (greater than 24/breaths per minute), serum albumin less than 3.3 g/dl), serum bicarbonate level less than 21 mmol/L, a high procalcitonin level (greater than 2.0 ng/mL), and a cross reactive protein level of greater than 20 mg/L at baseline.

28. *Answer:* B

Rationale: Anemia is characterized by grades. Grade 1 is an Hgb < lower limit of normal (LLN)—10.0 g/dL. Grade 2 is an Hgb <10.0 to 8.0 g/ dL. Grade 3 is an Hgb <8.0 g/dL, transfusion indicated, and Grade 4 is an Hgb <6.2 to 4.9 g/ dL, with life-threatening consequences requiring immediate intervention.

CHAPTER 41

1. *Answer:* B

Rationale: The subcutaneous tissue is composed of adipose tissue, which serves as an insulator to temperature changes, cushion to trauma, and an energy reservoir. The dermis is highly vascular with afferent sensory nerve receptors, which provides nutritional support to the avascular layer. The epidermis is the avascular outer layer, which serves as a barrier to prevent water loss and renews itself continuously through cell division. The inner connective tissue is the dermis layer.

2. *Answer:* B

Rationale:. Antihistamines disrupt the action of histamines in the brain that result in drowsiness. Corticosteroids orally can cause an increase in appetite, weight gain, insomnia, fluid retention, and mood changes. Capsaicin topically can cause warmth, stinging, or burning at the application site. Calamine lotion side effects include itching, redness, and irritation.

3. *Answer:* A

Rationale: Using alcohol wipes will dry the skin and create a potential risk for skin breakdown, and should be avoided. Gentle cleansing with tepid water and mild soap and protecting the area with a skin barrier will prevent skin breakdown. Handwashing is always important.

4. *Answer:* B

Rationale: Graft-versus-host disease can occur as a reaction to a bone marrow transplant. The donated bone marrow or peripheral blood stem cells view the recipient's body as foreign, and the donated cells/bone marrow attack the body, resulting in a serious skin rash. Skin grafting is a surgical procedure that involves removing skin from one area of the body and moving it, or transplanting it, to a different area of the body. A patient would not experience graft-versus-host disease as a reaction to a skin graft. Melanoma is a tumor of melanin-forming cells, especially a malignant tumor associated with skin cancer. Malnutrition relates to decreased protein stores.

5. *Answer:* D

Rationale: Acute radiation dermatitis may occur with all radiation therapy. The causative mechanism is free radical damage to tissue that can cause erythema, pain, dermal swelling, itching, and necrosis of the skin. Chemotherapy drugs activate immune complexes already circulating due to underlying collagen vascular disease process, causing a circular red scaly rash. This is found in allergic or immune complex reactions. Erythema multiforme rash involves extremities, including palms and soles. This is found in allergic or immune complex reactions. Thinning of skin, scarring and contractures, and telangiectasias are associated with chronic radiation dermatitis.

6. *Answer:* B

Rationale: A common dermatologic change associated with EGFR inhibitors is an acneiform rash of papules and pustules similar to acne although this rash contains no comedones. This acneiform rash typically involves the face, back, and upper chest. Onycholysis is manifested as a nail lifting from the bed. It is associated with paclitaxel, docetaxel, cyclophosphamide, doxorubicin, 5-fluorouracil (5-FU), and hydroxyurea. Capecitabine is associated with hand and foot syndrome. Cisplatin, hydroxyurea, and bleomycin can be associated with permanent hyperpigmentation of the gums.

7. *Answer:* C

Rationale: Photosensitivity related to certain chemotherapy agents makes the patient more sensitive to ultraviolet light. Solar-exposed areas may develop severe sunburn after only limited exposure to the sun. Photo enhancement occurs when the chemotherapy is given several days after sunburn, causing the sunburn to reappear in that area. Beau's lines appear as transverse lines in nails with bands corresponding to when drug was given. Paronychia is a skin infection around the fingernails or toenails. It usually affects the skin at the cuticle or up the sides of the nail as pain, swelling, and redness and can have abscesses.

8. *Answer:* A

Rationale: Symptoms related to chronic radiation dermatitis include thinning of skin, scarring and contractures, telangiectasias, and long-term skin sensitivity to irritants and environmental agents in the radiation treatment area. Acute radiation dermatitis is defined as the immediate dermatitis occurring in radiated areas with erythema, pain, dermal swelling, itching, and necrosis. Radiation recall dermatitis is defined as occurring in previously irradiated skin within 1 to 2 weeks after chemotherapy; erythema, edema, superficial ulcerations, and superficial skin sloughing. An allergic response where the drug touches the skin (erythema, local swelling, desquamation, blistering, necrosis possible) is defined as a contact allergy (through activated T-cells) and may not develop until 24 to 36 hours after initial contact with the allergen.

9. *Answer:* B

Rationale: A description of symptoms related to erythema multiforme (antigen–antibody complexes) is a rash with typical target lesions involving extremities, including the palms of the hands and the soles of the feet. This skin reaction can progress to a generalized rash. Itching, redness, and swelling within 1 hour after the infusion has begun are symptoms of an immunoglobulin E (IgE) mediated skin reaction. If life threatening, this skin reaction is termed as anaphylaxis and includes decreased blood pressure, decreased level of consciousness, and airway and breathing compromise. Radiation recall dermatitis occurs in previously irradiated skin within 1 to 2 weeks after

chemotherapy. The symptoms include erythema, edema, superficial ulcerations, and superficial skin sloughing. Vasculitis (from antigen–antibody complexes) is a skin reaction that involves generalized vascular inflammation with end organ damage.

10. *Answer:* C

Rationale: The skin reaction of immunoglobulin E (IgE) mediated is known to be caused by treatment with platinum derivatives (e.g., cisplatin, carboplatin). Itching, redness, and swelling within 1 hour after the infusion has begun are symptoms of an IgE. Acute radiation dermatitis may occur with any or all radiation therapy. The mechanism for the reaction is free radical damage to the tissue. Vasculitis (from antigen–antibody complexes) is caused by methotrexate exposure. Contact allergy skin reactions can come from a variety of sources, ranging from chemicals found in poison ivy, oak, and sumac, to materials found in clothing, jewelry, and shoes.

11. *Answer:* D

Rationale: J.T.'s skin reaction, which included symptoms of skin blistering, local swelling, and erythema, is a reaction to a contact allergy. Contact allergies develop after contact—usually with 24 to 48 hours—with a variety of substances, including chemicals found in poison ivy, oak, and sumac, snaps, contact from zippers, and metal-plated objects, contact with neomycin in antibiotic skin ointments, potassium dichromate, a tanning agent, and latex found in gloves and rubberized protective clothing. The source of the allergy most likely came from contact with latex. Food allergies are not a source of contact allergies; neither is radiation therapy. A reaction to a medication would result in a systemic response rather than a local response.

12. *Answer:* A

Rationale: Radiation recall dermatitis occurs in previously irradiated skin within 1 to 2 weeks after treatment with certain chemotherapy agents, including cetuximab, doxorubicin (Doxil, Adriamycin), docetaxel (Taxotere), gemcitabine (Gemzar), paclitaxel (Taxol), capecitabine, and 5-FU. Symptoms of radiation recall skin reaction include erythema, edema, superficial ulcerations, and superficial skin sloughing. Chronic radiation dermatitis is associated with the long-term effects of radiation therapy in port area, and is symptomatic of thinning of the skin, scarring and contractures, telangiectasias, and long-term skin sensitivity to irritants and environmental agents. A rash with typical target lesions involving extremities, including palms of the hands and soles of the feet, and can progress to generalized rash are symptoms of an immunoglobulin E (IgE) mediated skin reaction. Finally, flulike symptoms, which may progress to life threatening, is a symptom of serum sickness (antigen–antibody complexes).

CHAPTER 42

1. *Answer:* A

Rationale: Loss of skeletal muscle mass is the correct answer. Sarcopenia is defined as the subclinical loss of skeletal muscle mass and is commonly observed in patients with malignancy. The other options (bone marrow suppression, joint contractures, and muscle spasticity), even if present, do not fit the definition for sarcopenia.

2. *Answer:* D

Rationale: There are many factors that can contribute to the risk of developing musculoskeletal alterations but only option D (increased bed rest) is the correct answer. Complications of increased bed rest can lead to increased bone breakdown associated with diminished weight-bearing activities and atrophy of skeletal muscles due to physical inactivity. The use of medical marijuana, enteral tube feedings, and a vegetarian diet are not correct answers and not necessarily associated with muscle weakness.

3. *Answer:* B

Rationale: The correct answer is B. Assessment of this patient's functional abilities and signs and symptoms of disease has revealed a KPS of 50. A KPS reading of 50 requires considerable assistance and frequent medical care. The patient is not able to do self-care with effort (KPS of 80), nor is disabled and requires special care (KPS of 40). A patient who shows minor signs or symptoms of disease has a KPS of 90.

4. *Answer:* B

Rationale: Gait is the correct answer. Observation of the way a person walks and moves provides useful information about muscle strength and coordination. The other options help provide information about the patient's body build (habitus), personality, or state of mind (cleanliness and body language).

5. *Answer:* C

Rationale: The correct option is hypokalemia. Changes in normal levels of serum calcium, magnesium, phosphorus, potassium, and sodium are common after a treatment of chemotherapy and can have a profound effect on skeletal muscle contraction and strength and are generally decreased after cisplatin treatment. Hypokalemia is associated with muscle weakness and muscle cramps. Metabolic alkalosis occurs with a high bicarbonate level and can be associated with muscle spasms, not weakness. Hypochloremia, a low chloride level, is associated with fluid balance and can lead to dehydration. Hyperphosphatemia, a high phosphate level, is associated with dry skin, memory problems, seizures, and muscle cramps.

6. *Answer:* D

Rationale: Encouraging a patient to commit to a program of active range of motion exercises every 4 hours is correct. This nursing intervention helps preserve the patient's muscle strength and increase physical function. Active range of motion exercises on unaffected limbs and passive range of motion exercises on affected limbs are recommended at least three or four times per day. The patient's position should be changed every 2 hours rather than every nursing shift. Soft lighting is useful at night to help enhance vision, but not impaired mobility. A restraint vest is unlikely to be ordered for this patient.

7. *Answer:* D

Rationale: The Eastern Cooperative Oncology Group (ECOG) Performance Status ranges from scores of 0 to 5. With a score of 3, J.B. is capable of limited self-care, but is restricted to a bed or chair during half of his waking hours. Therefore, the correct answer is D. Patients with a score of 3 have some capacity for self-care but it is limited. For a patient who is completely unable to care for themselves, that is a score of 4, so answer A is incorrect. The patient who is fully active and able to carry on the normal activities that were performed prior to diagnosis rates a score of zero, so B is incorrect as well. The patient who is restricted from strenuous activity but can perform light housework, for example, or sedentary activities scores a 1 on the ECOG Performance Status score.

8. *Answer:* A

Rationale: The Eastern Cooperative Oncology Group (ECOG) Performance Status score of 1 means the patient is capable of performing light activities but is restricted in doing any strenuous physical activities. Patients restricted to a bed or chair during half of his waking hours and capable of limited self-care score a rating of 3. Patients who are fully disabled with no means to care for themselves rate a 4 on the scale, while a patient who is dead receives a rating of 5. The ECOG Performance scale ranges from 0 to 5.

9. *Answer:* C

Rationale: The electrolyte abnormalities the nurse might expect to find in the results is a change in his potassium levels. Potassium regulates heart function and helps maintain healthy nerves and muscles. Magnesium is another critical mineral and serves much of the same function as potassium. Chloride is important in regulating proper balance of bodily fluids, while calcium stabilizes blood pressure and helps build strong bones and teeth. Finally, phosphates interact closely with calcium.

CHAPTER 43

1. *Answer:* C

Rationale: Disease-related risk factors include peexisting neuropathies because of diabetes mellitus, human immunodeficiency virus infection, and preexisting vitamin B complex deficiency. Symptoms may include tingling of fingers and toes, jaw pain, foot drop, and muscular atrophy. Individual age under 60 years and anxiety and depression are not risk factors for neuropathies. Individual risk factors for neuropathy include age greater than 60 years and social issues, including malnutrition and alcohol abuse. A history of lumpectomy is not a major risk factor for neuropathies, but the incision may be sensitive to the touch.

2. *Answer:* A

Rationale: Neuropathies of the central nervous system (CNS) can lead to seizures, encephalopathy, and cerebellar dysfunction. Childhood epilepsy is not a factor in neurologic symptoms in a person with a diagnosis of cancer. Damage to PNS would have symptoms of numbness/tingling, not CNS symptoms. Anxiety and depression may be manifested as insomnia, fatigue, trouble concentrating, irritability, and restlessness.

3. *Answer:* C

Rationale: Medical management includes the use of mild analgesics and opioids. Anticonvulsants (e.g., gabapentin [Neurontin], pregabalin [Lyrica], and valproic acid [Depakote]) are used to alleviate painful peripheral neuropathies. A fentanyl patch is not mild nor is it appropriate for neuropathic pain. Steroids are not a treatment nor are antianxiety medications.

4. *Answer:* A

Rationale: Nursing management includes teaching patients about hand and foot care, including the use of massage and lotions. Exercise should be encouraged as should the use of assistive devices to promote safety and assist with mobilization and fine motor skills (not muscle strength). Patients should avoid excess stimulation of the skin.

5. *Answer:* B

Rationale: Protecting the patient's hands from cold is important as the neuropathy may prevent the recognition of dangerously cold temperatures. Hand-strengthening exercise helps promote independence. Although the prevention of infection is important, hand sanitizer can be drying, leading to small cuts and infection. A three point cane can assist with ambulation and would be important for a patient with neuropathy in the feet to promote safety. Refer to occupational and rehabilitation services, as indicated.

6. *Answer:* D

Rationale: Proprioception is perception or awareness of the position and movement of the body. A Romberg test can be used to evaluate balance and proprioception. To do the Romberg test, nurses should have the patient stand with their feet together, arms at their side, with eyes closed and observe the patient's movements. A slight sway is normal. A tuning fork vibration check and assessment of discrimination between sharp and dull shapes provides information about sensory function. Clonus is muscular spasm and it provides information about deep tendon reflexes.

7. *Answer:* B

Rationale: Assessing for discrimination between sharp and dull sensations is a procedure for assessing sensory function related to neuropathy. Observing for accurate movement of extremities is an assessment for proprioception, while having patients stand with their feet together, arms at their sides, with their eyes closed is part of the Romberg test and is classified as an evaluation for cerebellar and proprioception. Assessing for rapid alternating movement of hands is also classified as an evaluation method for cerebellar function and proprioception.

8. *Answer:* A

Rationale: An intervention to assist patients in improving mobility and self-care is developing an exercise and muscle-strengthening program. Other interventions include collaborating with physical and occupational rehabilitation services and using assistive devices to help with mobilization and fine motor needs. Answers B, C, and D are all examples of nonpharmacologic interventions to manage pain, anxiety, and depression, including offering the patient access to acupressure and acupuncture services, encouraging the patient to implement relaxation techniques, and referring the patient for biofeedback teaching.

9. *Answer:* D

Rationale: A nonpharmacologic intervention for symptoms such as pain, depression, and anxiety is to encourage the patient to take up relaxation techniques. Included are activities such as yoga, meditation, or guided imagery. Teaching the patient about the side effects of cancer and empowering the patient to communicate with her physician and caregivers regarding the severity of her symptoms are interventions to encourage the patient to participate in their own care. Since this patient is already sharing details of her symptoms, this intervention would not be needed. Providing assistive services for the patient in performing daily activities as needed is an intervention to assist with decreased mobility and diminished capacity for self-care.

CHAPTER 44

1. *Answer:* A

Rationale: Confusion may be a sign of electrolyte abnormalities. Patients having complications with nutritional therapy usually have diarrhea, not constipation, and tachycardia and normal respirations, not bradycardia and bradypnea.

2. *Answer:* C

Rationale: Cachexia is defined as progressive deterioration with muscle wasting that occurs when protein and calorie requirements are not met, greater than 5% involuntary weight loss has occurred over 6 months, poor quality of life (QOL), impaired functional status, muscle wasting, fatigue, and, ultimately, shortened survival. Malnutrition begins with changes in nutrient levels in the blood and tissues and can progress to organ malfunction. Depression is a risk factor developing cachexia. Anorexia is loss of appetite accompanied by decreased oral intake and is usually accompanied by other symptoms that exacerbate decreased food intake and progressive weight loss, with approximately 80% incidence in patients with cancer from diagnosis to advanced stages.

3. *Answer:* D

Rationale: Candies or lozenges will stimulate saliva production to keep the membranes moist and decrease risk of taste alterations. Patients should experiment with flavorings, perform oral hygiene before and after meals, and avoid alcohol.

4. *Answer:* A

Rationale: Multi-agent chemotherapy regimens are a risk factor for weight gain, especially those regimens that contain steroids. Adjuvant chemotherapy for breast cancer, not lung cancer, is a risk factor for weight gain. Immunotherapy and bisphosphate therapy do not present as an increased risk for weight gain. Hormonal, biologic medications such as interleukin-2 (IL-2) and steroids also lead to weight gain.

5. *Answer:* C

Rationale: Patients should consume cold foods to provide comfort, rather than hot foods. Soft and room temperature foods are also associated with improved oral intake. Oral hygiene should be done before and after meals, and pain medications should be given 30 to 60 minutes prior to eating to provide comfort from pain. Nystatin should be used after meals or at least 30 minutes prior to eating.

6. *Answer:* B
   Rationale: Dysgeusia is an unpleasant taste sensation, while a decrease in the acuity of taste is hypogeusesthesia, and the loss of taste is ageusia.

7. *Answer:* B
   Rationale: Participating in preparation of meals can stimulate taste by the aroma of foods. To avoid dry mucous membranes, patients should eliminate the intake of alcohol. Patients should chew gum before eating to change taste and food intake, and consumption of meat should be with gravy and sauces to keep membranes moist.

8. *Answer:* A
   Rationale: Electrolyte imbalances with hypercalcemia, hypokalemia, hyponatremia, and uremia have been found to be associated with loss of appetite.

9. *Answer:* D
   Rationale: Enteral feeding is given into the gastrointestinal (GI) tract. The naso-gastric tube is the only tube that is placed in the GI tract. A nephrostomy tube is placed in the kidney to drain urine. A urostomy tube is also placed in the kidney/ureter to drain urine. A tracheostomy tube is placed in the neck to establish a patent airway.

10. *Answer:* C
    Rationale: Non-Hodgkin's lymphoma is a risk factor for weight loss. Lung cancers and gastrointestinal cancers also put individuals at risk for weight loss. Chemotherapy regimens containing steroids, biologic medications like interleukin-2, and pleural effusions are all risk factors for weight gain.

11. *Answer:* D
    Rationale: Candidiasis is a known cause of taste alterations. Radiation therapy of the oral cavity can lead to thick saliva that alters taste sensation. Zinc deficiency caused by oncolytic agents that bind and chelate zinc results in loss of taste. Medications associated with taste alterations include cisplatin (Platinol), irinotecan (Camptosar), cyclophosphamide (Cytoxan), dacarbazine (DTIC-Dome), dactinomycin (actinomycin D, Cosmegen), mechlorethamine (nitrogen mustard, Mustargen), methotrexate (Mexate), vincristine (Oncovin), and fluorouracil (5-FU, 5-fluorouracil).

12. *Answer:* A
    Rationale: A nursing intervention for pneumothorax that is a complication arising from parenteral or nutritional therapy is determining that a chest radiography after insertion of subclavian catheter has been completed to verify placement. Pneumothorax may occur during subclavian catheter insertion, so it is important to observe the patient during insertion for chest pain, dyspnea, and cyanosis. Nurses must assure that a chest radiograph is completed and evaluated after insertion to verify placement.

Regulating infusion on a volumetric pump for accuracy is a nursing intervention for fluid overload. For a malpositioned catheter, nurses are recommended to monitor the catheter for migration from the superior vena cava to another vein, while making a notation of patient compliant of pain in the neck and shoulder, as well as swelling in the surrounding area. Checking each bottle or bag before and during infusion for color and clarity of solution is a nursing intervention for a contaminated solution leading to an infection.

13. *Answer:* B
    Rationale: A nursing intervention for preventing an air embolus, which is a complication arising from parenteral or nutritional therapy, is securing all IV tubing connections with tape to prevent disconnection. If air emboli are suspected, the nurse is recommended to clamp the tubing immediately and place the patient on left side in the Trendelenburg position. Observing for bright red blood pulsating from catheter is a nursing intervention for an arterial puncture. Infusing 10% dextrose in water solution peripherally or through other lumen of catheter at the same rate as with total parenteral nutrition (TPN) to prevent hypoglycemia is a nursing intervention for a clotted catheter. Finally, D is a nursing intervention for hypoglycemia. If a patient presents with hypoglycemia, a nursing intervention is to administer insulin in TPN, as ordered, monitor capillary blood glucose, monitor serum glucose levels, and observe for signs and symptoms of hypoglycemia. If sudden cessation of TPN occurs, infuse 10% dextrose in water solution peripherally at same rate as TPN. Per physician's order, administer 50 mL of 50% dextrose intravenously.

14. *Answer:* B
    Rationale: A nursing intervention for preventing contaminated equipment leading to an infection—a complication arising from parenteral or nutritional therapy—is changing all IV tubing per institutional or agency procedure, using aseptic technique, and avoid interrupting TPN for other infusions or blood collecting. Checking each bottle or bag before and during infusion for color and clarity of solution is a nursing assessment for contaminated solution that leads to infection. Infusing 10% dextrose in water solution peripherally or through other lumen of catheter at the same rate as with TPN to prevent hypoglycemia is a nursing intervention for a local infection. Proper dressing changes should also be completed using aseptic technique. Finally, a nursing intervention for hyperglycemia is a recommendation to check a patient's urine for sugar, ketones, and acetone every 6 hours.

15. *Answer:* C
    Rationale: Giving formula at room temperature is a nursing intervention for the prevention of abdominal distention, and for symptoms such as vomiting and diarrhea. Also, a nursing recommendation is to regulate infusion accurately over 20 minutes. When giving the formula at room temperature, the nurse may need to decrease the volume of the formula given to the patient. Diarrhea may be caused by the formula, by the patient being lactose intolerant, or by bacterial contamination, osmolality,

antibiotics, or *Clostridium difficile.* Giving continuous rather than bolus feeding is a nursing intervention for aspiration. Flushing the nasogastric tube with hot water or pulsating motions is a nursing intervention for contaminated equipment or clogged tube. Verifying proper placement via chest radiography and check placement each time using tube is a nursing recommendation for malpositioned tube.

16. *Answer:* D

Rationale: An example of a physical assessment strategy for a patient undergoing an overall nutritional assessment includes measuring a patient's weight and comparing it with their ideal body weight. Other physical assessment measures include skin turgor, muscle mass as measured by the patient's mid-arm circumference, and fat stores as measured by the thickness of the triceps skinfold. The measure of the patient's daily caloric intake and measures of blood pressure and heart rate are not part of the physical examination and are incorrect. Measures of serum prealbumin, total protein, and serum transferrin to assess protein stores are collected as part of a laboratory assessment of the overall nutritional assessment.

17. *Answer:* D

Rationale: An example of laboratory data that could be collected for a patient with cancer as part of an overall nutritional assessment is nitrogen balance. Nitrogen balance levels are collected to assess energy balance. Other aspects of laboratory testing include measuring serum prealbumin, total protein, and serum transferrin to assess protein stores, measuring hemoglobin and hematocrit index, and electrolyte levels. Measuring of allergic reactions to proteins in certain foods is a test to confirm allergies to foods such as peanuts or tree nuts, and is not part of an overall nutritional assessment. Skin turgor is part of a physical examination, and muscle mass is measured by the circumference of the mid-arm and another part of the physical exam.

18. *Answer:* C

Protein-calorie malnutrition caused by the metabolic effects of the tumor is a major cause of weight loss in oncology patients. Cancer cell division and growth are associated with increased protein metabolism and calorie use to meet the energy demands of malignant tumors. Patients may develop vitamin and mineral deficiencies due to inadequate intake of food. If liver and kidney function are adequate, most pharmacologic agents are metabolized normally. Malignant tumor metabolism is not associated with increased fat metabolism.

CHAPTER 45

1. *Answer:* B

Rationale: The patient is experiencing chronic cancer-related pain. Chronic cancer-related pain can be due to direct tumor involvement, diagnostic/therapeutic procedures, or cancer treatment and lasts longer than 3 months. Answer A is incorrect because the patient reports it is well-controlled. If the patient's baseline pain becomes uncontrolled and he has acute exacerbations

with movement, this would be defined as incident breakthrough pain. Insidious breakthrough pain occurs unpredictably. Answer C is incorrect as the pain is not acute. Acute pain is self-limiting and typically lasts less than 6 months. Answer D is incorrect. The patient does not show signs of visceral pain.

2. *Answer:* C

Rationale: The correct answer is C, visceral pain, which is often found in patients with pancreatic, hepatic, and gastrointestinal cancer, leading to distention, compression, and tumor infiltration into the abdominal tissue. Answer A is incorrect as somatic pain is well-localized and arises from the bone, joint, or connective tissue, and is described as sharp, throbbing, or as pressure. Sympathetically maintained pain is a type of neuropathic cancer pain caused by autonomic dysregulation; therefore, answer B is incorrect. Answer D is another type of neuropathic pain, caused by peripheral nerve injury.

3. *Answer:* D

Rationale: The correct answer is D. During modulation, neurons in the brainstem (pons and medulla) descend to the dorsal horn and release neuromediators, which inhibit the transmission of pain impulses at the dorsal horn. Opioids work at the dorsal horn by binding to receptors and preventing transmission of the pain signal to the higher brain centers. Answer A, transduction, is the initiation of the pain process where neurotransmitters are released at the time of injury, generating an action potential to relay the message to the central nervous system. Answer B, transmission, continues to relay the thalamus and other centers in the brain. Answer C, perception, is where the brain finally senses the pain impulse and triggers modulation.

4. *Answer:* C

Rationale: The correct answer is C, mucositis. While other pain syndromes can occur with head and neck cancer, almost 100% of patients undergoing combined radiation and chemotherapy develop mucositis and subsequent pain. Answer A, postsurgical head and neck cancer pain, can occur and increases without consistent mobility and range of motion following surgery. Lymphedema, answer B, is rare with head and neck cancers. Sinusitis, answer D, is not an associated symptom with this therapy.

5. *Answer:* A

Rationale: The correct answer is A, postherpetic neuralgia, which is characterized by burning, aching, and shock-like pain and often occurs as a sequelae to shingles due to immunosuppression from chemotherapy. Answer B is incorrect, as patients are not at increased risk of CIPN when immunosuppressed. Answer C is incorrect because lymphedema, although painful, is due to surgical disruption of the lymph channels, not chemotherapy. Answer D, CRPS, is a centrally generated pain syndrome caused by autonomic dysregulation but is not related to immunosuppression.

6. *Answer:* D

Rationale: The World Health Organization's analgesic ladder recommends the use of an opioid and possibly an analgesic adjuvant for moderate pain. Answer D is the best answer that incorporates an opioid/acetaminophen combination and is given as needed for intermittent pain. Answer A, acetaminophen, only contains a nonopioid analgesic. Answer B, morphine, is used for severe pain and is not a good choice because of the metabolites, M3G and M6G, that can accumulate in patients with renal compromise. Answer C, the fentanyl patch, is used for severe pain; additionally, the patient has intermittent pain and does not require around-the-clock analgesia at this time. The patient may also be opioid naïve, and fentanyl is contraindicated in opioid-naïve patients.

7. **Answer:** A

Rationale: The risk of addiction with opioids is correct; therefore, acknowledging the problem is important. However, nurses should clarify the definition of addiction and reinforce the importance that opioids have on the pain management plan. Answer B is incorrect as addiction can be a concern in some patients. Answer C is incorrect, because an increase in pain is likely due to advanced disease. Tolerance is a physiologic state of adaptation whereby the repeated exposure to a drug results in diminished effect of the drug over time and a possible need to increase the drug dose to achieve the same level of effect. Answer D is incorrect as patients on chronic opioids may experience withdrawal. This is separate from addiction and is a physiological phenomenon.

8. **Answer:** D

Rationale: Pain is a complex phenomenon and requires assessment of all domains. The perception that pain is a punishment is an existential concern; patients have reported feeling that they are punished by God or punished because of their life choices. This concern requires additional assessment and attention. Fear of addiction often involves a lack of understanding about the definition of pain. This is a cognitive-psychological concern. Depression is another psychological concern, and the fatigue is a potential physical manifestation of the pain leading to this concern. Lack of mobility is both a physical and social concern as patients may be limited in both their physical and social life.

9. **Answer:** D

Rationale: The correct answer is D. A psychological concern when conducting a comprehensive pain assessment is taking note of a patient's history of mental illness, including such conditions as anxiety and depression. Answer A is incorrect. A patient's financial hardship due to the cost of pain medication is a social concern. The influence of how religion and prayer assist a patient in coping with pain is a spiritual or existential concern; therefore, answer B is incorrect. Answer C is also incorrect. How a patient perceives traditional medicine is also a spiritual or existential concern.

10. **Answer:** C

Rationale: The correct answer is C. A social concern when conducting a comprehensive pain assessment is how the family caregiver responds to a patient's pain. Is the caregiver accepting and supportive of the patient's pain, or do they feel the patient is exaggerating? How

a caregiver responds to a patient's pain has a strong impact on the level of care. Answer A is incorrect. The patient's experience with coping with pain in the past is a psychological concern as past experience will shape how they react to current or future pain. The patient's willingness to try nontraditional medicine, such as complementary and alternative therapies, is also a psychological concern. Answer B thus is incorrect. Answer D is incorrect. The role of a spiritual community in a patient's ability to cope with pain is a spiritual or existential concern.

11. **Answer:** D

Rationale: The correct answer is D. The patient's level of cognition, including any signs of confusion or delirium, is a psychological concern when conducting a comprehensive pain assessment. The role of pain in the everyday life of the patient and the amount of support a patient receives, either with family or through the community, are both examples of social concerns. Therefore, answers A and C are incorrect. Answer B is also incorrect. The definition of how a patient differentiates pain and suffering is a spiritual or existential concern.

12. **Answer:** D

Rationale: The correct answer is D. The "P" stands for Provocation/Palliation. Provocation refers to what caused the pain and palliation refers to what relieves the pain. Answers A, B, and C—pain, position, and proximity—are all incorrect and not part of the acronym for the pain assessment known as PQRST. The rest of the acronym is as follows. "Q" stands for quality of pain. How does the pain feel? The "R" in the acronym stands for region or radiation. In this case, the patient is asked where the pain is located and if the pain radiates. The "S" stands for severity. Patients are asked to rate their pain on a scale of 0 to 10. Finally, the "T" is timing. Is the pain constant or intermittent?

CHAPTER 46

1. **Answer:** B

Rationale: Compression of the tracheobronchial tree may occur from bronchospasm, laryngeal swelling from hypersensitivity reactions related to chemotherapy, and/or biotherapy treatments or superior vena cava syndrome. Abnormal fluid accumulation of fluid within the lung is due to the development of a pneumothorax, hemothorax, hydrothorax, or empyema. An alveolar hemorrhage is most often as the result of an autoimmune disorder and is not a hypersensitivity symptom. Bronchitis is an inflammation of the lungs and is not a hypersensitivity reaction.

2. **Answer:** D

Rationale: To maximize safety, the patient should be encouraged to use supplemental oxygen and assistive devices such as a cane or a walker as needed with ambulation to prevent hypoxia. Keeping the temperature warm may cause dehydration, which could lead to difficulty breathing. Cool temperatures and drinking plenty of fluids are encouraged. The patient should keep active. This may improve quality of life, and may lower fatigue and depression, as well as improve muscle strength.

3. *Answer:* D

Rationale: An inflammation process affects the interstitial lung parenchyma, which can cause an infectious and noninfectious lung injury. The release of hormones and signaling an antigen response are not causes of immunotherapy-induced pulmonary toxicity. Proportionate amounts of drugs and the volume of the drug administered do not contribute to immunotherapy-induced pulmonary toxicity.

4. *Answer:* C

Rationale: Dyspnea is the cardinal sign of pneumonitis. Pneumonitis is an inflammation of the lung tissue. Other symptoms include nonproductive cough, malaise, fatigue, and fever. Dyspnea may develop over weeks to months, but may also develop quickly, within a few hours, and may also occur years following drug exposure. An elevated heart rate and the development of crepitus are not signs of pneumonitis.

5. *Answer:* B

Rationale: The chemotherapy agent may be discontinued, or the dose may be reduced for prompt resolution. While rest is desirable, strict bedrest is not required. Physical activity and breathing exercises should be those that promote oxygenation throughout the lungs. Monitoring of EKGs and ECHO are required to monitor for cardiac toxicity. An ABG may be required if the patient is hypoxic; however, serial ABGs are not required.

6. *Answer:* C

Rationale: On assessment, clubbing of the fingers due to chronic hypoxemia, cyanosis, pallor, jugular vein distention, upper extremity swelling, and venous congestion in the chest may be found in patients with dyspnea. Palpation of a carotid artery pulse on assessment is normal. If the lower extremities were swollen that could indicate congestive heart failure. A ventilation rate (respiratory rate) of 20 is normal.

7. *Answer:* A

Rationale: Benign pleural effusions may be caused by increased negative pressure in the pleural space, or atelectasis. Spontaneous hemopericardium is the rupture of blood into the pericardial sac. The formation of pustules is not a cause of pleural effusion. Direct extension of primary tumor to the pleura is a cause of malignant, not benign, pleural effusions.

8. *Answer:* C

Rationale: On auscultation, egophony caused by lung consolidation and fibrosis is often found in persons with a pleural effusion. Egophony is an increased resonance of voice sounds heard within auscultating the lungs. Diminished or absent breath sounds will be found, rather than rhonchi and rales, which are typically heard with pneumonia. A tracheal shift is common in pneumothorax. Dullness to percussion is typically found in pleural effusion.

9. *Answer:* D

Rationale: Therapeutic aspiration using an intrapleural chemical agent such as talc is the most efficacious, evidence-based treatment. Indwelling pleural catheters are used to manage pleural effusions, not peritoneal catheters. A VATS (video-assisted thoracoscopic surgery) is also a form of pleural effusion management. Both chemotherapy and radiation therapy may be effective in tumors that are responsive such as lymphoma or small cell lung cancer (SCLC).

10. *Answer:* D

Rationale: Bevacizumab is associated with the pulmonary and radiologic abnormalities of bilateral ground-glass opacities and consolidation with the pattern of lung involvement classified as hemoptysis. Bortezomib is linked to bronchiolitis, which is associated with hyperinflation and air trapping. Alpha-interferon is associated with bronchiolitis, and includes air flow obstruction, airway hyperreactivity, and hyperinflation. Erlotinib is associated with interstitial pneumonitis and is categorized as diffuse, patchy, and ground-glass opacities.

11. *Answer:* A

Rationale: Sorafenib is associated with pulmonary and radiologic abnormalities associated with acute pneumonitis. Indications of acute pneumonitis includes diffuse patchy ground-glass opacities and diffuse reticular pattern. Other agents associated with acute pneumonitis are bortezomib, cetuximab, dasatinib, erlotinib, everolimus, gefitinib, gemcitabine, idelalisib, imatinib, irinotecan, pemetrexed, piritrexim, procarbazine, rituximab, sunitinib, temozolomide, and temsirolimus. Busulfan is associated with bronchiolitis and is indicated by hyperinflation and air trapping. Isolated acute chest pain is associated with etoposide, as is doxorubicin.

12. *Answer:* B

Rationale: An empyema is an abnormal accumulation of infected fluid or pus in the pleural space and is generally treated with systemic antibiotics. Radiation therapy is done to reduce obstructions caused by lung tumors. Epinephrine is used to treat anaphylaxis, while oxygen is used to treat anaphylaxis or the patient who is hypoxemic.

13. *Answer:* C

Rationale: Bleomycin in combination with radiation therapy places a patient at high risk for pneumonitis. Answers in A, B, and D present options that are not associated with this patient's therapy regimen.

CHAPTER 47

1. *Answer:* B

Rationale: The definition of a sleep-wake disturbance is an actual or perceived disturbance in night sleep with resulting daytime impairment. Sleep-wake disturbances can include insomnia, sleep-related breathing problems, circadian rhythm disorders, and excessive sleepiness. These issues often occur in combination with fatigue, anxiety, and depression. An active biobehavioral process is the definition of sleep, while a transient inability to initiate or maintain sleep describes insomnia. Circadian rhythm disorders are included as part of sleep-wake disturbances.

2. *Answer:* A

Rationale: Antihistamines can be used to help patients fall asleep. They may be preferred if concerned about cross-dependence. Antihistamines should be used with caution for older adults. Antipsychotics have a sedating effect but should be considered as a last course of treatment due to the drug's serious side effect profile. Alpha adrenergic receptor blockers relax muscles, but do not help patients fall asleep. Antidepressants are effective if used for insomnia, associated with depression.

3. *Answer:* D

Rationale: Patients should be encouraged to make their bedrooms restful, free of distractions like televisions, tablets, and cell phones, and should try to keep their rooms cool and dark. Patients should try to avoid caffeine after 12:00 pm, due to caffeine's stimulating effect. Patients should develop a routine of only going to bed when sleepy at about the same time each night and waking at the same time each day.

4. *Answer:* D

Rationale: Enjoying an afternoon nap may impact his ability to fall asleep and stay asleep. Risk factors for sleep-wake disturbances include daytime naps, use of caffeine and or nicotine close to bedtime, lack of daily exercise, and lack of a regular bedtime routine. By waking up at the same time each morning, limiting use of caffeine to the morning hours, and exercising each day, the individual is making a routine conducive to sleep.

5. *Answer:* C

Rationale: The sleep-wake cycle consists of two phases. The two cycles are rapid eye movement (the active phase) and non-rapid eye movement (quiet or restful phase). These phases repeat with each cycle lasting approximately 90 minutes. Four to six cycles occur during a 7- to 8-hour sleep period. There is not an awakening phase.

6. *Answer:* D

Rationale: Although it is important to check a patient's sleep cycle at each of the time points given, D is the best answer, as sleep assessments should be done throughout the patient's entire duration of treatment and should coincide with any changes in health status. Sleep assessment should not be limited to the initial assessment or after their first cycle of chemotherapy and at the end.

7. *Answer:* D

Rationale: Pain in the patient's hip describes a physical stressor. Physical stressors can play a role in sleep-wake disturbances and should be assessed and treated appropriately to minimize their effect on the sleep-wake cycle. Concern over losing his job and feeling anxious and afraid of what the future holds all describe psychological stressors.

8. *Answer:* B

Rationale: Polysomnography is a diagnostic tool to diagnose sleep-wake disturbances such as sleep-related breathing disorders and limb movement disorders. An EEG assesses electrical energy in the brain and is often helpful when evaluating seizure activity. The NCCN distress thermometer looks at distress. Lack of sleep can lead to a higher level of distress, but it is not a diagnostic test. Assessment of the characterization of sleep, including bedtime routine, time to sleep, and sleep duration, should be assessed but they are not part of a diagnostic test.

CHAPTER 48

1. *Answer:* A

Rationale: Disseminated intravascular coagulation (DIC) occurs when an underlying disorder, such as malignancy, inappropriately activates coagulation pathways. With DIC, intravascular thrombi formation is widespread throughout the body leading to end organ damage and organ failure. Ongoing consumption of platelets and coagulation factors results in hemorrhage. End organ damage and hemorrhage is not due to lack of available hemoglobin and typically occurs in more than one part of the body. The thrombi often are intra versus extravascular.

2. *Answer:* D

Rationale: In addition to pallor, petechiae, tachycardia, tarry stools, joint pain, stiffness, and hemoptysis, other symptoms of DIC are often a result of bleeding and clotting. They could include jaundice, hematomas, acral cyanosis, bleeding at sites of invasive procedures, ecchymosis, visual disturbances, hypotension, dyspnea, tachypnea, hemoptysis, changes in the color and temperature of extremities, tarry stools, hematemesis, abdominal pain, hematuria, joint pain and stiffness, headache, and mental status changes.

3. *Answer:* A

Rationale: Activation of the coagulation cascades seen in disseminated intravascular coagulation (DIC) is often precipitated by an underlying disorder that causes excessive activation of coagulation, such as malignancies, including acute and chronic leukemia, and solid tumors, especially cancers of the prostate, lung, breast, and stomach. Infection, trauma, burns, sepsis, pregnancy, and liver disease can also precipitate DIC. Identifying and managing the underlying precipitating cause often corrects the DIC. Supportive treatment of DIC may include transfusion of platelets, fresh frozen plasma, cryoprecipitate, and anticoagulants, as appropriate. Development of DIC is not associated with genetic changes.

4. *Answer:* A

Rationale: Thrombotic thrombocytopenic purpura (TTP) is a blood disorder characterized by clotting in small blood vessels of the body, resulting in a low platelet count. Thrombi in the small vessels may also cause thrombocytopenia, microangiopathic hemolytic anemia (MAHA), neurologic abnormalities, fever, and possibly organ damage. Platelet counts are usually low instead of high. The thrombi in the small vessels also cause thrombocytopenia not anemia.

5. *Answer:* A

Rationale: Plasma exchange therapy is the most common method for treating thrombotic thrombocytopenic purpura (TTP). Other blood products may be used if replacement is needed. Antibiotics and fluid restriction are not typical therapies to treat TTP. IV fluids may be used in some cases for volume replacement. Drugs that may prompt TTP are discontinued. Gene therapies for hereditary TTP are under investigation.

6. *Answer:* A

Rationale: Malignancy is the most common cause of SIADH, especially small cell lung cancer. Nonmalignant causes of SIADH include nervous system disorders, pulmonary disorders, and HIV. Drug-induced causes can occur with medications such as antidepressants or chemotherapeutic agents such as vinca alkaloids (i.e., vincristine, vinblastine).

7. *Answer:* C

Rationale: A patient with SIADH would not have an increased urine output, but rather a decrease in urination due to hypersecretion of arginine vasopressin (AVP) that inhibits urine formation. Decreased serum sodium, normal serum potassium, and signs of mental status changes, including headache, decreased mentation, and personality changes, are all typical SIADH symptoms. SIADH most commonly produces symptoms within the neurologic and gastrointestinal systems, associated with the presence of hyponatremia.

8. *Answer:* D

Rationale: Taxanes (e.g., paclitaxel, docetaxel) are associated with increased risk for hypersensitivity reactions. Paclitaxel infusions include premedication to prevent hypersensitivity reactions, as well as a longer infusion time. Symptoms of a hypersensitivity reaction may include flushing or rash, fever, bronchospasm, urticaria, hypotension, edema, angioedema, hemolysis, vasculitis, nephritis, arthritis, graft rejection, contact dermatitis, formation of granulomas, or a feeling of impending doom.

9. *Answer:* B

Rationale: Anaphylaxis is an acute, potentially fatal, multiorgan system reaction caused by the release of chemical mediators from mast cells and basophils. It involves prior sensitization to an allergen with later re-exposure, producing symptoms via an immunologic mechanism. Thrombotic thrombocytopenic purpura is a blood disorder characterized by the formation of thromboses in small blood vessels of the body that can possibly lead to organ damage. DIC is caused by extensive intravascular thrombi resulting in end organ damage and hemorrhage due to the consumption of platelets and coagulation factors. Sepsis can be a life-threatening organ dysfunction caused by impaired regulation of the patient's response to infection, involving pro- and antiinflammatory responses. Neither sepsis nor DIC is caused by the release of chemical mediators from mast cells and basophils.

10. *Answer:* A

Rationale: Currently, first-line therapy pharmacologic for anaphylaxis is epinephrine. Additional helpful pharmacologic treatments can include inhaled beta agonists, IV fluids, corticosteroids, and H1 receptor antagonists.

11. *Answer:* D

Rationale: M.A. is at increased risk for infection leading to sepsis because she is older than age 65, has cancer, and has a compromised immune system related to the presence of neutropenia resulting from her chemotherapy treatments. Neutropenic fever, defined as a temperature >100.4°F, may be an early sign of sepsis. Sepsis is life-threatening organ dysfunction caused by impaired regulation of the patient's response to infection, involving pro- and antiinflammatory responses. Septic shock is a subset of sepsis causing profound metabolic, cellular, and circulatory compromise leading to hypotension that requires vasopressors to maintain mean arterial pressure. Septic shock has a greater potential for mortality than sepsis, with a rate greater than 40%. Confusion may also be present as sepsis progresses and in septic shock. Patients may experience tachycardia, not bradycardia and hypotension, not hypertension. Thrombocytopenia is associated with an increased risk of bleeding.

12. *Answer:* A

Rationale: A white blood cell count with a left shift (increased release of immature neutrophils into the blood, typically indicating infection) may be one abnormal lab value of a patient who is experiencing sepsis. Additionally, abnormal laboratory values include a suspected or documented infection. Leukocytosis or leukopenia may be present. There may be a prolonged PT or aPTT. Arterial hypoxemia, decreased platelets, decreased fibrinogen, hyperglycemia, increased lactic acid, positive blood cultures, and elevated creatinine >0.5 mg/dL are also sometimes present in sepsis. Abnormal laboratory values indicative of septic shock (in addition) include elevated liver functions, elevated lactate, urine output <0.5 mL/kg per hour for at least 2 hours without hypovolemia, increased creatinine >2.0 mg/dL, anemia, thrombocytopenia <100,000 cells/μ, and hypoglycemia.

13. *Answer:* C

Rationale: Tumor lysis syndrome (TLS) is an oncologic emergency in which large amounts of tumor cells are rapidly destroyed, spilling their cellular contents into the systemic circulation, potentially resulting in serious complications that can manifest as electrolyte abnormalities including hyperuricemia, hyperkalemia, hyperphosphatemia, and hypocalcemia. TLS can occur within 6 hours of cancer therapy initiation. Newer targeted treatments for cancer may also cause TLS.

14. *Answer:* A

Rationale: Prevention of tumor lysis syndrome (TLS) will likely include administering IV hydration 24 to 48 hours prior to treatment initiation for high-risk patients to facilitate renal perfusion and increase urine output minimizing the risk of uric acid and calcium phosphate deposition in the renal tubules. Prior to their initial cytotoxic treatment, patients at risk of TLS receive medication prophylaxis with uric acid lowering agents, such as allopurinol and rasburicase. Rapid lysis of massive amounts of malignant cells results in the release of the intracellular contents into the circulation causing electrolyte disturbances (i.e., hyperkalemia, hyperphosphatemia, and hyperuricemia), which need to be managed. Oncology nurses need to identify and report symptoms of TLS as soon as possible. Assessment includes high acuity monitoring including ECG changes, intake and output, daily weights, and indications for the need for kidney dialysis. Restriction of potassium rich foods and educating patients and their significant others concerning TLS and TLS interventions are other nonpharmacologic management strategies.

15. *Answer:* C

Rationale: Hypercalcemia of malignancy is an abnormally high level of calcium corrected for albumin (>10.5 mg/dL) and is the most common oncologic emergency occurring in 20% to 30% of all cancer patients. Tumor lysis syndrome (TLS) is an oncologic emergency in which large amounts of tumor cells are rapidly destroyed, spilling their cellular contents into the systemic circulation, potentially resulting in serious complications that can manifest as electrolyte abnormalities. TLS can occur within 6 hours of cancer therapy initiation. Newer targeted treatments for cancer exhibit TLS. Syndrome of inappropriate antidiuretic hormone (SIADH) is a condition in which antidiuretic hormone (ADH), in activated form called arginine vasopressin (AVP), is inappropriately triggered despite the presence of normal or increased fluid balance. This results in hyponatremia and hypo-osmolality. In the oncology setting, ADH can be inappropriately produced by cancer. Disseminated intravascular coagulation (DIC) is a systemic disorder of coagulation. Within DIC, extensive intravascular thrombi cause end organ damage and hemorrhage due to the consumption of platelets and coagulation factors

16. *Answer:* A

Rationale: Tumors associated with hypercalcemia of malignancy include breast, lung, prostate, multiple myeloma, lymphoma, and hematologic malignancies. Other risk factors include hyperparathyroidism, vitamin D intoxication, chronic granulomatous disorders, and some medications including diuretics and lithium.

17. *Answer:* B

Rationale: Symptoms of hypercalcemia depend on the severity. Gastrointestinal symptoms include anorexia, abdominal cramping, loss of appetite, nausea, vomiting, pancreatitis, and peptic ulcer. Neurologic symptoms include restlessness, difficulty concentrating, lethargy, confusion, seizures, and coma. Muscular symptoms include fatigue and generalized weakness, ataxia, and pathologic fractures. Renal symptoms include frequent urination, nocturia, polydipsia, and renal failure. Cardiovascular symptoms include orthostatic hypotension, shortened QT, ventricular arrhythmia, and ST segment elevation.

18. *Answer:* C

Rationale: Denosumab is a monoclonal antibody that decreases bone resorption. It is utilized in patients unable to receive bisphosphonates. Denosumab is not excreted through kidneys and therefore may be used in patients with renal insufficiency. This agent is also used in patients who are refractory to bisphosphonate therapy. Bevacizumab is used to treat metastatic cancer. Infliximab (Remicade) is used to treat rheumatoid arthritis, ankylosing spondylitis, psoriatic arthritis, psoriasis, Crohn's disease, and ulcerative colitis. Pembrolizumab is used to treat melanoma and other cancers.

19. *Answer:* D

Rationale: Urgent medical management of sepsis includes intravenous fluid resuscitation; fluids are not withheld. All the other treatment options are correct: sources of infection are controlled (i.e., removal of infected lines, draining abscesses), empiric antibiotic therapy with one or more antibiotics are administered within the first hour of presentation, vasopressor therapy is ordered to maintain an MAP of 65 mm Hg and urine output of >0.5 mL/kg per hour.

20. *Answer:* B

Rationale: Signs and symptoms of anaphylaxis include urticaria and angioedema. Pain or itching around intravenous insertion sites describes a localized hypersensitivity reaction. Feelings of fatigue are common in patients with cancer but are not indicative of anaphylaxis.

CHAPTER 49

1. *Answer:* B

Rationale: The cranium is a rigid, nonexpandable chamber that contains brain tissue, blood, and cerebrospinal fluid (CSF) that are maintained within a narrow range of intracranial pressure (ICP). Any increase in the volume of one of these components causes the ICP to increase. An increase of ICP >20 mmHg in adults is considered pathologic. Increased intracranial pressure in this patient with breast cancer results from metastatic tumor deposits that increase the volume of brain tissue and occupy space in the intracranial cavity. Neurologic changes resulting from increased ICP may range from subtle to severe. It is possible that head injury could lead to increased intracranial pressure, but in this patient, it is more likely that the presence of brain metastases that occupy space within the cranium is the cause of the increased intracranial pressure. Vitamin deficiency and increased hormone production are not associated with increased intracranial pressure.

2. *Answer:* D

Rationale: Patients with lung cancer have increased risk for metastases to the brain. The entire brain may be irradiated prophylactically to destroy any metastatic cells that may be present and are too small to be seen on imaging. Brain irradiation increases the risk of developing increased intracranial pressure. Early signs and symptoms of intracranial pressure may be subtle and may include headache that is worse in the mornings and is aggravated when bending over or during Valsalva maneuvers. The patient may also experience nausea, vomiting, and weakness. The presence of dehydration may be associated with weakness, but headache in the mornings or with bending or during Valsalva maneuvers are unlikely. The signs and symptoms the patient is experiencing are not indicative of seizures or dementia.

3. *Answer:* D

Rationale: ICP monitoring via intraventricular, intraparenchymal, subarachnoid, or epidural site is the most reliable method to diagnose ICP, with the goal being to keep ICP less than 20 mmHg and cerebral perfusion between 60 and 75 mmHg. While PET with CT scan is a method of diagnosing ICP, it is not reliable. Bone marrow biopsy is not a test used to diagnose ICP. Labs for glucose and protein do not diagnose ICP; however, CSF examination is used if leptomeningeal metastasis or meningitis is suspected.

4. *Answer:* C

Rationale: The most effective method to rapidly decrease ICP is hyperventilation, which causes vasoconstriction and decreased cerebral blood volume and ICP. H.C. would need to be sedated and intubated and ventilated to a partial pressure of carbon dioxide (PCO2) between 26 and 30 mmHg. The effects of hyperventilation are short-lived. While radiation therapy to the head may be used to shrink metastatic tumor in the brain in some patients, this treatment would be contraindicated for H.C. because brain RT is the causative factor of her increased intracranial pressure. Systemic biotherapy administration is not an effective method to rapidly reduce ICP. Administration of chemotherapy or targeted agents intrathecally is a treatment; however, it is not a rapid means of reducing ICP. Injection of steroids into the cervical spine is not a method to reduce ICP.

5. *Answer:* A

Rationale: The nurse should monitor the patient for any changes indicating decreasing cardiac output, such as decreased urinary output, changes in vital signs, and changes in mentation. Patients should avoid the prone position or activities that exert pressure on the abdomen. The patient's head of bed should be elevated to about 30 degrees. Endotracheal suctioning should be minimized.

6. *Answer:* D

Rationale: The diagnostic procedure of choice for evaluating spinal cord compression is an MRI of the entire spine as multiple sites of metastasis may exist. Positron emission tomography is both sensitive and specific but less available than MRI and is not recommended to be used alone for diagnosis or treatment guidance. Diagnostic radiology films of the thoracic spine may show bone abnormalities and soft tissue masses in that area but miss the rest of the spine and are not used to diagnose or rule out spinal metastasis. Computerized tomography of the spine is used as an alternative when MRI unavailable or contraindicated but is less sensitive than MRI.

7. *Answer:* B

Rationale: Patients diagnosed with spinal cord compression (SCC) should be instructed to assess for signs of compromised feelings or sensations. Patient should report any changes in sensory or motor function, as well as sexual dysfunction, which may indicate sensory deficits. Mobility should be based on findings of stable or unstable spine and patient should maintain a safe level of independents with the limits of the SCC. The nurse should monitor for progression of motor or sensory deficits, including bowel patterns and frequency. Loss of appetite is not a symptom of SCC. It is unlikely that diuretics would be ordered because urinary retention or incontinence may be a feature of autonomic dysfunction.

8. *Answer:* C

Rationale: When obstruction of the superior vena cava (SVC) occurs, there is decreased venous return to the heart from the head, neck, thorax, and upper extremities, and hemodynamic compromise occurs from mass effect on the heart. SVC occurs because of compression or obstruction of the vessel, such as by tumor, lymph nodes, or thrombus. Thrombosis may concomitantly occur but is not the cause of superior vena cava syndrome (SVCS). Myocardial infarction is not a cause of SVCS.

9. *Answer:* D

Rationale: The presence of non–small lung cancer, especially in the right lung, accounts for the most cases of SVCS. When obstruction of the superior vena cava occurs, venous blood return to the heart from the head, neck, thorax, and upper extremities is compromised and characteristic symptoms of SVCS develop. Symptoms include dyspnea, sensation of head fullness, headache, blurred vision, nasal stuffiness, hoarseness, dysphagia, nonproductive cough, chest pain, and orthopnea (the need to sleep in an upright position). Symptoms are more pronounced in the morning and improve after being in an upright position after a few hours. Sinusitis and pneumonia may have similar symptoms; however, symptoms usually do not improve. Churg-Strauss syndrome is a rare disorder caused by blood vessel inflammation.

10. *Answer:* B

Rationale: The signs of orange-brown, malodorous feculent emesis are signs of a distal small intestine obstruction or colonic obstruction. Rapid-onset, bitter, bile-stained emesis that may be projectile would be a sign of a proximal small intestine obstruction. Signs of a small bowel obstruction include more severe nausea and vomiting. Non-bile colored, sour emesis with undigested food would be a sign of gastric outlet obstruction.

11. *Answer:* C

Rationale: Fluid accumulation in the pericardial sac may occur secondary to increased permeability of cardiac capillaries caused by chemotherapy or biotherapy. Coronary artery disease and leakage of fluid into the chest from the pneumothorax do not cause fluid to accumulate in the pericardial sac. Inaccurate insertion of a central line may puncture the pericardial sac and cause fluid accumulation in the pericardial sac.

12. *Answer:* A

Rationale: Surgical management includes colectomy with primary anastomosis with or without ostomy. Hyperosmolar agents and methylnaltrexone are treatments for constipation. Insertion of a biliary stent is not a surgical procedure to treat bowel obstruction.

13. *Answer:* D

Rationale: Checkpoint inhibitor immunotherapy is associated with increased risk of pneumonitis. Pneumonitis may be an adverse event of several of the checkpoint inhibitor agents including PD-1/PD-L1 inhibitors, as well as many other biotherapy agents. Systemic hyperthermia is an alternative treatment for cancer and is not a risk factor for a patient developing pneumonitis. Pneumonitis is not a typical side effect of platinum-based chemotherapy. Dendritic cell-based treatment works by boosting the immune system and is not a factor for developing pneumonitis. Another major risk factor for pneumonitis is radiation therapy to the chest.

14. *Answer:* C

Rationale: The patient's symptoms most likely indicate bowel perforation. Patients may be able to pinpoint the precise time of bowel perforation, noting a sudden relief of pain, followed by more severe pain. In addition, the patient's recent abdominal surgery increases the risk of bowel perforation. A post-surgical ileus is not considered a risk factor for bowel perforation. Patients receiving pain medication short term to manage postoperative pain will not become addicted to pain medication.

15. *Answer:* C

Rationale: While radiation therapy is the primary treatment for SVCS for patients with SCLC, the urgency of this patient's admission makes percutaneous intravascular stent placement the most effective treatment to restore blood flow and resolve symptoms. Chemotherapy is also a treatment; however, it should follow the patient's initial urgent treatment. Surgical resection is rarely used due to the effectiveness of stent placement.

16. *Answer:* D

Rationale: Pneumonitis is the correct answer. Pneumonitis due to chest radiotherapy may occur between 4 and 12 weeks after completion of radiation therapy. Factors that may contribute to risk of pneumonitis include undergoing combination therapy, as well as immunotherapeutic agents such as rituximab for treatment of her lymphoma. Symptoms may include low-grade fever and hypoxia. Myocardial effusion and cardiac tamponade are not correct because patients do not typically present with a low grade fever. While patients with superior vena cava syndrome often present with dyspnea, the other symptoms of chest pain and low grade fever are not common.

17. *Answer:* B

Rationale: The patient is at risk for developing cardiac tamponade due to his history of cardiovascular disease, diagnosis of mesothelioma, and treatment with doxorubicin (which may cause cardiotoxicity), and more than 4000 cGy of radiation to the chest. While the patient's diagnosis of mesothelioma and complaints of dyspnea may put the patient at risk for SVCS, symptoms of SVCS are usually more pronounced in the morning and improve or disappear after being upright for several hours. Radiation recall, which is a severe skin reaction that occurs in the radiation treatment field when certain chemotherapy drugs are administered during or soon after radiation therapy to the involved area, is not accurate. The patient is not at risk for developing cardiomyopathy based on the data provided.

18. *Answer:* C

Rationale: Patients with a chest malignancy, especially lung cancer, have an increased risk of developing superior vena cava syndrome (SVCS). The SVC is an easily compressed low-pressure vessel that is located in the mediastinum surrounded by several fairly rigid structures. SVCS may occur because of compression or obstruction of the SVC by tumor mass, enlarged mediastinal lymph nodes, or thrombus formation. The presence of a right-sided lung tumor accounts for the most cases of SVCS. Plaque deposition in the carotid artery, pulmonary embolism, and myocardial infarction are not associated with the development of SVCS.

19. *Answer:* C

Rationale: The most common presenting symptom of spinal cord compression (SCC) is back pain. New onset back pain in a patient with a history of cancer is the hallmark presentation of SCC. Pain can occur before the development of any neurologic symptoms. The common progression of symptoms in SCC is pain, motor weakness, sensory loss, motor loss, and autonomous dysfunction.

20. *Answer:* C

Rationale: Obstruction of the superior vena cava causes jugular vein distention and edema of the face, neck, upper thorax, breasts, and upper extremities. Abdominal distension and fever are not associated with superior vena cava syndrome (SVCS). Tachycardia, not bradycardia, usually occurs with SVCS. Cheyne-Stokes respirations are not indicative of SVCS.

CHAPTER 50

1. *Answer:* B

Rationale: Body image is based upon how a person feels about their body's actual or perceived appearance and/or change in function. While others' perceptions—including friends, family, and strangers—might influence the patient's perception of physical change, the patient's perception is the sole focus of the concept of body image.

2. *Answer:* D

Rationale: Nurses can educate patients about treatment and potential body image changes so they can anticipate and prepare for changes as much as possible. Body image is not affected by contact with long-lost relatives. Antidepressants, a pharmacologic intervention, may be recommended in combination with psychotherapy if body image distress is impactful to well-being, prolonged, and unresponsive to nonpharmacologic management. Grief does not follow a timeline.

3. *Answer:* A

Rationale: Chemotherapy-induced hair loss is total and includes eyelashes, nose hair, and pubic hair. Hair loss typically starts 2 weeks after chemotherapy treatment, may occur over a day to weeks, and occurs later when the patient is treated with low dose of chemotherapy. Hair regrowth usually starts 6 to 8 weeks after completion of treatment. Hair may come back slowly, thinner, or take up to a year to regrow.

4. *Answer:* C

Rationale: Altered body image issues are a concern for both males and females. Young individuals may be at higher risk for altered body image than older adults. Body image satisfaction is not dependent on time since diagnosis.

5. *Answer:* B

Rationale: WHO classifications of alopecia: grade 0—no alopecia; grade 1—minimal hair loss; grade

2—moderate, patchy hair loss; grade 3—complete alopecia but reversible; grade 4—irreversible alopecia.

6. *Answer:* A

Rationale: Moon face is a potential body image change associated with the use of high-dose corticosteroids. Weight gain is more likely than weight loss with high-dose corticosteroids. Corticosteroids are not associated with neuropathic pain or cachexia.

7. *Answer:* B

Rationale: Body image disturbance can result in psychological distress manifesting in changes in role and changes in sexuality, such as wife/mother, husband/father. Coping often occurs by avoidance. The reactions of others can lead to increased distress. Depending on the change, body image changes and disturbances are a long-term concern for some patients. Body image changes may lead to decreased self-confidence and depressive thoughts.

8. *Answer:* D

Rationale: There is no evidence that scalp cooling increases scalp metastases. There are two types of scalp cooling that include automatic (start 30 to 45 minutes before and 20 to 150 minutes after) and manual (start 30 minutes before). The effectiveness of scalp cooling is based on the type of chemotherapy treatment, contact with scalp, hair type, and liver function. One side effect is headache that can be mitigated with acetaminophen.

CHAPTER 51

1. *Answer:* D

Rationale: Caregiver burden is defined as the emotional, physical, social, financial, and spiritual impact perceived by a caregiver that is influenced by multiple patient and caregiver comorbidities and symptoms. A continuum of health care activities for someone unable to independently care for themselves describes caregiving, not caregiver burden. Support and health management for the well-being of another person describes caregiving, not caregiver burden. A time-sensitive, life-changing commitment and experience describes caregiving, not caregiver burden.

2. *Answer:* C

Rationale: The CARE (Caregiving, Advise, Record, and Enable) Act requires hospitals to record a family caregiver name and to notify the caregiver when the patient is discharged. CARE requires hospitals to record caregivers, not ambulatory settings. The Credit for Caring Act supports family caregivers who work. This act helps address the financial challenges of family caregiving and assists family caregivers to stay in the workforce and be more financially secure and gives eligible family caregivers the opportunity to receive a tax credit for 30% of the qualified expenses above $2000 paid to help a loved one, up to a maximum credit amount of $3000.

3. *Answer:* D

Rationale: Younger persons report higher level of emotional distress. Females are at a greater than two-fold rate of caregiver burden when compared to men. Lower education is associated with the highest levels of caregiver burden. Cohabitation with the care recipient is associated with higher levels of caregiver burden.

4. *Answer:* A

Rationale: Cardiometabolic risk is a physiological factor that puts caregivers with poor health at a higher risk of experiencing problems. Weight loss, not gain, is a clinical or physical outcome and not a physiological factor. Sleep deprivation, not too much sleep, is a clinical or physical outcome and not a physiological factor. Social isolation is a psychosocial risk factor, not a physiological factor.

5. *Answer:* B

Rationale: To elicit information about health perceptions, the nurse would include questions regarding medical problems, prognosis, and goals of care. Cognitive status would include questions such as, "Is the patient cognitively impaired?" Caregiving needs would include questions such as, "Is the care recipient totally dependent 24/7?" and are about the caregiver, not the care recipient. Caregiver values would include questions about the caregiver, not the care recipient.

6. *Answer:* A

Rationale: An aging and growing population has made caregiving a major public health concern. Enabling the caregiver to learn new skills is often cited as a positive aspect and is not the reason for a major public health concern. Caregiving is associated with economic burden but is not the reason for a major public health concern. Caregiving can impact relationships but is not the reason for a major public health concern.

7. *Answer:* C

Rationale: The caregiver mainly provides day to day care and activities of daily living (ADLs). The caregiver is typically uncompensated. Being a caregiver involves significant amounts of time and energy for months or years and is normally not time limited. The caregiver may be involved with financial demands but is not accountable to cover costs.

8. *Answer:* D

Rationale: Dependency creates an environmental stressor that can cause depression in both the caregiver and the recipient. A secondary caregiver provides support for the caregiver and recipient and is a positive aspect for the caregiver. Resilience is a positive characteristic of the caregiver. Documentation is not required for the caregiver, but the caregiver must know who to call if the plan of care for symptom control is not working.

9. *Answer:* B

Rationale: The health care team should provide continuous therapeutic communication with caregivers. Therapeutic communication is important at the onset of the caregiving experience and at the advance care planning appointment, but it needs to be done continually as needs change. Therapeutic communication with caregivers should be continuous and not rely on the patient alone.

10. *Answer:* B

Rationale: The Caregiver Strain Index measures burden through factors such as employment, finances, physical, social, and time aspects, and includes 13 screening items. The Caregiver Reaction Assessment looks at caregiver burden through self-esteem, lack of family support, and impact on finances, schedule, and caregiver health, and includes 24 items. The Caregiver Burden Scale has 15 items and examines burden through patient needs, caregiver tasks, and caregiver burden. Finally, the Zarit Burden Interview has 22 items and examines burden through health, psychological well-being, finances, social life, and relationships with the impaired person.

11. *Answer:* C

Rationale: The caregiver profile would include the following information: educational background of the caregiver, whether the caregiver is employed, and if the caregiver has dependents who require care as well. Assessment of the caregiver relationship would include the following: what is the caregiver's relationship to the patient and how long has the caregiver been in this role. Assessment of other caregivers would include whether there are other family members or friends involved in providing care and if there are paid caregivers (e.g., home health aides) involved. Assessment of the physical environment would include the following: does the care recipient's home have grab bars and other adaptive devices and necessary equipment to assist with care, if the care recipient is homebound, other concerns (i.e., laundry, grocery shopping, meal preparation, and medication pick-ups from the pharmacy), if there is a readily accessible bathroom on the same floor that the care recipient spends most of the day, presence of stairs, and if the care recipient is a pet owner and if they can handle pet care.

12. *Answer:* D

Rationale: The Family Medical Leave Act is a federal law that allows employees to take up to 12 weeks of unpaid leave per year to care for themselves, or for a seriously ill family member, or for a new child without losing their jobs or health care insurance. The Recognize, Assist, Include, Support, and Engage Family Caregivers Act of 2017, or the RAISE Family Caregivers Act, provides for the establishment and maintenance of a family caregiving strategy. The CARE (Caregiver Advise, Record, and Enable) Act enables family caregivers to provide safe and effective home care to older adults, requires hospitals to record family caregiver name with hospital admission, the hospital is required to notify the caregiver when the patient is discharged and provides instructions of medical tasks for transitions of care. The Credit for Caring Act supports family caregivers who work, helps address the financial challenges of family caregiving and assists family caregivers to stay in the workforce and be more financially secure, and gives eligible family caregivers the opportunity to receive a tax credit for 30% of the qualified expenses above $2000 paid to help a loved one, up to a maximum credit amount of $3000.

CHAPTER 52

1. *Answer:* A

Rationale: Social determinants of health (SDOH) are the circumstance in which people are born, live, work,

play, learn, worship, and age and comprise five domains: (1) economic stability, (2) neighborhood and built environment, (3) education access and quality, (4) health care access and quality, and (5) social and community context. The availability of Federally Qualifying Health Centers and county public health vaccine programs are components of the health care access and quality domain. Section 8 housing availability is part of the neighborhood and built environment.

2. *Answer:* C

Rationale: Structural racism refers to practices that disproportionality distribute and sustain access to power and resources between groups assigned to different racial categories. These practices are normative, often legal practices that are engrained into society. Structural racism is also sometimes called systemic or institutionalized racism. Restricted access to care would be an example.

3. *Answer:* D

Rationale: Socioeconomic factors, environmental conditions, and health behaviors determine about 80% of a person's health. A focus on social risks is needed in health care because these hazards are associated with decreased treatment compliance, poor health outcomes, and increased care costs. Nurses should develop an understanding of how the SDOH are impacting a patient, when advising them to engage in healthy behaviors (e.g., physical activity, healthy diet, and cancer screening).

4. *Answer:* C

Rationale: Up to 48% of cancer survivors report financial toxicity due to out-of-pocket expenses. Financial toxicity leads to poor cancer treatment completion rates and increased medical problems. Patients may need to prioritize paying for basic needs of food and shelter over seeking medical care. Because nearly 50% of oncology patients report financial toxicity, oncology nurses need to assess for and connect patients with resources to mitigate financial toxicity.

5. *Answer:* A

Rationale: The neighborhood and built environment refer to the location and physical aspects that one interacts with where they live and influences access to transportation, healthy food, and safe spaces for physical activity. Transportation influences the distance and availability of bus lines and routes to grocery stores and public and medical services. Health literacy is part of the education quality and access domain. Social isolation and racism are part of the social and community context domain. The quality of the schools are part of the assessment of education access and quality.

6. *Answer:* B

Rationale: About 20% of people in the United States do not have broadband internet. People without broadband are not able to use telehealth, and policies that require a camera to be used for telehealth may further limit access for those with poor Internet connectivity.

7. *Answer:* D

Rationale: Health literacy (i.e., the extent to which individuals can understand information to inform their health-related decisions) impacts patient's decision-making and outcomes. Patients with high literacy levels may have low health literacy. Health literacy does not refer to only the written word. Health literacy encompasses all forms of information transfer.

8. *Answer:* C

Rationale: It is recommended that patient education materials be written at a 6th-grade reading level. However, most educational materials are written above the 8th-grade reading level because of the complexity of the content. Oncology nurses should review and clarify patient education materials with the patient and family.

9. *Answer:* A

Rationale: The PREPARE: Protocol for Responding to and Assessing Patient's Assets, Risks, and Experiences contains 15 questions that identify needs related to housing, food, transportation, utilities, childcare, employment, education, finances, and personal safety. The WellRx Questionnaire contains 11 questions that identify needs related to food insecurity, housing, utilities, income, employment, transportation, education, substance abuse, childcare, safety, and abuse. Available in English or Spanish. The OCHIN is designed for social determinants assessment integrated through the electronic health record. Includes items from the PREPARE tool. The YCLS (Your Current Life Situation) contains nine questions designed to identify needs recommended by the Institute of Medicine. Also includes an additional item bank for a more detailed assessment.

10. *Answer:* D

Rationale: The Harvard IAT is a self-assessment test a nurse can complete to understand bias. The practice of cultural humility is a lifelong process of self-reflection and self-critique whereby the individual not only learns about another's culture, but one starts with an examination of her/his own beliefs and cultural identities. The AHC HRSN (Accountable Health Communities Health-Related Social Needs) is a patient assessment tool, not a personal assessment of the nurse. It contains 10 questions to help identify patient needs around housing instability, food insecurity, transportation problems, utility help needs, and interpersonal safety. Also includes eight supplemental questions to assess financial strain, employment, family and community support, education, physical activity, substance abuse, and mental health and disabilities. Oncology nurse navigators can comprehensively assess patient needs using the ONN Patient Assessment. Nurses can look up resources for a patient near their home by using the neighborhood navigator tool from the EveryONE project that identifies resources by zip code.

CHAPTER 53

1. *Answer:* A

Rationale: Culture is defined as the customary beliefs, social forms, material traits, and characteristic features of everyday existence shared by people of a racial, religious, or social group in a particular place or time. Diversity is the situation of being composed of differing elements, especially the inclusion of people of different races or cultures in a group. Race is a social construct based on expressed phenotype (observable characteristics such as skin tone or hair texture) in which people are categorized based on external, selective, and arbitrary physical features. Ethnicity reflects cultural heritage as defined as historical, cultural, contextual, and geographic experiences of a specific community or population. An ethnic group may comprise more than one racial group.

2. *Answer:* C

Rationale: Race is identified in social foundations and ethnicity is identified in cultural foundations. Ethnicity is based in the identity of a wide racial diversity, whereas race is based in the phenotype of a culture. Race is a social construct based on expressed phenotype (observable characteristics such as skin tone or hair texture) in which people are categorized based on external, selective, and arbitrary physical features. Ethnicity reflects cultural heritage as defined as historical, cultural, contextual, and geographic experiences of a specific community or population.

3. *Answer:* A

Rationale: Race: a social construct in which groups of people are clustered according to shared physical traits, and having no basis in one's biological, anthropological, or genetic composition. Ethnicity reflects cultural heritage; historical, cultural, contextual, and geographic experiences of a specific community or population.

4. *Answer:* C

Rationale: The "thumbs up" gesture is considered as a vulgar connotation in some cultures and is discouraged. However, it is appropriate to fold your hands in your lap, thereby avoiding pointing or gesturing with the hands, which is unacceptable in some cultures. Planting your feet on the floor is appropriate as exposing the soles of the feet is offensive in some cultures. It is appropriate to stand 2 feet away from the patient or caregiver as closeness of personal space may be seen as intrusive and violating in some cultures.

5. *Answer:* B

Rationale: Pursuit of basic needs (food and shelter) takes priority over seeking care for a cancer diagnosis or treatment unless symptoms prohibit basic activities of daily living. Poverty-stricken populations do not have adequate access to quality health care, and they may not undergo cancer screening. These populations are at higher risk of developing cancer due to higher exposure to poor nutrition, workplace carcinogens, and modifiable risk factors. Although lack of access to quality care and poor nutrition and environmental exposures are risk factors for malignancy, they do not necessarily lead to late stage detection of malignancy. Persons experiencing poverty must make choices about basic needs, and food and shelter will take priority over health care.

6. *Answer:* D

Rationale: Patients will forego cancer screening if they have a fatalistic view of a cancer diagnosis, with cancer being synonymous with certain death and they believe that nothing can be done to change their fate if they are, indeed, diagnosed with cancer. The other responses focus on cultural response to treatment not screening. Some cultures rely on traditional healers and will forego diagnosis and treatment under conventional models of health and wellness. Distrust of the conventional U.S. medical system may play a role in inconsistent cancer prevention, screening, or treatment. Ignorance of the cancer treatment process is usually an issue among immigrants. Some patients may be suspicious of clinical trials for treatment because of historical unethical treatment of some members of their/racial ethnic group.

7. *Answer:* B

Rationale: Spirituality is the relationship or connection to the sacred, giving a broader meaning and purpose that is experienced through personal or communal devotions, or through meditation, art, nature, or ceremony. Religion describes an organized system of faith and worship, while culture consists of customary beliefs, social forms, material traits, or characteristic features of everyday existence shared by people of the same religious group. Ethnicity is the historical, cultural, contextual, and geographic experiences of a specific community or population.

8. *Answer:* B

Rationale: When something or someone is considered as sacred, it is connected to a higher power, and venerated as such through established norms, rituals, and traditions. Sacred, however, does not necessarily connote religious, as something sacred can be outside of a traditional religion. For instance, in certain Native American traditions, medicine is seen as protected knowledge that is passed down from generation to generation, not associated with a specific religion, but is knowledge that is granted by a higher power and therefore sacred. Spirituality gives "meaning and purpose" in a higher power and may inspire feelings of hope and resolution. Spirituality, though, is not necessarily tied to religion or to a "sacred" item. Belief can be defined as trust or faith and does not necessarily denote a belief in a higher power or in anything that is sacred.

9. *Answer:* D

Rationale: An oncology nurse may access a patient's and caregiver's spiritual needs by practicing deep listening. Deep listening is the practice of listening to learn and requires the listener to temporarily suspend judgment or preconceived notions. The idea is to openly receive new information, whether the news is good, bad, or indifferent. From a nursing assessment standpoint, deep listening would allow the patient to express personal feelings about spirituality without fear of judgment, while allowing the nurse to more accurately assess the spiritual needs of the patient or caregiver. Consulting pastoral services does not occur during the assessment phase but can be done during nursing management of spiritual needs. Prayer and reading from scripture are also not activities done during assessment, but, when appropriate during the trajectory of care, can be done by nurse, patient, and family as a sincere, genuine gesture of compassion. In addition to deep listening, other recommendations for nursing support include holding a presence, bearing witness, and practicing compassion.

10. *Answer:* B

Rationale: For some cultures, avoiding eye contact is a way of showing respect. Although eye contact in some cultures can be seen as a source of comfort and support, and a way to establish a personal connection between two people, in other cultures eye contact may be seen as intrusive. The potential relationship to depression cannot be determined without further interaction. The other choices are also incorrect.

11. *Answer D*

Rationale: Gender identity includes transgender, nonbinary, cisgender, and intersex. Sexual preference includes heterosexual, homosexual, lesbian, gay, bisexual, asexual, pansexual, and queer.

CHAPTER 54

1. *Answer:* A

Rationale: Primary approaches to cancer-related distress include psychotherapeutic interventions such as CBT, psychotherapy, group therapy, psychoeducation, and counseling. Although an anti-anxiolytic may be considered, it is generally not indicated every 4 hours, and hydrotherapy, as well as benzodiazepines, are not first recommendations for primary treatment of cancer-related distress.

2. *Answer:* C

Rationale: Co-existing risk factors or sequelae of distress may give rise to psychiatric disorders, such as post-traumatic stress disorder (PTSD). Symptoms may include forgetfulness, avoidance or fight/flight behaviors, emotional lability, angry outbursts, numbing, insomnia, and agitation. These symptoms should be evaluated by a psychiatric professional. Although this patient may have anxiety, treatment with an anti-anxiolytic will not effectively manage treatment of PTSD, which are the symptoms this patient is exhibiting, and there is no prior history of mental illness or unusual behavior. The patient has not stated that they want to stop therapy so a hospice referral may not be appropriate until the patient has the PTSD evaluated.

3. *Answer:* C

Rationale: Medications, fever, electrolyte imbalance such as vitamin B12 deficiency, sodium or potassium imbalance, anemia, and sepsis may all produce effects that mimic and cause depression. Hypoglycemia is more commonly associated with anxiety than hyperglycemia, which is more commonly associated with fatigue. Well-controlled HTN is not a cause of depression, anxiety, or nervousness. Hypercalcemia, not hypocalcemia, is associated with depression.

4. *Answer:* B

Rationale: SSRI medications should be taken regularly as they take time to reach full effect (months), may interact with herbal supplements, and should not be discontinued without the supervision of the prescriber as abrupt discontinuation may precipitate withdrawal and associated adverse events. If a patient on an SSRI feels suicidal, they should seek emergency care.

5. *Answer:* A

Rationale: Loss of personal control is a source of distress in pediatric cancer patients, just as in adult cancer patients. Clinicians should allow pediatric patients to make decisions between choices provided to them by their health care team, and to participate in the decision-making process as developmentally appropriate to help address this source of distress. Parents serve as decision-makers but pediatric patients should be offered choices whenever possible to decrease distress. Distraction can be helpful, but it will not promote a sense of personal control. For the pediatric population, clinicians should provide opportunities to make choices and express concerns through play and expressive arts (e.g., art therapy).

6. *Answer:* A

Rationale: Education is useful in preventing and addressing psychologic distress and impaired coping and empowers patients in decision-making. Early screening and use of evidence-based interventions, as well as ruling out physiologic causes of distress, anxiety, or depression, improves outcomes. Referral to social work may be indicated through early screening but should not be automatically implemented. Complete avoidance of difficult subjects would further delay identification and addressing areas of impaired coping and would not be helpful.

7. *Answer:* A

Rationale: Cancer-related distress should be identified and screened early with every patient. There are many interventions specific to distress that may be utilized even in the absence of co-existing psychiatric diagnoses. The National Comprehensive Cancer Network (NCCN) recommends that patients be screened early and then routinely to identify the level and source of their distress so that further evaluation can be completed. Even after an initial screening, if symptoms appear, patients should be rescreened. While asking the patient's family about the patient's distress may provide insight, it does not consider the patient's point of view that is necessary in determining if the patient is experiencing cancer-related distress.

8. *Answer:* D

Rationale: An ambivalent emotional relationship to the deceased increases risks for complicated grief, as does perceiving death as preventable, or having co-existing psychosocial issues, medical conditions, or legal or financial issues. A deep emotional relationship to the deceased, a large family support network, or an expected death are not risk factors for complicated grief.

9. *Answer:* D

Rationale: Highest levels of emotional distress are reported in patients with lung cancer. Higher levels of distress are often seen in patients in advanced stage of disease, poor pain control, ineffective emotional and practical support, financial and job insecurity, changes in roles such as in occupation, within family, between friends, altered physical capacity and cognitive functioning, and developmental life tasks disrupted by diagnosis and treatment.

10. *Answer:* A

Rationale: Medications associated with an increased risk of anxiety include the following: corticosteroids, neuroleptics causing akathisia, thyroxine, bronchodilators, antihistamines, decongestants, beta-adrenergic stimulants, and opioids that induce hallucinations. Angiotensin

receptor blocker common side effects include upper respiratory infections, dizziness, back pain, diarrhea, fatigue, low blood sugar, and chest pain. Side effects of angiotensin-converting enzyme (ACE) inhibitors include cough, headache, fatigue, and dizziness. Common side effects of beta blockers include dizziness, weakness, fatigue, cold hands and feet, dry mouth, skin, or eyes, headache, diarrhea, or constipation.

11. *Answer:* B

Rationale: Reactive depression is defined as a normal response to a precipitating event or situation such as a diagnosis of cancer and its associated treatment. Reactive depression is not more common in any specific age group. Side effects of corticosteroids commonly include anxiety and insomnia. Persons who have experienced domestic violence are at risk for posttraumatic stress disorder (PTSD).

12. *Answer:* D

Rationale: There is typically a reluctance to express emotions when an individual is experiencing a loss of control. Overt or covert statements that suggest an individual is experiencing a loss of control include expressed frustration or dissatisfaction with care, as well as anger or criticism toward staff. Objective characteristics of loss of personal control include refusal or reluctance to participate in decision-making, in activities of daily living (ADLs), and a reluctance to express emotions. Behavioral responses may include apathy, resignation, withdrawal, uneasiness, anxiety, and aggression. Excessive house cleaning would not represent reluctance to engage in ADLs. Asking frequent questions about therapy and complimenting staff are not indicators of loss of control.

13. *Answer:* A

Rationale: Although a 5- to 9-year-old tries to consider loss from a concrete and logical point of view, loss is often perceived as a punishment for a bad behavior or action. Two- to 5-year-old children view loss as temporary and may express little distress or fear of not being loved. Nine- to 12-year-old children usually have a realistic perception of loss and often view it as a separation from the loved one. Twelve- to 18-year-olds look at loss in both abstract and realistic ways, and often consider loss to be a threat to their own independence.

14. *Answer:* B

Rationale: Cognitive symptoms associated with grief include a lack of concentration, distractibility, preoccupation with loss, searching for meaning, intrusive thoughts, or psychiatric symptoms. Physical signs and symptoms include fatigue, headache, shortness of breath, gastrointestinal complaints, sleep disturbance, and cardiac symptoms. Psychological responses include shock, denial, guilt, anger, hostility, ambivalence, sadness, shame, depression, preoccupation, ruminating, anxiety, or dulled senses. Socially there may be dependency on or avoidance of others and occupational lapses. Spiritual manifestations might include searching for meaning or a change in personal views or beliefs. Hyperactivity and increased energy are not common manifestations of grief.

15. *Answer:* B

Rationale: Emotion-focused is directed toward changing one's own emotional reaction. In the example,

209

the patient is trying to change his emotional reaction with the help of a therapist and peer support. Problem-focused coping aims to remove the stressor, which is being addressed with treatment with chemotherapy. Meaning-focused coping occurs when the individual derives meaning and peace from the stressful experience. Primary appraisal coping is based beliefs, values, and goals. Secondary appraisal coping is based on one's belief and conception of being able to reduce or minimize the threat.

16. *Answer:* A

Rationale: Symptoms of anxiety include feelings of suffocation, dizziness, and fatigue or exhaustion. Palpitations and eating disturbances are also signs of anxiety, but a feeling of worthlessness or guilt is generally associated with depression. Crying easily and bouts of insomnia are also a sign of depression, while difficulty swallowing is a sign of anxiety. Finally, a sense of impending doom and becoming easily overwhelmed are all symptoms associated with anxiety. Exhibiting outward signs of psychomotor agitation is a sign of depression. Other symptoms of anxiety include becoming persistently tense, a feeling of being unable to relax, worrying, easily excitable, exhibiting poor concentration or attention, and having a sense of indecisiveness. Another well-known sign of anxiety is experiencing panic attacks, which can become acute in some patients.

17. *Answer:* D

Rationale: Symptoms of depression include decreased energy and recurrent thoughts of death and suicide. A change in appetite—either weight gain or weight loss—is also associated with being depressed, while being easily overwhelmed is a sign of anxiety. Being unable to relax is a sign of anxiety, while insomnia is exhibited in both patients with anxiety and depression. Having a sense of impending doom is a sign of anxiety. Experiencing hypersomnia, particularly daily hypersomnia or regular hypersomnia, is one of the signs of depression.

18. *Answer:* D

Rationale: H.K.'s report of sleeping until the afternoon should be a signal to her nurse that she is suffering from hypersomnia. Sleeping for long periods of time, especially on a regular basis, pushes beyond the boundaries of cancer-related fatigue and can be a sign of depression. Becoming highly agitated and easily overwhelmed is a sign of anxiety. Having trouble swallowing and often feeling suffocated is also a sign of anxiety, as is also complaining of a sense of impending doom. Hypersomnia is one of five symptoms that a clinician should watch out for when deciding whether to refer a patient for further evaluation. Other signs include a change in appetite or weight gain, insomnia, psychomotor agitation, or retardation that is noticeable to the naked eye, a decrease in energy, feelings of worthlessness or guilt, difficulty concentrating or making decisions, and recurrent thoughts of death or thoughts (or plans) of suicide. Any five of these symptoms should alert the nurse to refer for an evaluation of a more serious mental condition.

19. *Answer:* C

Rationale: An example of an objective symptom is a measurement of weight loss or gain. Other objective symptoms include the patient showing a flat or depressed affect, the patient crying, exhibiting slow speech, and psychomotor excitation or retardation. Subjective symptoms include report of depressed mood, report of insomnia, and reports by the patient of feeling worthless or guilty. Other subjective symptoms include social withdrawal, feelings of fatigue, difficulty concentrating, thoughts of death and ideas of suicide, irritability, and sleep complaints without an underlying physical cause.

20. *Answer:* B

Rationale: The HADS assessment tool is a 14-item scale (7 questions dealing with anxiety and 7 questions dealing with depression). The NCCN Distress Thermometer has a scale of 0 (no distress) to 10 (severe distress) measurement, with accompanying simple questions identifying source of distress. For the NCCN Distress Thermometer, the recommendation is that a score of 4 or more triggers further physician or nurse evaluation, referral to psychosocial services, or both. The HADS tool has a score ranging from 0 to 21 (0 to 3 per question) to evaluate anxiety or depression levels. Answer D of 0 to 25 (0 to 5 per question), is an incorrect range.

21. *Answer:* A

Rationale: Distress is impacted by developmental stage, phase of disease, past coping skills, and available resources, which is why careful and ongoing assessment is important. Patients will not necessarily self-identify as experiencing distress, and the manifestations are different in each patient. Understanding the impacting factors influences treatment, which is not necessarily the same for all patients. Distress is not a universal response to the diagnosis of cancer and frequently requires intervention. According to recommendations from the National Comprehensive Cancer Network (NCCN), a patient score of 4 or higher requires further evaluation and intervention as appropriate.

22. *Answer:* D

Rationale: Withdrawal or social isolation could be symptomatic of clinical depression and deserves further evaluation. The other options—from crying to being preoccupied with the deceased—represent normal grief responses, especially early in the grieving process.

CHAPTER 55

1. *Answer:* B

Rationale: The PLISSIT model consists of the provider creating a safe space for patients to talk about sexual concerns (i.e., giving *permission*), giving targeted and specific *limited information* about the patient's concerns, offering targeted (*specific information*) interventions to treat the patient's concerns, and referring to a specialist as needed for *intensive therapy*.

2. *Answer:* D

Rationale: Nonpharmacologic interventions for sexual concerns typically include skills-based learning targeting communication and relationship dynamics. Couple's counseling can include marital therapy and cognitive existential couple therapy. Other nonpharmacologic interventions include implementing exercise to decrease fatigue and improve libido, pelvic floor rehabilitation, cognitive stress management, and considering changes in positioning. Eros therapy uses an FDA-approved device to increase blood flow to the clitoris and requires a prescription, and herbs and lubricant oil are considered pharmacologic agents that can potentially disrupt the body or be harmful.

3. *Answer:* A

Rationale: If the provider believes the patient is "too old or too young" to have concerns about sexuality, is terminally ill, or does not have a partner, they may fail to ask about issues related to sexuality. Providers should not assume that if there was a discussion about sexuality during the initial assessment that no further discussion is needed, because as treatment plans unfold, further questions may develop. Providers should never assume that patients do not want to discuss sexuality. Other reasons why health care providers may fail or hesitate to discuss issues related to sexuality include personal cultural and religious beliefs, lack of time, believing that treatment is more important than sexuality, feeling it is not their responsibility, and lack of knowledge about how to discuss sensitive issues or available resources.

4. *Answer:* C

Rationale: Gentle massage and caressing and kissing are generally considered safe for immunocompromised patients. Rectal intercourse puts patients at risk for infection if tears occur during coitus just as vaginal stimulation without lubrication increases risk of vaginal tears and subsequent infection. Stimulating nipple or penile rings when thrombocytopenic could increase the risk of bleeding.

5. *Answer:* C

Rationale: Those who experience infertility report lower sexual satisfaction and functioning (leading to poorer quality of life), and for 29% of patients, affects treatment decision-making. This is why preserving fertility is a key survivorship issue that needs to be addressed at diagnosis. Discussions of potential threats to fertility and family planning should be initiated prior to starting cancer therapies so as to allow for the most options for fertility preservation.

6. *Answer:* A

Rationale: Chemotherapy and radiation therapy can cause long-term sexual changes in 30% to 100% of survivors and can occur years after treatment. For women, menopausal symptoms, such as changes to the atrophic, urogenital, and vaginal areas, decreased vaginal lubrication, vaginal stomatitis, dyspareunia, sleep, mood, body image alterations, loss of sense of femininity, decreased libido, and weight gain can impact sexuality. Libido is often decreased. Women undergoing chemotherapy can engage in sexual intercourse, but they should be aware of the potential risk of shared body fluids when within 3 days of chemotherapy. Women should not engage in intercourse if they are experiencing immunosuppression or thrombocytopenia because of the risk of vaginal or other tissue tears increasing the risk of bleeding or infection. Vaginal dryness, not increased vaginal secretions, are a side effect of menopause.

7. *Answer:* D

Rationale: Serum anti-Mullerian hormone (AMH), a direct biomarker for ovarian aging, is a better predictor of menopausal transition than age, and follicle count or ovarian volume, but only in women over the age of 25. Serum AMH may not be helpful in adolescent and young adult childhood survivors as ovarian reserve is most robust in women's 2nd decade of life.

8. *Answer:* C

Rationale: There are no strict guidelines regarding when to begin attempting to conceive, but, in general, the recommendation is to wait 1 year because the greatest risk of recurrence tends to be within the first 12 months. If a woman expresses a desire to conceive at or after this time, providers should evaluate if she has physically and psychologically recovered following her treatment, that long-term side effects will not negatively impact her pregnancy and determine whether she is at low risk for recurrence.

9. *Answer:* D

Rationale: In the "5 A's" discussion model to enhance sexual health communication, the **"advise"** step is to normalize symptoms and acknowledge the problems. To bring up the topic is to **ask.** Asking about sexual functioning and using standardized assessments, if needed, is to **assess.** To provide information and resources and refer as needed is to **assist.** The last step in the "5 A's" assessment is to **arrange** (providing follow-up to check on how the patient is doing).

10. *Answer:* D

Rationale: A potential change that could affect sexuality or sexual functioning in either male or female patients with cancer being treated with steroids is reduced sexual function and sexual desire. Hyperglycemia as a result of steroid use can result in reduced sexual function and decreased sexual desire, erectile dysfunction in men, thinning of the vaginal wall, and orgasm dysfunction in women. The other changes—alopecia to include the loss of pubic hair, peripheral neuropathy symptoms that affect sexual functioning, and infertility—can all manifest in patients as a result of chemotherapy treatment.

11. *Answer:* A

Rationale: A potential side effect of pelvic radiation therapy in a male patient with prostate cancer that would affect his sexual functioning is vascular or nerve damage causing temporary or permanent erectile dysfunction (ED). Pelvic radiation can also cause men to have absent or weak orgasm, painful ejaculation, and decreased volume of ejaculation. Brachytherapy used to treat prostate cancer causes ED in 6% to 61% of patients. Chemotherapy treatments have been known to cause retarded or inhibited ejaculation and decreased or loss of libido. Immunotherapy treatments can cause flu-like symptoms that could affect libido, as well as mouth sores that could impact sexual behavior.

12. *Answer:* C

Rationale: A potential change that could affect sexuality or sexual functioning in a female patient with cancer receiving chemotherapy treatments is vaginal stomatitis. Other symptoms of chemotherapy that affect female sexuality include premature menopause, decreased libido, body image changes, decreased vaginal lubrication, dispensability and capacity, and dyspareunia. Decreased vaginal elasticity/stenosis is a side effect of pelvic radiation therapy. Other changes include decreased vaginal lubrication, hardened clitoris, dyspareunia, vaginal sensation changes, and vaginal atrophy/vault shortening. In general, this type of therapy can also create a concern for the "safety" of the partner. Chronic constipation should not affect sexual functioning. Chest pain and shortness of breath are typically caused by immunotherapy and can affect sexual behavior in an adverse manner.

13. *Answer:* A

Rationale: Preservation of fertility in both male and female patients with cancer should be the initial priority as options later into the process may become more restricted. The nurse should initially focus on listening to the patient, not providing details regarding impact of the treatment, and the options that are available. The patient's concerns regarding their own survival need to be addressed but combined with a frank discussion about the viability of future fertility. This discussion includes methods of fertility preservation prior to treatment and talk of adoption and other issues, as needed.

CHAPTER 56

1. *Answer:* B

Rationale: *Oncology Nursing Society: Scope and Standards of Practice* describe the expectations for oncology nursing practice across various care settings. For each standard, criteria for demonstrating competence are provided at the RN level that apply to all nurses who provide care to patients with cancer or practice in an oncology setting. Additional standards that apply to graduate-level prepared nurses and advanced practice registered nurses are included for some standards. The *Standards of Oncology Nursing Education* were developed to guide educators in the oncology nursing setting and schools of nursing about preparing nurses to care for cancer survivors across many settings. The ASCO/ONS Chemotherapy Administration Safety Standards are interprofessional standards outlining best practices for reducing errors related to chemotherapy processes. The nurse recruiter represents the institution's job specification, not origin of professional standards.

2. *Answer:* B

Rationale: Nursing standards of practice and professional performance (NSPPP) set expectations for competent nursing practice and serve as powerful guides for ensuring evidence-based, quality nursing care and provide direction to nurses and their employers related to

expectations and development of competence. As a nurse educator, the nurse is focused on policy and development for the entire staff, not individual professional growth. Staff may or may not agree with a policy, but such policies should be based on standards and evidence-based practice. The nurse educator may also be responsible for continuing education of the staff, but when working on a policy she is looking at NSPPP and promoting evidence-based practice.

3. *Answer:* C

Rationale: The ASCO/ONS Chemotherapy Administration Safety Standards are interprofessional standards that outline best practices to reduce the risk of error during the process of chemotherapy provision. They are not tiered but interprofessional. These standards address appropriate staff and policies, planning, consent and education for patients and caregivers, ordering, preparing, administrating by parenteral and oral routes and documentation and monitoring adherence, side effects, and complications. They do not include information for locating clinical trials or information for patients/public to understand efficacy/side effects of chemotherapy.

4. *Answer:* D

Rationale: A side-by-side comparison of current documentation practices with the standards for documentation can identify gaps and potential areas for improvement. *ONS Nursing Documentation Standards for Cancer Treatment* describe nursing documentation requirements for persons with a diagnosis of cancer undergoing cancer treatment and requiring supportive care and reflect the minimal elements to include documentation about people undergoing treatment for cancer. They address chemotherapy and biotherapy administration, radiation therapy, blood and marrow transplantation, oncologic surgery, central venous access devices, blood product transfusion, and extravasation management. Ease of locating policies will not necessarily result in appropriate documentation. A consultant could review policies, but without a side-by-side comparison it is not clear if the documentation is appropriate and meets the requirements of the standard. The compliance department may be more concerned with coding and reimbursement.

5. *Answer:* B

Rationale: Standards of Oncology Practice include the following components: assessment, diagnosis, outcomes identification, planning, implementation, coordination of care, health teaching and health promotion, and evaluation. Standards of Oncology Professional Performance include the following components: ethics, culturally congruent care, collaboration, communication, leadership, education, evidence-based practice and research, quality of practice, professional practice evaluation, resource utilization, and environmental health.

6. *Answer:* C

Rationale: The full definition for standards for professional nursing practice, as stated by the American Nurses Association (ANA), is an "authoritative statements of the duties that all registered nurses [RNs], regardless of role, population, or specialty, are expected to perform competently" (ANA, 2015a, p. 3). According to the Institutes of Medicine (IOM), clinical practice guidelines are defined as "statements that include recommendations intended to optimize patient care that are informed by a systematic review of evidence and an assessment of the benefits and harms of alternative care options" (IOM, 2011, p. 15). Therefore, any statement with a recommendation is not defined as a standard. Finally, the standards of professional nursing are meant for all nurses, including, and not limited to, subspecialties.

7. *Answer:* B

Rationale: The definition for the education component in the Standards of Professional Performance is the oncology nurse seeks and expands personal knowledge and competence that reflect the current evidence-based state of cancer care and oncology nursing and contributes to the professional development of peers, assistive personnel, and interprofessional colleagues. Collaboration is defined as the oncology nurse partners with the patient and family, the interprofessional team, and community resources to optimize cancer care. The definition of evidence-based practice and research is the oncology nurse integrates relevant research into clinical practice and identifies clinical dilemmas and problems appropriate for study while supporting research efforts. Finally, resource utilization is defined as the oncology nurse considers factors related to safety, efficiency, effectiveness, and cost in planning and delivering care to patients.

8. *Answer:* C

Rationale: Oncology Navigation Standards of Professional Practice do not mandate affiliation with oncology nurse practitioners in providing patient care. The standards are designed to enhance the quality of professional navigation services provided to people impacted by cancer. The Standards note that navigators advocate with and on behalf of people at risk for cancer, cancer patients, survivors, families, and caregivers to protect and promote the needs and interests of people impacted by cancer. The Standards encourage navigator participation in the creation, implementation, and evaluation of best practices and quality improvement in oncology care. The Standards promote navigator participation in the development, analysis, and refinement of public policy at all levels to best support the interests of people impacted by cancer and to protect and promote the profession of navigation. The Standards emphasize that navigators educate all stakeholders, including physicians, about the essential role of navigators in oncology systems

CHAPTER 57

1. *Answer:* D

Rationale: A nonpayment for complications model exists when EBP is not followed, which supports pay for performance. EBP has not been implemented throughout the United States or globally consistently. EBP supports pay for performance initiatives. Evolution of evidence is not limited, but instead evolves on a continual basis.

2. *Answer:* A

Rationale: P = Patient population of interest. I = is not Improvement, but Intervention or issue of interest. O = is not Opportunity, but Outcomes. T = is not Theory, but Time Frame. C = Comparison Intervention or Control Group

3. *Answer:* A

Rationale: Level 1 is the highest level of evidence on which to base practice change. Level 1 is a systematic review of randomized control trials (RCTs). Level 2 is single-site RCT studies. Level 5 is a systematic review of descriptive or qualitative studies. Level 7 is the lowest level of evidence on which to base practice change; it is an expert opinion.

4. *Answer:* C

Rationale: Practice changes should first be implemented or piloted in one or two practice areas to ensure feasibility, sustainability and outcomes. Incorporation into a policy may take place after the pilot. Publishing may take place after the pilot. Review by the IRB would take place before research starts if patients are involved.

5. *Answer:* B

Rationale: EBP is most valuable when clinical practice is changed and the impact of the practice on patient outcomes is communicated effectively and adopted. Information about outcomes should be disseminated such as through grand rounds, professional journals, and national conferences, but impact on clinical practice and patient outcomes are most important and valuable components of EBP.

6. *Answer:* D

Rationale: Qualitative research is used to describe or explore phenomena or gain understanding into some aspect of the patient/provider care experience. Characteristics of qualitative research are that it is process-focused, subjective, and not generalizable. Types of qualitative research include descriptive, survey, phenomenology, and content analysis. Quantitative research to describe relationships between variables, examine cause and effect, and identify facts. Characteristics of quantitative research are that it is outcome-focused, objective, and may be generalizable. Types of quantitative research include quasi-experimental, experimental, and correlational.

7. *Answer:* D

Rationale: A systemic review of randomized control studies (RCT) studies is the highest level of evidence on which to base practice change. Single-site randomized control studies (RCT) studies are considered at a level 2 of evidence. A single descriptive study or qualitative study is a level 6, while a case or cohort study is a level 4. Other levels include quasi-experimental studies (level 3), systematic review of descriptive or qualitative studies (level 5), and expert opinion (level 7) and the lowest level on which to base practice change.

8. *Answer:* B

Rationale: Starting journal clubs, ongoing evidence-based practice (EBP) education, and access to key databases is an example of creating a sense of inquiry and creating an EBP culture, which is also the first step in

213

the multistep process of using evidence to support clinical practice. Identifying a problem or trigger is a second step in the process, which can be either problem-focused or knowledge-focused. Searching and critiquing the literature for relevant studies and identifying of information and stakeholders needed to solve the problem are steps later in the process.

CHAPTER 58

1. *Answer:* D
Rationale: Focus groups are used for community assessment before the development of targeted patient education programs and materials. Individual assessment would involve specific questions for that exact person to understand specific educational needs of that individual person. Caregiver assessment would involve specific questions related to care delivery or the needs of the caregiver. Survivors would be an individual assessment with specific questions for the survivor.

2. *Answer:* B
Rationale: M = Measurable. S = Specific. A = Attainable. R = Realistic. T = Timely

3. *Answer:* C
Rationale: Performance analysis of information from quality improvement, incident reports, and other data, such as infection control data, are used in the evaluation phase. Development of the teaching plan uses principles of adult learning elements. Determination of teaching objectives is stating the goals of education. Content identification is within the teaching plan development phase.

4. *Answer:* D
Rationale: "List four vegetables with high-fiber content" includes specific outcome criteria. It is specific about what (vegetables with high fiber content) and specific about the number (four). This outcome is measurable. "Understand nutritional impact on body" is vague, not an objective outcome. It is not clear what constitutes understanding and nutritional impact. "Prepare low-fat foods" is vague, not an objective outcome, as it does not identify what prepare means (once, twice, without assistance etc.). "Maintain adequate sodium intake" is vague, not an objective outcome, as it is not specific as to what constitutes adequate sodium intake and it is not clear what maintains means (1 week, 1 month, 6 months, etc.).

5. *Answer:* A
Rationale: Diagnostic methods are routinely used in testing nurses' and other staff members' competency and knowledge base in specific areas. Patients are assessed using specific questions related to the needs of the patient. Caregivers are assessed using specific questions related to their needs or the needs of the recipient of their care. The community is assessed using specific methods, such as a survey, checklist, or interviewing a focus group.

6. *Answer:* A
Rationale: Social learning theory encompasses learning by watching and imitating others. Cognitive learning theory is an internal process that requires attention, thought, and reasoning. Behavioral learning theory is based on observable behaviors that are reinforced to increase the strength of the behavior. Humanistic learning theory encompasses the uniqueness of all individuals and is a learner-directed approach.

7. *Answer:* C
Rationale: Adult learning theory is described as someone who is self-directed, independent, and problem-centered, which includes the internet search example. Operant conditioning is also known as behavioral learning and is based on observable behaviors that are reinforced to increase the strength of the behavior. Motivational theory is focused on how human behavior is activated. Pedagogy (teaching children) is the opposite of andragogy (adult learning).

8. *Answer:* C
Rationale: Motivational learning is activated through internal and external cues. The foundation of motivational learning is studying the processes that explain the "why" and the "how" human behavior is activated and directed through external and internal cues. An internal cue could be an inner drive to stop smoking for a person's health or to "be there for my family." An external cue could be the cost of cigarettes or having to work around a nonsmoking policy in a person's workplace. Social learning theory revolves around watching and learning from the behavior of others. Cognitive learning is an internal process that requires attention, repetition, and ultimately, retention. Humanistic learning theory is a learner-directed approach, with a foundation based upon the theory that everyone is unique and learn in different ways.

CHAPTER 59

1. *Answer:* C
Rationale: State Boards of Nursing (BoN) provide oversight of nursing practice by enforcing the state nurse practice act to protect the health, welfare, and safety of the public. The National Council of State Boards of Nursing (NCSBN) develops the National Council Licensure for Registered Nurses (NCLEX) examination. The NCSBN also encourages and facilitates consistency among state boards of nursing. Nurse practice acts define nursing role, titles, and scopes of practice. The NCLEX is the licensing examination, not a regulating body. The NCLEX is a standardized exam that each state board of nursing uses to determine whether or not a candidate is prepared for entry-level nursing practice.

2. *Answer:* B
Rationale: The Affordable Care Act (ACA) provides coverage to Americans with preexisting conditions (cancer is a preexisting condition). The ACA also mandates insurers to offer dependent coverage for children to age 26 regardless of if they are in college. The ACA prohibits annual and lifetime limits on coverage. The ACA prohibits arbitrary withdrawals of insurance coverage, mandates essential health services (such as screening examinations or vaccination), and allows four tiers of benefit coverage from low to high monthly premiums and out-of-pocket costs.

3. *Answer:* D

Rationale: Oncology-specific accreditation and certification agencies and programs include the Oncology Nursing Certification Corporation (ONCC), American College of Surgeons–Commission on Cancer (ACS-COC) and the Quality Oncology Practice Initiative (QOPI). The QOPI, which is associated with the American Society of Clinical Oncology, is a quality program designed for outpatient-oncology practices to promote self-assessment and improvement. The QOPI uses over 190 evidence-based quality measures and generates individual performance scores by practice, site, and provider, as well as benchmarked scores comparing all participating practices. The Joint Commission accredits and certifies health care organizations and programs for meeting specific performance and quality standards. The NIH is a federally funded biomedical research agency. CMS administers the Medicare program and works in partnership with state governments to administer Medicaid and other related programs.

4. *Answer:* C

Rationale: Approximately 3% of cancer survivors file for bankruptcy, which requires legal consultation. Insurance and prescription coverage would be insurance company issues, and social workers, navigators, and patient advocates can often assist with obtaining coverage and reimbursement. Many cancer survivors face employment discrimination that would require legal services; a promotion is not employment discrimination.

5. *Answer:* B

Rationale: Breach of duty is defined as a failure to meet an acceptable standard of care. Malpractice is a deviation from a professional standard of care. Negligence is a deviation from the acceptable standard of care that a reasonable person would use in a specific situation. Proximate cause is a cause that directly produces an event and without which the event would not have occurred.

6. *Answer:* D

Rationale: Common causes of litigation against nurses include issues associated with lack of informed consent, improper operation of a medical device, not following standards of care, failure to communicate appropriately, inadequate or inappropriate patient assessment, inadequate teaching, lack of patient advocacy, medication errors, inappropriate delegation or supervision, inadequate documentation, and working while impaired. Following standard of care is not a litigation risk. Communicating effectively/appropriately is not a litigation risk factor nor is advocating for patients.

7. *Answer:* D

Rationale: Communicating clearly when educating patients and families is an example of the development of interpersonal communication, while fostering positive relationships with patients and their families can minimize risk of malpractice. When a nurse has clearly explained and educated a patient on, for example, treatments, their potential side effects, and how to effectively manage those side effects, the nurse improves the level of patient care, but also lessens the chances for malpractice

or disciplinary risk later in the patient's journey, since the patient has been well-educated and informed. Attending continuing education programs, obtaining specialty certifications, and becoming involved in patient advocacy programs are examples of maintaining knowledge and skills, another strategy in minimizing personal risk for nurses.

8. *Answer:* B

Rationale: The correct answer is negligence. Negligence is the deviation from the acceptable standard of care that a reasonable person would use in a specific situation. Malpractice, on the other hand, is a deviation from a professional standard of care. The two terms are often confused and the line between them is thin, but distinct. Defamation involves harming the reputation of someone by making false statements to a third person. Breach of duty, unlike malpractice and negligence, is the failure to meet an accepted standard of care.

9. *Answer:* C

Rationale: Malpractice is the deviation from a professional standard of care. Examples of medical malpractice include a misdiagnosis or a failure to diagnosis. Negligence is the deviation from the acceptable standard of practice. An example of negligence in nursing is misusing equipment or perhaps taking a personal phone call in the middle of a patient's treatment. Slander is defined as making a defamatory statement expressed in a transitory form, especially speech. Duty is a care relationship between a patient and provider.

10. *Answer:* A

Rationale: The Oncology Nursing Society's Practice Standard named "Statement on the Scope and Standards of Oncology Nursing Practice Generalist and Advanced Practice" is described as the scope of oncology nursing practice, standards of care for RNs and advanced practice RNs, and professional performance issues. Options B, C, and D describe other ONS Practice Standards. Option B describes *Standards of Oncology Education: Patient/Significant Other and Public (4th ed.).* Option C describes Survivorship Care Standards for Accreditation. Option D is the ONS Standard for Educating Nurses Who Administer Chemotherapy and Biotherapy.

CHAPTER 60

1. *Answer:* A

Rationale: Increased technology and availability of life support measures increases the likelihood of aggressive care longer, contributing to concerns of overtreatment. Effective collaboration between the physician and nurse about treatment and a request by the patient to continue treatment would not cause moral distress in the nurse. Helping the patient complete an advance directive would not cause moral distress. Nurses who lack knowledge and time to help the patient make an autonomous decision might put the nurse at risk for moral distress.

2. *Answer:* C

Rationale: Informed consent ensures the patient has adequate understanding of the risks, benefits, alternatives,

215

and consequences of treatment. Completing the entire treatment plan and guaranteeing cure of his disease are not provisions of the informed consent. The informed consent consists of risks and benefits. Therefore, there may be risks of treatment that may cause harm to the patient. The informed consent process ensures the patient has an adequate understanding of risks, benefits, alternatives, and consequences of treatment and supports autonomy and human dignity. Informed consent touches on issues of beneficence, justice, and veracity.

3. *Answer:* A

Rationale: Advocating for patients is part of the provision of promoting, advocating, and protecting the rights, health, and safety of the patient. The other answers are part of the provisions of the code that establishes boundaries of duty and loyalty, delineating nursing's responsibilities toward social justice, health policy, and advancement of nursing as a science and profession.

4. *Answer:* C

Rationale: Deontology is the theory that argues that an action's goodness is derived from intention and certain actions are intrinsically right or wrong. Utilitarianism is the theory that what is good is what will result in the most benefit for most people. Ethical egoism is the theory that it is always good to promote one's own good, and divisibility is not any ethical principle.

5. *Answer:* B

Rationale: In shared decision-making, the patient chooses treatment options in conjunction and with guidance from the physician. Informed consent ensures the risks and benefits of treatment and supports an autonomous decision. Power of Attorney involves allowing another person to make decisions, and combined decision-making is not a type of decision-making.

6. *Answer:* D

Rationale: The ethical principle that is defined by the duty to not harm others is nonmaleficence. Nonmaleficence, in nursing terms, can mean ensuring that the benefits of treatment outweigh the potential harm. Beneficence is doing good or doing what is of benefit. However, this term is often shaded in grey, for what is good for one person may not be of benefit to another person, so trying to act with beneficence may prove ethically challenging for some nurses. Autonomy is showing respect to an individual for their right to choose or their right to self-determination. Autonomy in nursing, according to the American Nurses Association, stems from a core value of giving a patient their dignity. Justice, as it relates to medical and nursing care, is allowing each patient, no matter their life circumstances or morality, access to the same resources.

7. *Answer:* D

Rationale: Justice is allocating the same resources to each patient, no matter their socioeconomic status, race, religion, or moral standing. In nursing care, that means making available the same level of care or treatment to the rich and the poor, the morally just, and those who have committed crimes. It is the same resources for all. Ensuring the benefits of a patient's treatment outweighs the harm is an example of nonmaleficence. Showing

compassion toward a patient in a nurse's care is an example of beneficence, while respect for a person's right to choose their own destiny, or, in medical terms, their own plan of care, is an example of autonomy.

8. *Answer:* B

Rationale: Step 3 in identifying ethical concerns is to analyze the problem using ethical theories or approaches. In this step, nurses are to discuss what principles, codes, laws, or perspectives are relevant. Exploring practical alternatives is the fourth step. Nurses are to discuss possible courses of action, with the goal of an action that is ethically reasonable and most likely to achieve the desired outcome with the least harm. Gathering the information and obtaining the facts is the first step in the process towards identifying ethical concerns. Finally, the last step in the process (Step 5) is evaluating the process and outcome. Debriefing sessions with those involved are critical for exploring whether the problem was adequately resolved, and for discussing implications for future similar situations. In Step 1, the nurse gathers information from key participants and obtains the facts to understand the multiple complex perspectives of the ethical problem. In Step 2, the nurse identifies the type of ethical problem that exists.

9. *Answer:* C

Rationale: The concept of everyday ethical comportment refers to practice-based knowledge, skills, and reasoning that nurses can learn through lived clinical experiences of caring for patients and developing an ethical sense of what is right and good. Nurses can take responsibility and ownership for their professional behaviors, words, and practice. This type of conduct is exemplified by the concept of everyday professional comportment and includes attributes of mutual respect, harmony in beliefs and actions, commitment to colleagues and patients, and collaboration. Respect for the autonomy of others is part of the ethical principal of autonomy that stems from the core value of dignity. Identifying the type of ethical problem that exists and defining what makes this an ethical problem is Step 2 in identifying and addressing ethical concerns. Considering social determinants of health to develop group interventions for vulnerable populations is part of addressing health disparities and inequities.

10. *Answer*: A

Rationale: Self-care in nursing is a priority to promote mental health, build resilience, and decrease burnout. Nurses need to identify and practice self-care strategies to mitigate the effects of the multiple stressors they experience while working on the front lines of health care. Self-care practices are a joint responsibility of individual nurses and health care organizations. Taking responsibility and ownership for their professional behaviors, words, and practice is the type of conduct exemplified by the concept of *everyday professional comportment*. Acting on concerns about patients' decision-making abilities is part of rational autonomy: When seriously ill patients make decisions considering the values and preference of their family members in addition to or instead of their own values. When indicated, any concerns about the patient's decision-making ability should be evaluated using a formal assessment of capacity. Using social media platforms to learn and conduct research is part of nursing education.

CHAPTER 61

1. *Answer:* B

    Rationale: Barriers to building a collaborative relationship include a lack of clearly defined, distinct domain of influence, a lack of understanding regarding scope of practice, overlapping and changing domains of practice that produce competition, lack of recognition of knowledge and expertise of a profession, and legal responsibilities. Interdisciplinary team meetings provide an opportunity for collaboration and team building among professionals. Developing and initiating change of shift reporting practices promotes nurse to nurse collaboration.

2. *Answer:* C

    Rationale: Certification helps assure the public that the certified nurse has the knowledge and qualifications needed to practice in his or her clinical area of nursing. It is not a guarantee of increased pay although some employers do acknowledge the value of certification with increased pay or promotion. It is not mandated for re-licensure or by the (Board of Registered Nursing) BRN.

3. *Answer:* C

    Rationale: The Plan-Do-Study-Act (PDSA) model is used in quality improvement studies. It typically seeks to answer three fundamental questions, which include identification of the goal, determining how a change will be recognized as an improvement, and what changes will result in improvement. It typically occurs in settings and situations where everyday care occurs. The PICOT question format is a consistent approach and strategy for developing answerable, researchable questions. P stands for Population/patient; I stands for Intervention/indicator (Variable of Interest). C stands for Comparison/control; O stands for Outcome; and T stands for Time it takes for the intervention to achieve an outcome or how long participants are observed. SMART goal stands for Specific, Measurable, Achievable, Relevant, and Time-Bound. Defining these parameters as they pertain to the goal helps ensure that your objectives are attainable within a certain time frame. The PLISSIT model consists of the provider creating a safe space for patients to talk about sexual concerns (i.e., giving permission), giving targeted and specific limited information about the patient's concerns, offering targeted (specific information) interventions to treat the patient's concerns, and referring to a specialist as needed for intensive therapy.

4. *Answer:* B

    Rationale: The Institute of Medicine (IOM) provides a national focus on knowledge regarding safety and setting national safety goals and tracking their progress. Institutions should develop and implement safety systems and development of a "culture of safety" where safety is an explicit organizational goal. Recognizing and removing faulty equipment helps promote safety. Certification helps assure that the nurse has knowledge and qualification for practice in a specific area, but it does not assure that medical errors will not occur. Sitting on an evidence-based care committee may increase awareness of potential problems but does not necessarily prevent individual medical errors. Reading nursing journals may increase knowledge about nursing practice but the specific content may not be at reducing medical errors.

5. *Answer:* C

    Rationale: There are several types of errors. This is a preventive error. Preventive errors stem from inadequate risk assessment (falls, suicide, infection, etc.). Diagnostic errors include a wrong diagnosis or a delay in diagnosis. Treatment errors include errors in administering or an avoidable delay in treatment. Other types of errors include communication or equipment failure.

6. *Answer:* D

    Rationale: The implementation of policies and procedures that promote a culture of safety is an important step. Confidential, nonpunitive investigatory processes involving peers is an effective strategy. Staff training in event prevention strategies is important as is effective and efficient response to identified issues.

7. *Answer:* B

    Rationale: Patient family advisors (PFAs) are recognized by the Joint Commission as essential in supporting organizational performance improvement. Engaging PFAs in decisions around health care delivery where possible leads to measurably improved outcomes in quality and safety. Their participation provides insight regarding an organization's strengths and where opportunities for improvement reside. They provide valuable input on policy, procedure, and practices that patients and their caregivers find helpful in staying engaged in their plan of care.

8. *Answer:* C

    Rationale: The American Rescue Plan Act of 2021 lowers health care premiums for millions of Americans, eliminating premiums for some who participate in the health insurance marketplace established in 2016. The Affordable Care Act (or "Obamacare") was passed in 2010 and resulted in an estimated 30% of traditional Medicare payments going through alternative payment models like bundled payments and accountable care organizations. The goal was to make accessible, affordable cancer care to reduce disparities and reform traditional fee-for-service payment reimbursements to new payment models. The Affordable Care Act included the Individual Mandate, stating that individuals must sign up for health insurance or face a tax penalty, but this was repealed in late 2017. Medicaid is a state-run program.

CHAPTER 62

1. *Answer:* B

    Rationale: Compassion fatigue is a state of physical and emotional distress, or apathy that results from caring for those experiencing pain or is a result of the constant demands of caring for other. For example, those patients seen on an inpatient oncology unit or in a busy infusion area are populations with constant demanding care needs.

217

Exhaustion, cynicism, and inefficacy from chronic job stress are symptoms of burnout. Compassion fatigue is often correlated with burnout, but there are differences. C and D are not syndromes relating to any problem.

2. *Answer:* C
   Rationale: Caring for high acuity patients and working under high levels of stress with a large caseload on an inpatient unit such as those on a bone marrow transplant unit over a long period of time can cause compassion fatigue. Other risk factors include nurses who are young and single with less than 10 years of experience in nursing. Overconfidence is not a risk factor; having a high level of self-judgment imposed by either the nurse or the employer puts the nurse at risk for developing compassion fatigue.

3. *Answer:* B
   Rationale: Scheduling a day at a spa is a way of managing compassion fatigue because the nurse is doing something for herself and exhibits self-care. Other self-care activities include good nutrition and sleep. Staying out late and binge drinking are not ways of managing self-care. This may be a behavioral sign of compassion fatigue. Adequate sleep is recommended; however, lying in bed for weeks at a time is not. Getting the adequate amount of sleep along with exercise is a better way of taking care of oneself. Verbalizing feelings to friends, family, and coworkers may offer support. Speaking to facility social workers or chaplains may also provide counseling and support.

4. *Answer:* C
   Rationale: Burnout occurs over a prolonged period of time and is due to chronic job stressors. Individuals with burnout may experience cognitive, emotional, or physical exhaustion, feelings of detachment and distancing from work, including social interactions. They may also have feelings of incompetence and being overwhelmed. Compassion fatigue is emotional and physical distress due to the prolonged demands of caring for high acuity individuals or those in pain. Chronic fatigue syndrome is an unexplained medical disorder. Cognitive disorders are related to cognitive disabilities and may include confusion and poor judgment.

5. *Answer:* C
   Rationale: While the Maslach Burnout inventory is an assessment tool used for diagnosing compassion fatigue, the Professional Quality of Life Scale (ProQOL) uses subscales including assessing for secondary stress disorder, burnout, and compassion satisfaction. The tool is easy to use and score and is the most commonly used. The secondary scales provide more extensive assessment data. The Mental Status exam and Montreal Cognitive Assessment scale are frequently used to assess cognitive changes in individuals.

6. *Answer:* D
   Rationale: Making time for prayer and meditation is an example of a self-reflection exercise that a nurse can try as part of self-care management. Spending time in prayer or in mediation is a good way to center thoughts and allow for self-reflection. Indulging in a massage, spending time exercising (recommend three to four times weekly for 20 to 30 minutes), and enjoying a hobby, listening to music, humor, and enjoying nature are all activities that emphasize self-care.

7. *Answer:* C
   Rationale: Mindfulness-based interventions include activities that focus a person's attention on the present experience, becoming more aware of one's physical, mental, and emotional condition, in a way that is nonjudgmental. Mindfulness has been shown to be effective at reducing stress. The interventions can be offered individually or in a group setting. Establishing good nutrition and eating well, as well as scheduling preventive and medical care appointments, are examples of emphasizing self-care. Sending cards to the family, reminiscing about time spent with patients, and sometimes attending the funeral of patients with whom there has been a close bond, are self-reflective exercises.